Other Titles in This Series

Kieran Murphy • Fergus Robertson
Editors

Michael J. Lee • Anthony F. Watkinson
Series-Editors

Interventional Neuroradiology

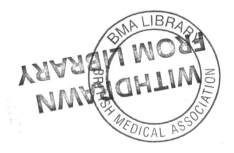

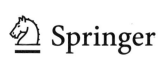

Editors
Kieran Murphy
Department of Radiology
University Health Network
Mount Sinai Women's College Hospital
Toronto, Ontario
Canada

Fergus Robertson
Department of Neuroradiology
National Hospital for Neuroradiology
and Neurosurgery
London, UK

Series Editors
Michael J. Lee
Department of Neuroradiology
Beaumont Hospital and Royal College
of Surgeons of Ireland
Dublin
Ireland

Anthony F. Watkinson
Department of Neuroradiology
The Royal Devon and Exeter Hospital and
University of Exeter Medical School
Exeter
UK

ISBN 978-1-4471-4581-3   ISBN 978-1-4471-4582-0   (eBook)
DOI 10.1007/978-1-4471-4582-0
Springer London Heidelberg New York Dordrecht

Library of Congress Control Number: 2013954560

To Helen, Finley, and Orla – my home team.
Fergus Robertson

To my long suffering family –
Rulan, Ronan, and Anya, the most
interesting people I know – thank you.
Kieran Murphy

Preface from the Book Editors

Interventional neuroradiology is the most rewarding field in medicine today. Where else can a physician change the course of a patient's life in minutes? It is a challenging career that makes demands on the hearts and minds of all of us engaged in it. It requires great self-control and technical virtuosity. It takes confidence but demands humility. Our field today is built on the shoulders of the great practitioners like Terbrugge, Lasjaunias, Rufenacht, and Molyneux, and the inventiveness of Guglielmi, Palmaz, Deramond, and Theron. In this book, you will find your colleagues have taken the time to share with you their best knowledge to save you from the errors and mistakes that they have made and that they will always remember. We thank our colleagues for their significant contributions and hope that you find this a worthwhile addition to the books you keep in your angio suites, to be referred to at times of need.

A final thought, when wondering if you should put in more TPA, or another coil, listen to that little voice in your head that is saying, "You can always do more, you can never do less" and remember that despite your best intentions, bad outcomes happen. If you work in a bomb factory and bombs go off, you were doing your best.

Toronto, ON, Canada   Kieran Murphy
London, UK   Fergus Robertson

Preface from the Series Editors

Interventional radiology treatments now play a major role in many disease processes and continue to mushroom with novel procedures appearing almost on a yearly basis. Indeed, it is becoming more and more difficult to be an expert in all facets of interventional radiology. The interventional trainee and practicing interventional radiologist will have to attend meetings and read extensively to keep up to date. There are many IR textbooks which are disease specific, but incorporate interventional radiology techniques. These books are important to understand the natural history, epidemiology, pathophysiology, and diagnosis of disease processes. However, a detailed handbook that is technique based is a useful addition to have in the cath lab, in the office, or at home where information can be accessed quickly, before or even during a case. With this in mind, we have embarked on a series of books which will provide specific information on IR procedures. Textbooks on Angioplasty and Stenting, Transcatheter Embolization, Biopsy and Drainage, and Tumor Ablative Techniques have already been published. The specialized fields of Neuro and Pediatric Interventional Radiology warrant textbooks in their own right. The final book to complete the series will focus on Emergency Procedures in Interventional Radiology.

We have chosen two editors, who are experts in their fields, for each book. One editor is European and one is from North America so that the knowledge of IR techniques detailed is balanced and representative. We have tried to make the information easy to access using a consistent bullet point format with sections on clinical features, anatomy, tools, patient preparation, technique, aftercare, complications, and key points at the end of each chapter. A short recommended reading list is included.

These technique-specific books will be of benefit to those Residents and Fellows who are training in interventional radiology and who may be taking subspecialty certificate examinations in interventional radiology. In addition, these books will be of help to most practicing interventional radiologists in academic or private practice. We hope that these books will be left in the interventional lab where they should also be of benefit to ancillary staff, such as radiology technicians/radiographers or nurses, who are specializing in the care of patients referred to interventional radiology.

We hope that you will use these books extensively and that they will be of help during your working IR career.

Exeter, UK   Anthony F. Watkinson
Dublin, Ireland   Michael J. Lee

Acknowledgments

We gratefully acknowledge all our coauthors for sharing their experience and knowledge and the staff at Springer for all their work on this book.

Kieran Murphy
Fergus Robertson

Acknowledgements

Contents

Part IX   Spine Intervention

Editor and Author Affiliations

Forward

Gil Gonzalez, MD Department of Neuroradiology, Massachusetts General Hospital, Boston, MA, USA

Series Editors

Michael J. Lee, MD, EBIR Department of Neuroradiology, Beaumont Hospital and Royal College of Surgeons of Ireland, Dublin, Ireland

Anthony F. Watkinson, BSc, MSc (Oxon), MBBS, FRCS, FRCR, EBIR Department of Neuroradiology, The Royal Devon and Exeter Hospital and University of Exeter Medical School, Exeter, UK

Volume Editors

Kieran Murphy, MB, FRCPC, FSIR Joint Department of Medical Imaging, UHN Mount Sinai WCH, Toronto, ON, Canada

Fergus Robertson, MA, MBBS, MRCP, FRCR Department of Neuroradiology, National Hospital for Neuroradiology and Neurosurgery, Queen Square, London, UK

Contributors

David H. Abramson, MD Department of Surgery, Memorial Sloan-Kettering Cancer Center, New York, NY, USA

Ronit Agid, MD, FRCPC Department of Medical Imaging, Division of Neuroradiology, Toronto Western Hospital, University of Toronto, Toronto, ON, Canada

Tommy Andersson, MD, PhD Department of Neuroradiology and Clinical Neuroscience, Karolinska University Hospital and Karolinska Institute, Stockholm, Sweden

Marcus Bradley, BSc, MBBS, MRCP, FRCR Department of Neuroradiology, Frencham Hospital, Bristol, UK

Scott E. Brodie, MD, PhD Department of Ophthalmology, Mount Sinai Hospital, New York, NY, USA

James Chen, BS Division of Interventional Neuroradiology, The Johns Hopkins Hospital, Baltimore, MD, USA

Andrew Clifton, MA, MRCP, FRCR Department of Neuroradiology, Atkinson Morley Wing, St. George's Hospital, London, UK

Rufus Corkill, MBBS, BSc, FRCS, FRCR, MSc Department of Neuroradiology, Level 1, John Radcliffe Hospital, Oxford, UK

Ira J. Dunkel, MD Department of Pediatrics, Memorial Sloan-Kettering Cancer Center, New York, NY, USA

David Fiorella, PhD, MD Department of Neurosurgery, Cerebrovascular Center, Stony Brook University Medical Center, Stony Brook, NY, USA

Y. Pierre Gobin, MD Department of Neurosurgery, Weill Cornell Medical College of New York Presbyterian Hospital, New York, NY, USA

Edward D. Greenberg, MD Division of Interventional Neuroradiology, Department of Neurosurgery, New York Presbyterian Hospital-Weill Cornell Medical Center, New York, NY, USA

Gianluigi Guarnieri, MD Department of Neuroradiology, AORN Cardarelli, Naples, Italy

Roberto Izzo, MD Department of Neuroradiology, AORN Cardarelli, Naples, Italy

Sudhir Kathuria, MD Division of Interventional Neuroradiology, Department of Radiology, The Johns Hopkins Hospital, Baltimore, MD, USA

Peter Keston, MB, ChB, MRad, FRCR, FRCS Department of Neuroradiology, Western General Hospital, Edinburgh, Scotland

Wilhelm Kuker, MD, PhD, FRCR Department of Neuroradiology, John Radcliffe Hopsital, Oxford, UK

Robert Lenthall, MBBS Department of Diagnostic Imaging, Nottingham University Hospital NHS Tower, Nottingham, UK

Jeremy Madigan, MB, ChB, FRCR Department of Neuroradiology, St. Georges Hospital, Tooting, London, UK

Brian P. Marr, MD Ophthalmic Oncology Service, Memorial Sloan-Kettering Cancer Center, New York, NY, USA

Lucy A. Matthews, BMBS, MRCP Department of Neuroradiology, John Radcliffe Hospital, Oxford, UK

Matthew Mattson, MD, MRCP, FRCR Department of Radiology, Barts and The London NHS Trust, London, UK

John S. Millar, MRCP, FRCR Department of Neuroradiology, Wessex Neurological Center, University Hospital Southamptom, Southampton, UK

Kevin Murphy, MB, Bch, BAO, MRCS Department of Radiology, Cork University Hospital, Cork, Ireland

Mario Muto, MD Department of Neuroradiology, AORN Cardarelli, Naples, Italy

Peter Kim Nelson, MD Department of Radiology and Neurosurgery, NYU: Langone Medical Center, New York, NY, USA

Mary Newton, MD Department of Anesthesia, The National Hospital for Neurology and Neurosurgery, London, UK

Geoffrey D. Parker, BMBS, FRANZCR Department of Radiology, Royal Prince Alfred Hospital, Camperdown, NWS, Australia

Andy Platts, MBBS, FRCS, FRCR Department of Radiology, Royal Free Hospital, London, UK

Lissa Peeling, MD Department of Neurosurgery, Cerebrovascular Center, Stony Brook University Medical Center, Stony Brook, NY, USA

Mani Puthuran, MD, FRCR Department of Neuroradiology, The Walton Centre for Neurology and Neurosurgery NHS Trust, Liverpool, UK

Martin G. Radvany, MD Division of Interventional Neuroradiology,
The Johns Hopkins Hospital, Baltimore, MD, USA

Prem S Rangi, MB, ChB Department of Radiology, The Royal Free Hospital,
London, UK

Shelley Renowden, BSc, MRCP, FRCR Department of Neuroradiology,
Frenchay Hospital, Bristol, UK

Andrew Shawyer, BSc, MBBS, FRCR Department of Interventional Radiology,
Barts and the Royal London, London, UK

Jessica Spence, MD Department of Medical Imaging, Division
of Neuroradiology, Toronto Western Hospital, Toronto, ON, Canada

Chris Taylor, BSc (Hons), MBBS, MRCP, FRCA, FFICM
Department of Neuroanesthesia and Neurocritical Care, The National Hospital
for Neurology and Neurosurgery, London, UK

Gerald Wyse, MB, Bch, BAO, MRCPI, FFRRCSI Department of Radiology,
Cork University Hospital, Cork, Ireland

Fabio Zeccolini, MD Department of Neuroradiology,
AORN Cardarelli, Naples, Italy

Part I

Basic Skills

Diagnostic Cerebral Angiography and Groin Access and Closure

Kevin Murphy and Gerald Wyse

Abstract

A full clinical history, physical examination, and review of the study indication should be performed prior to every cerebral angiogram. Perform noninvasive imaging initially with magnetic resonance (MR), computed tomography (CT), and/or CT/MR angiography. Closely review all imaging and laboratory data prior to invasive angiography.

Keywords

Diagnostic cerebral angiography • Groin access • Closure • MR • CT • History and physical

Diagnostic Evaluation

A full clinical history, physical examination, and review of the study indication should be performed prior to every cerebral angiogram. Perform noninvasive imaging initially with magnetic resonance (MR), computed tomography (CT), and/or CT/MR angiography. Closely review all imaging and laboratory data prior to invasive angiography.

K. Murphy, MB, Bch, BAO, MRCS (✉) • G. Wyse, MB, Bch, BAO, MRCPI, FFRRCSI
Department of Radiology, Cork University Hospital, Cork, Ireland

K. Murphy, F. Robertson (eds.), *Interventional Neuroradiology,*
Techniques in Interventional Radiology,
DOI 10.1007/978-1-4471-4582-0_1, © Springer-Verlag London 2014

Indications for Performing a Diagnostic Cerebral Angiogram

Despite the advances of CT and MR angiography, invasive diagnostic cerebral angiography still has a broad number of indications. Today cerebral angiograms are commonly performed to access dynamic process such as AV shunts or following intracranial interventions such as coil embolization of aneurysms. Cerebral angiography can be performed to further investigate patients with:

- Stenosis or occlusion
- Aneurysm
- Vascular malformations
- Vasculitis
- Vascular tumors
- Previous intracranial intervention

Contraindications

Absolute

- History of anaphylaxis to iodinated contrast
- Patient informed refusal

Relative

- Coagulopathy
- Contrast allergy
- Abnormal renal function
- Uncontrolled hypertension
- Decompensated heart failure
- Pregnancy

Patient Preparation

Nil by mouth for 6–8 h preferable
Peripheral IV access
Correct coagulopathy and other contraindications where possible

Relevant Aberrant Anatomy

Familiarity with common vascular anatomy is essential. Understanding of the common aberrant or variant anatomy is critical to avoid misinterpretation.

Common Arch Variants

- "Normal" (70 %).
- Common left common carotid and innominate origin (termed "bovine" arch) (13 %).
- Left common carotid arises from the innominate (9 %) (also termed "bovine" arch).
- Left vertebral artery directly from arch (5 %).
- Left brachiocephalic trunk (2.7 %).
- Aberrant right subclavian (0.5 %).

Common Intracranial Variants

- Complete circle of Willis (20–25 %)
- Hypoplasia of one or both posterior communicating arteries (PComs) (34 %)
- Hypoplastic/absent A1 segment of the anterior cerebral artery (ACA)
- Origin of posterior cerebral artery (PCA) from the internal carotid artery (ICA) with and absent or hypoplastic P1 segment (17 %) (fetal PCom or fetal circulation)
- Infundibular dilatation of the PCom origin (10 %)

Preprocedure Medications

Sedation of the patient is not routinely required. An oversedated patient can be difficult to neurologically assess, and an acute complication may be missed. In addition noncompliance from a sedated patient may lead to a poor quality or even nondiagnostic study.

Procedure

Access

A common femoral artery (CFA) groin approach, the right groin in particular, is favored for access. The femoral artery is easily compressed post procedure and is associated with a low puncture site complication rate even in the setting of antiplatelet agents.

Fig. 1 JB-1, Berenstein, Sim1, and SIM 2 catheters

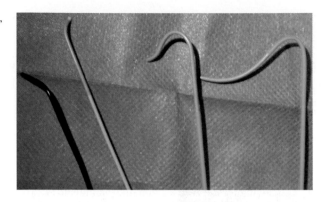

Radial access continues to grow in popularity for coronary procedures. Compression with a wrist brace negates the need for prolonged supine bed rest post procedure. Although useful for ipsilateral vertebral artery access, this approach is not ideal to access all four vessels during a cerebral angiogram. Brachial and axillary access may be used but are associated with higher puncture site complication rates.

The authors recommend the use of a "micro" access set (21-gauge access needle with a short 0.018″ wire and a 4-French sheath). Alternatively, a standard 18-gauge needle with 0.035″ wire can be used.

- Routine fluoroscopy to accurately locate the center of the femoral head is recommended.
- Infiltration of local anesthetic (1–2 % lignocaine).
- A subsequent single-wall puncture with a 21-gauge needle is performed with a small skin insertion to aid sheath insertion.
- Ultrasound guidance should be readily available and is a valuable adjunct.
- Long sheaths 25 cm or more are useful in the setting of diseased or tortuous iliac vessels.

Immediately after sheath insertion a femoral angiogram should be performed. This leads to early discovery of arterial injury or dissection. It also ensures that the puncture site is appropriate for insertion of a closure device.

After gaining access to the (right) common femoral artery, the following are routinely used:

- Short 4-French sheath
- 4-French 100-cm Berenstein catheter (Fig. 1)
- 0.035″ hydrophilic angled glide wire
- Closed system pressurized saline flush (Fig. 2)

A 5-French system can also be used.

A wide variety of different selective end-hole catheters may be utilized. An unfolded aorta or tortuous anatomy may require two different catheters. Operator preference varies from basic hockey-stick-style catheters to more complex tip shapes. Commonly used

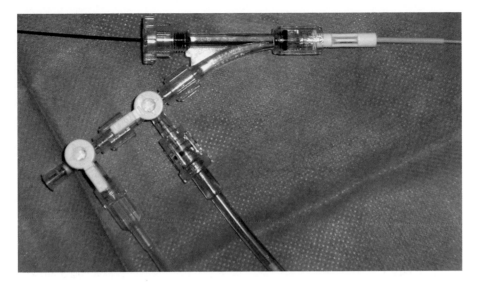

Fig. 2 Closed system with adaptor, contrast pump connection, and saline flush

catheters for cerebral angiography include Bernstein, Headhunter, Sim 1, Sim 2, JB-1, and Vert catheters or equivalent (Fig. 1).

Regular flushing of the catheter is essential during cerebral angiography to prevent clot formation and a possible embolic complication. Always use a double-flush and meniscus-to-meniscus technique. Closed continuous flush systems enable a single operator to perform a cerebral angiogram without an assistant. Continuous saline flushing prevents clot formation in the catheter. Meticulous examination of these closed flush systems is required to ensure the system is free of air. Operator inexperience or unfamiliarity with such systems can lead to devastating air embolism. Opinions and practices regarding these closed flush systems vary widely.

Angiography

A complete cerebral angiogram includes angiograms in at least two views of both carotid bifurcations, the intracranial circulation from both common carotid arteries, the vertebral arteries, and the posterior circulation. 3D DSA assessment of the artery of interest is usually performed. Additional angiograms relating to the clinical indication can be performed as well as relevant magnified branch assessments.

Intraprocedural Medications

Routine heparin use for cerebral angiography is optional. Heparin should be used in patients at high risk of thrombosis.

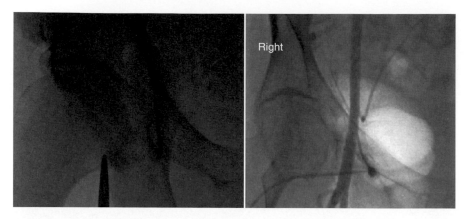

Fig. 3 Accurate pre-puncture localization as well as low-dose angiogram (fluoroscopy loop) of the right CFA is advised to ensure safe puncture and sheath placement

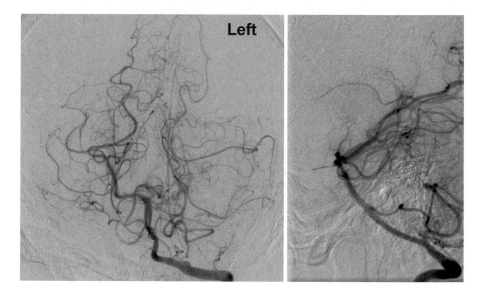

Fig. 4 Normal two plane vertebral angiogram

Performing the Procedure

Accurate pre-puncture localization as well as low-dose angiogram (fluoroscopy loop) of the right CFA is advised to ensure safe puncture and sheath placement (Fig. 3).

Angle the tube with 20–30° of LAO may assist in cannulation of the carotids and the left vertebral arteries from the arch. Fluoroscopy techniques such as roadmap or fluoro fade can be of assistance.

An occipitofrontal-type frontal plane view in conjunction with a true lateral view is advisable for ICA analysis (Fig. 4). Vertebral analysis is best assessed with a true lateral in association with a fronto-occipital/Towne's frontal plane projection (Fig. 5). Always review the clinical indication and the angiograms obtained before removing the sheath

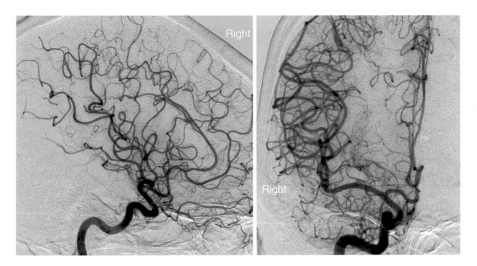

Fig. 5 Normal two plane ICA angiogram

Groin Closure

The two broad alternatives to close a CFA arteriotomy are the employment of manual compression or the use of a vascular closure device (VCD). When manual compression is utilized, nonocclusive pressure should be applied to the arteriotomy puncture site for at least 10 min post procedure. When a large caliber sheath has been used or when the patient is anticoagulated, this length of time is insufficient and a longer duration of pressure and observation is needed. It is advised that the patient lies supine for 4 h if closure is with manual compression. The patient should be examined for the presence of distal pulses, hematoma, and pseudoaneurysm formation at the site of puncture. A wide choice of VCDs is available and broadly fit into the following categories of device:

- Passive external pad or patch which enhances manual compression
- Suture devices which close the arteriotomy
- External extravascular collagen plug or nitinol clip

Vascular closure devices are utilized in 30–50 % of all angiograms worldwide. The complications associated with the use of VCDs are comparable to manual compression (3–5). Closure devices have the advantage of earlier hemostasis and earlier mobilization. Both of these are advantageous when the patient is anticoagulated or coming out of a general anesthetic. The risk of groin infection and possibly the need for puncture site surgery are marginally greater with VCDs. However, overall, the differences between VCDs and manual compression are not statistically significant. The cost of these devices should also be considered. The most popular closure devices on the market are shown in Table 1. A statistically significant difference in efficacy and complication rate does not exist between these commonly used closure devices.

Angio-Seal™, ProGlide/Perclose™, and StarClose™ dominate the market at present. Device deployment for these three closure methods is shown in Figs. 6, 7 and 8.

Table 1 Commonly used closure devices

Device	Manufacturer	Device type
Angio-Seal®	St. Jude Medical	Bovine collagen
VasoSeal®	Datascope	Bovine collagen
Duett Pro®	Vascular Solutions	Collagen/thrombin
Exoseal	Cordis	PGA plug
Perclose®	Abbott Vascular	Suture
ProGlide®	Abbott Vascular	Suture
X Site®	Datascope	Suture
FemoSeal®	Radi Medical	Collagen
SuperStitch®	Sutura Inc.	Suture
EVS®	Medtronic	Titanium staple
StarClose®	Abbott Vascular	Nitinol clip
SoundSeal®	Therus/Boston Scientific	Ultrasound (passive)
Boomerang®	Cardiva Medical	Tamponade (passive)
Mynx®	AccessClosure	Tamponade (passive)

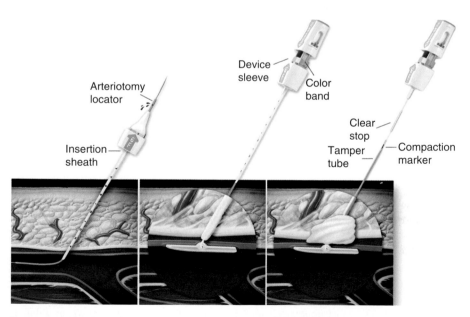

Fig. 6 Schematic of Angio-Seal™ deployment (Courtesy of St. Jude Medical)

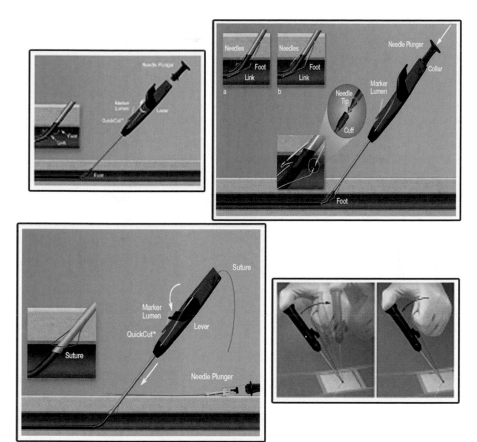

Fig. 7 Schematic of ProGlide™ deployment (Courtesy of Abbott Vascular)

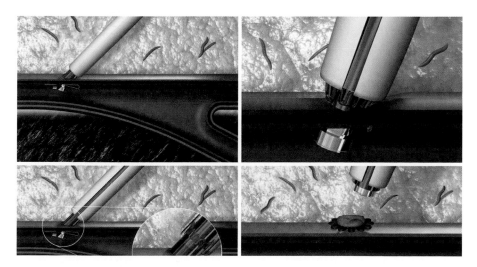

Fig. 8 Schematic of StarClose™ deployment (Courtesy of Abbott Vascular)

Post-procedure Care

- Assess neurological status post procedure.
- Monitor groin and vitals frequently (e.g., every 15 min × 1st hour, every 30 min × 2nd hour, and once in 3rd hour).
- Bed rest for 2–4 h, depending on method of closure.
- Clear and concise instructions should be provided to the patient regarding activities and restrictions.
- Follow-up should be planned prior to discharge and is essential to ensure long-term patient well-being.

Complications from Diagnostic Cerebral Angiography

Groin

- Hematoma (2.5–5 %)
- Pseudoaneurysm (0.4–0.9 %)
- Infection (0.5–0.9 %)
- Limb ischaemia (0.2–0.4 %)
- Requirement for surgery (0.2–0.6 %)

General

- Allergy (<0.04 %)
- Renal failure (depending on preexisting factors)

Neurological

- Transient neurological deficit (0.3–0.4 %)
- Non-transient neurological deficit (<0.01 %)
- Asymptomatic cervical dissection (0.3–0.4 %)

Key Points

- ⟩ Perform and review all noninvasive imaging initially.
- ⟩ Correct relative contraindications where possible.
- ⟩ Always check the groin pre puncture and check sheath position once in place
- ⟩ Always review the clinical indication and angiograms before removing the sheath.
- ⟩ Manual compression is the gold standard to close an arteriotomy.

Suggested Reading

1. Biancari F, D'Andrea V, Di Marco C, Savino G, Tiozzo V, Catania A. Meta-analysis of randomized trials on the efficacy of vascular closure devices after diagnostic angiography and angioplasty. Am Heart J. 2010;159(4):518–31.
2. Circle of Willis. Contributed by Dr Frank Gaillard. 2008. http://radiopaedia.org/articles/circle_of_willis.
3. Das R, Ahmed K, Athanasiou T, Morgan RA, Belli AM. Arterial closure devices versus manual compression for femoral haemostasis in interventional radiological procedures: a systematic review and meta-analysis. Cardiovasc Intervent Radiol. 2011;34(4):723–38. Epub 2010 Oct 29.
4. Dawkins AA, Evans AL, Wattam J, Romanowski CA, Connolly DJ, Hodgson TJ, Coley SC. Complications of cerebral angiography: a prospective analysis of 2,924 consecutive procedures. Neuroradiology. 2007;49(9):753–9. Epub 2007 Jun 27.
5. Layton KF, Kallmes DF, Cloft HJ, Lindell EP, Cox VS. Bovine aortic arch variant in humans: clarification of a common misnomer. AJNR Am J Neuroradiol. 2006;27(7):1541–2.
6. Nikolsky E, Mehran R, Halkin A, Aymong ED, Mintz GS, Lasic Z, Negoita M, Fahy M, Krieger S, Mousse I, Moses JW, Stone GW, Leon MB, Pocock SJ, Dangas G. Vascular complications associated with arteriotomy closure devices in patients undergoing percutaneous coronary procedures: a meta-analysis. J Am Coll Cardiol. 2004;44(6):1200–9.

Diagnostic Spinal Angiography

Peter Keston

Abstract

Spinal angiography encompasses both transarterial catheter digital subtraction angiography and, increasingly, magnetic resonance- and computed tomography-based techniques for noninvasive imaging of spinal blood vessels.

Keywords

Spinal catheter angiography • AVF • AVM • Myelopathy

Introduction

- Spinal angiography encompasses both transarterial catheter digital subtraction angiography and, increasingly, magnetic resonance (MR)- and computed tomography (CT)-based techniques for noninvasive imaging of spinal blood vessels.
- We will discuss the clinical indications for spinal vascular imaging.
- Imaging of spinal blood vessels is technically demanding due to their small size, large number, and anatomical complexity.
- We will review the vascular anatomy of the spinal cord and vertebral column and discuss diagnostic spinal angiography (DSA) techniques with an emphasis on minimizing risk and maximizing diagnostic accuracy.
- Specific clinical scenarios require modification of angiographic technique, and these will be elaborated.

P. Keston, MB, ChB, MRad, FRCR, FRCS
Department of Neuroradiology, Western General Hospital, Edinburgh, Scotland
e-mail: peter.keston@luht.scot.nhs.uk

K. Murphy, F. Robertson (eds.), *Interventional Neuroradiology,*
Techniques in Interventional Radiology,
DOI 10.1007/978-1-4471-4582-0_2, © Springer-Verlag London 2014

Spinal Vascular Anatomy

Spinal Cord

Arterial

- One anterior spinal artery (ASA) and two posterior arteries (PSA).
  - ASA gives circumferential (coronal) and penetrating (sulco-commissural) branches and supplies much of the central grey matter.
  - PSAs supply posterior and posterolateral cord.
- ASA is formed cranially from branches of each vertebral artery and is also supplied by several segmental branches.
  - Arise from segmental artery and follow the ventral nerve root.
  - In the thoracolumbar spine the supply is dominated by the arteria radicularis magna (Adamkiewicz artery).
- PSAs are formed from branches of the vertebral arteries or PICA vessels and are also supplied by radicular branches of the segmental arteries.
  - More numerous segmental arterial supply, following the dorsal nerve roots
  - Extensive collateralization between sides
- ASA and PSAs anastomose around the conus and through coronal arteries on the surface of the spinal cord.

Venous

- Venous drainage by the perimedullary venous plexus.
- Plexiform but concentrated in posterior and anterior groups and along the lines of the dorsal and ventral root entry zones on each side.
- Perimedullary veins drain via radicular veins to the epidural venous plexus and superiorly to the pontomesencephalic veins around the medulla and brainstem.
- No valves.

Vertebrae and Paravertebral Soft Tissues

- Arterial supply is by segmental vessels with well-developed intersegmental and contralateral anastomosis. Each segmental vessel gives supply to:
  - Vertebral body
    - Proximal occlusion can cause hemivertebral infarction which may be evident with magnetic resonance imaging (MRI).
  - Foraminal branches
    - Supply dura and dural arteriovenous fistula (DAVF) and radicular vessels to spinal arteries.
  - Intercostal arteries
    - Potential anastomosis with internal thoracic and lateral thoracic arteries

— Posterior branches
- To posterior elements of each vertebra and adjacent erector spinae muscles where collateral vessels crossing the midline may replicate the shape of the Adamkiewicz vessel as they loop up over the spinous process.
- Venous drainage is by a plexus of epidural veins which freely anastomose with a plexus of paravertebral veins. The radicular veins and basivertebral veins drain directly into this plexus.

Indications for Spinal Angiography

Myelopathy

Diagnose/Exclude Spinal Dural Arteriovenous Fistula (sDAVF) (Figs. 1, 2, and 3)

- Increased perimedullary venous pressure with cord venous ischemia.
- Progressive, often stepwise, myelopathic symptoms commonly pain.
- Most frequent in middle age males.
- Coexistent spinal degenerative disease often blamed (diagnostic delay).

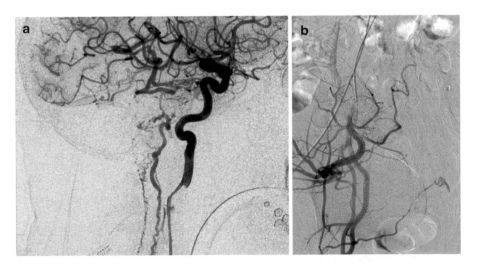

Fig. 1 Two patients presenting with spinal cord symptoms. Myelopathic changes and enlarged perimedullary veins were evident on MRI. Complete spinal angiography must include the intracranial vessels and the pelvic vessels. (**a**) A right petrous apex dural AV fistula has caused venous high flow stenosis, and venous drainage has is now via the ipsilateral basal vein and from there to give retrograde flow in the contralateral basal vein, pontomedullary venous plexus, and finally to the spinal perimedullary veins. (**b**) Patient known to have spina bifida occulta. The lateral sacral artery supplies a DAVF at the spina bifida defect. This was not evident with a pelvic flush aortogram series and was only visualized with a selective internal iliac injection

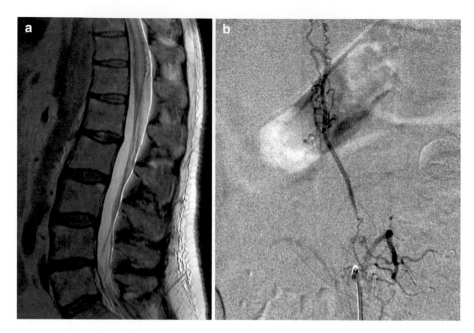

Fig. 2 Typical magnetic resonance imaging (MRI): (**a**) and DSA (**b**) appearances of a spinal DAVF. The combination of cord edema, mild cord swelling, and abnormally enlarged perimedullary veins is strongly indicative of a spinal vascular abnormality. The DSA reveals the arterial supply from a small radicular branch (*), the fistula (+), and the draining vein (x) which follows the nerve root to reach the perimedullary venous plexus

- MRI – usually swollen/edematous (occasionally hemorrhagic) lower cord and conus (irrespective of the fistula site) and prominent vessels in spinal subarachnoid space.
- MRI appearances overlap with other causes of cord swelling, including spinal cord infarction, tumor, and demyelination.

Spontaneous Intraspinal Hemorrhage

- Spontaneous intraspinal hemorrhage is rare in the absence of a coagulation disorder or a history of spinal instrumentation.
- Spinal arteriovenous abnormalities are a recognized cause of spontaneous epidural, subdural, and subarachnoid hemorrhage.
- Spinal angiography should be considered in patients with intracranial subarachnoid hemorrhage where cerebral angiography has been normal, particularly if there is a heavy posterior fossa/foramen magnum blood load.
- Structural (and possibly angiographic) MR imaging is desirable prior to undertaking DSA.

Planning for Surgery/Embolization

- Vascular spinal tumors are surgically challenging to treat, and preoperative embolization reduces operative time and blood transfusion requirement.

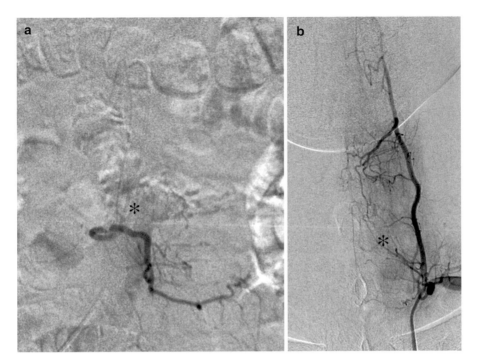

Fig. 3 Care is needed with every injection. (**a**) Patient presented with rapidly progressive paraparesis. MRI suggested cord ischemia but possible abnormal perimedullary vessels also noted. The DSA at T12 on the left revealed a tight stenosis of the radicular vessel and the Adamkiewicz artery (*) taking origin distal to the stenosis. Atheromatous disease is more frequently encountered at the vessel origins, and even careful catheterization may cause vessel occlusion. Avoid excessive catheter and wire manipulation. (**b**) Proximal injection in the left thyrocervical trunk reveals a large radiculomedullary artery (+) taking origin from the origin of the ascending cervical artery. Inadvertent trauma with a guidewire could have disastrous consequences

- Diagnostic angiography is indicated to map the vascular supply to the tumor deposit prior to surgery, and plan preoperative embolization.
- Surgery to the lower thoracic/upper lumbar spine or to the adjacent aorta risks occlusion of the Adamkiewicz vessel. Angiography is indicated to localize the segmental vessel which gives rise to Adamkiewicz.

Diagnostic Spinal Angiography

Cross-Sectional Angiographic Imaging

Spinal vascular lesions fall into the differential diagnosis in a relatively large number of patients where there is evidence of myelopathy and possibly abnormal spinal vascularity on cross-sectional CT/MRI. It may be desirable to establish the exact position of the artery of Adamkiewicz prior to embarking on major spinal or thoracic vascular surgery. Comprehensive spinal DSA is not always appropriate in these circumstances due to the inherent risk of spinal cord ischemia. Safer, but less sensitive, spinal angiography can be obtained with noninvasive cross-sectional techniques.

CT Angiography

- Multi-slice scanners have improved acquisition times, contrast, and spatial resolution.
- Low sensitivity for spinal vascular lesions due to proximity of bony structures.
  − Bone subtraction techniques are improving and may further improve sensitivity.
- Low risk and well tolerated.
- Large radiation dose to cover whole spine.

MR Angiography

- Contrast-enhanced elliptically centered acquisition.
- Low spatial resolution but very good contrast resolution now possible.
  − Moderate sensitivity for spinal vascular lesions.
- Some difficulty studying patients with myelopathy due to involuntary movements.
- Low risk.
- Time resolved studies can now be performed with promising results – may aid localization of level of shunt allowing more targeted catheter angiography.

Cone Beam CT

- Modern angiographic equipment can be used to obtain cross-sectional imaging during aortic contrast injection.
- Very good spatial and contrast resolution (very high arterial contrast concentrations can be achieved with aortic injection).
- Invasive but risk lower than selective angiography and better tolerated.
- Sensitivity in detection of spinal vascular lesions not well established but likely to be significantly better than with CT or MRI.
- Can be used in combination with selective injections to clarify complex vascular anatomy.

Spinal Digital Subtraction Angiography (SDSA)

Techniques

Consent

Fully informed consent

- Statement of the reason for performing the test.
- Statement of expected benefit.
  - Increased diagnostic accuracy
  - Planning for treatment
  - Exclusion of potentially curable diagnosis
- Explanation of the possibility of spinal cord infarction leading to paraplegia and incontinence.
  - Risk is difficult to quantify but is in the order of 1 % – higher in patients with known atheromatous disease or underlying systemic vascular abnormality.
- List the risks related to arterial access, use of contrast agents, and thromboembolic complications, and discuss the need for cerebral angiography with its inherent risk of stroke.
- Provide written information.
- Best practice is to allow time to "cool off" between consent and procedure.
- Consent to be obtained by the operator in person.
- Record details in the patient's files.

Preparation

- Check renal function (eGFR) – potential for large contrast doses.
- Urinary catheter should be considered in all cases as long cases and often preexisting urinary dysfunction.
- Prophylactic intravenous antibiotic therapy recommended prior to catheterization if there is a history of urinary symptoms.
- Consider fasting for 12 h prior for general anesthetic and will reduce bowel gas shadowing.
- Bowel preparation with oral or rectal agents has been advocated to reduce artifact.
- Intravenous cannula should be placed.
- Cardiac and oxygen saturation monitoring is essential.

- General anesthesia (GA) improves image quality.
  - Eliminates involuntary movements in patients with cord pathology.
  - Avoids respiration artifact.
  - Keep anesthetic and monitoring equipment out of the field of view.
  - Explain that repeated respiration holds will be required.
- Local anesthesia can be used.
  - Cooperative patients.
  - Avoid the use of intravenous sedation – patient cooperation is essential.
  - Coach patient about breath holding before you get started.
  - It may be necessary to stage the examination in an awake patient, particularly if vessel selection is difficult.
- Intravenous (IV) hyoscine or IV glucagon may be used to paralyze the bowel and reduce artifact.

Radiography

- This is a high radiation dose study. Take all possible steps to minimize your patient's, your staff's, and your own dose:
  - Single AP plane almost always adequate.
  - Keep collimation relatively tight – also improves image quality.
  - Use pulsed fluoroscopy at a low frame rate.
  - Slow image acquisition (1 frame/s) is acceptable for most vessels.
    - Thoracic and lumbar radicles are small and have slow flow when catheterized.
    - Ensure that it is possible to extend a run to at least 30 s (preferably at 0.5 or 0.33 frames/s) for attempting to image the venous phase when the Adamkiewicz vessel is identified.
  - Appropriate radiation protection.
- Accurate recording of levels is essential.
  - Skin markers/opaque ruler can be used, but be aware that they "move" in respect to the vertebrae due to parallax (worse if placed at the patient's back) and due to respiration phase and patient movement (worse if placed at the front).
  - Markers can overlap vessels if placed too near the midline.
  - Establish vertebral body anatomy and anomalies in numbers of segments from spinal MRI.
  - Find an angiographic "baseline."
    - Identify the superior mesenteric artery or a renal artery and establish its level by correlation with cross-sectional imaging.
    - Use this as a fixed reference point for numbering vertebrae
    - Confirm this by counting up from lumbosacral junction and down from T1.
  - Select a field of view which covers five vertebrae starting at a known level.
  - Avoid any table movement until all vessels in that section of the spine have been studied.

— The catheter tip can then be used as a fixed reference point to move to the next section up or down.

— The vessels are numbered by the segmental level supplied, not by the vertebral body opposite which they arise – *Tip*: the hemivertebral blush tells you which vertebra.

— Ensure that all segmental arteries are studied.

Catheter Selection

This is very subjective, but some general observations hold true:

- Radicles are cranially directed in the thoracic spine but progressively more caudally directed towards the lower lumbar spine. A forward-facing catheter (e.g., cobra shape) works well in the thoracic spine, but a retroflexed (Simmons 2 or 3) catheter shape may be better in the lumbar region. Look at the angulation of the vessel origins as you study each level.
- Good shape retention and torquability are essential: consider 5 F or even 6 F catheters.
- The radicles are small: larger catheters increase the vessel dissection risk. Try to find a catheter with a supportive body but soft, tapered tip. It may be necessary to use a 4 Fr catheter if the radicles are very small. These have poor shape retention and poor tolerance to repeated torque maneuvers so consider a fresh catheter after each few runs.
- It is useful to have pigtail and straight tip catheters available for aortic runs.
- Use a retroflexed catheter to study the internal iliacs and have your preferred cerebral catheters available for studying the intracranial circulation and cervical vessels.

Techniques for Vessel Selection

- Position the catheter in the aorta at the level to be studied.
- Ensure that the tip is not impacted in the vessel wall.
- Rotate clockwise to determine the tip position (tip moves right to left implies that it is pointing forwards and vice versa).
- The right-sided segmental vessels arise from the posteromedial aortic wall on the right. The left-sided vessels generally arise from the posterior wall close to the midline.
- Start "searching" with the catheter tip just below the level of the pedicles.
- When you have selected a vessel, a small increase in forward pressure (or tension if using a retroflexed catheter shape) is helpful to engage in the vessel origin although.
- Care is needed to prevent ostial dissection and reactive vessel spasm
- Inject contrast using an angiographic run: avoid unnecessary contrast administration under fluoroscopy to minimize the dose and to prevent a standing column of contrast in the vessel (the catheter tip often occludes arterial inflow).

Tips

- Each segmental vessel tends to lie in line with its cranial and caudal neighbors, approximately one vertebral body height above or below.
- The contralateral vessel generally arises at the same craniocaudal level as its counterpart.
  - It is common for there to be a small infundibulum from which both segmental vessels arise, and it may be possible to move from right to left without completely disengaging the catheter and merely torquing and re-engaging in the other vessel.
  - Always disengage the catheter tip atraumatically before moving on – pull out a forward-facing catheter and push out a retroflexed one.
  - Start cranially (caudally if a retroflexed catheter is required) and select each vessel on one side in series before moving to the other side.
- If there is a "missing" vessel:
  - Use a straight tip catheter to perform an aortic run.
    - The contrast layers at the back of the aorta fill several segmental vessels in one injection.
    - Compare with cross-sectional angiography if available – aberrant or conjoined vessels are not unusual.
  - Do not rely on aortic injections to exclude DAVF.
    - Always try for a selective injection.

Vessels to Study

For a complete spinal angiogram:

- Subclavian arteries
- Vertebral arteries (catheter tip must be proximally placed)
- Thyrocervical and costocervical trunks
- Each segmental vessel
- Median sacral artery
- Internal iliac vessels
  - Lateral sacral arteries

A comprehensive cerebral angiogram should be included if there is any suggestion of abnormality involving the cervical or posterior fossa structures.

Artery of Adamkiewicz

- T8 to L2 and more often on the left.
- Characteristic hairpin loop configuration.
- Analyze ASA carefully to exclude enlargement or abnormally high flow.
  - May indicate cord arteriovenous malformation (AVM) out with field of view

- Extended run to look for venous phase.
  - Wide craniocaudal field of view.
  - Delayed or absent indicates AVM/AVF draining to perimedullary veins.
  - Early indicates cord AVM with shunting and early venous drainage.
  - Normal phase with no distension of the perimedullary veins indicates that there is venous hypertension, and AVM/AVF is less likely.
- Do not leave the catheter in place after injection.
  - Restricts flow due to proximal vessel occlusion
  - Can cause cord ischemia
  - Alters the normal hemodynamics and will prevent the normal flow of contrast to the perimedullary veins

Found a Vascular Lesion?

- Targeted run AP, LAO, RAO, and lateral if possible.
- Three-dimensional DSA if possible.
- Double check that good quality runs are available for each segmental vessel for two levels above and below.
- Ensure that Adamkiewicz/ASA has been positively identified.
- For cervical lesions it may be possible to study the ASA by using a nondetachable balloon to temporarily occlude the vertebral just distal to the ASA origin and injecting the vertebral proximal to this.
- Analyze the venous drainage to exclude intracranial involvement/venous stenotic disease and venous ectasia – all predispose to subarachnoid hemorrhage.

Complications

- Spinal Cord Infarction
  - Occlusion or embolism in spinal radicular vessel
  - Can cause primary infarct in the arterial territory or "watershed" infarct at the edge of the territory
  - Cord swelling and T2 hyperintensity: can take a day or more to become apparent on MR
  - Diffusion restriction
  - Occasional microhemorrhage
- Other Vessel Injury
  - Segmental vessels
  - Aorta
  - Puncture site
  - Cerebral vessels

- Bleeding Complications at Puncture Site
  - Groin hematoma
  - Pseudoaneurysm
  - Retroperitoneal hemorrhage
- Bacteraemia/Septic Shock
  - Traumatic urinary catheterization in patient with urinary retention/infection
- Contrast or Drug reactions
- Incomplete Study/Poor Technique
  - Missed diagnosis

Key Points

> Spinal angiography is challenging and requires a thorough knowledge of spinal arterial and venous anatomy.
> Spinal vascular pathologies are complex and may be difficult to find and delineate.
> A careful, considered, and systematic approach is key to a successful study.
> An exhaustive examination of all potential vessels supplying the neuroaxis and its linings may be necessary.

Suggested Reading

1. Hurst RW, Rossenwasser R. Neurointerventional management: diagnosis and treatment. 2nd ed. London/New York: Informa Healthcare; 2012.
2. Lasjaunias P. Surgical neuroangiography. Berlin/New York: Springer; 2001.
3. Pearse Morris P. Practical neuroangiography. Philadelphia: Lippincott Williams and Wilkins; 2007.
4. Thron AK. Vascular anatomy of the spinal cord: neuroradiological investigations and clinical syndromes. Wien/New York: Springer; 1988.

Vascular Access: Guide Catheter Selection, Usage, and Compatibility

Jeremy Madigan

Abstract

Success in neurovascular interventions often depends upon achieving a stable position with an appropriately chosen guide catheter. Procedures can easily fail or be unnecessarily prolonged because of poor guide catheter selection or compromised catheter position. An ever-increasing array of products means the neurointerventionalist must have a clear understanding of the basic principles of the guide catheter properties, selection, and appropriate usage.

Keywords

Vascular access • Guide catheter • Selection • Usage • Compatibility • Neurovascular intervention • Adverse consequence • Vessel damage • Complications • Prolapse • Microcatheter position • Safety

Introduction

- Success in neurovascular interventions often depends upon achieving a stable position with an appropriately chosen guide catheter.
- Procedures can easily fail or be unnecessarily prolonged because of poor guide catheter selection or compromised catheter position.
- An ever-increasing array of products means the neurointerventionalist must have a clear understanding of the basic principles of the guide catheter properties, selection, and appropriate usage.

J. Madigan, MB, ChB, FRCR
Department of Neuroradiology, St. Georges Hospital, Tooting, London, UK
e-mail: jeremy.madigan@stgeorges.nhs.uk

K. Murphy, F. Robertson (eds.), *Interventional Neuroradiology,*
Techniques in Interventional Radiology,
DOI 10.1007/978-1-4471-4582-0_3, © Springer-Verlag London 2014

Potential adverse consequences of poor guide catheter selection and placement include:

- Vessel damage, thromboembolic, and/or hemodynamic complications
- Inability to track microcatheters, balloons, stent delivery devices, etc.
- Prolapse of the guide lower into the neck or aortic arch at a crucial moments, often with the loss of a hard won microcatheter position.

General principle: the more distal the position that can be *safely* achieved with the guide catheter, the better.
Patient or technical factors contributing to choice of guide catheter include:

Patient Factors
- Size of vessel
- Vessel tortuosity: iliac/aortic/neck vessel
- Height of the patient
- Calcifications
- Patient morphology (short, fat hypertensive patients with no neck who used to be taller)

Technical Factors
- Access rigidity versus distal positioning
- Required internal lumen for planned procedure/potential rescue maneuvers
- Necessity for flow arrest (e.g., test-occlusion or mechanical clot retrieval)

More general factors relating to guide catheter selection often come down to personal choice or experience. Generally desirable properties in a guide catheter include:

- Soft atraumatic distal tip
- Stiff/sturdy proximal shaft for support
- Multiply graded transitions in rigidity from proximal to distal ends
- Large internal lumen relative to the outer diameter (thin wall profile), but without excessive compromise of wall weakness/tendency to kink

In reality, most guide catheters present a compromise between the above properties, and the selection of a guide catheter for any given case may depend on the most important properties required.

With the above factors taken into consideration, the following are questions to ask when selecting a guide catheter for a specific case:

- Can it be safely navigated into the vessel without occluding flow and without undue risk of causing dissection or severe spasm?
- Will it accommodate all of the equipment planned for use in the case?
- What case-specific complications might be anticipated, and will the guide catheter accommodate (separately or concurrently) any additional catheters/balloons/stents etc. that might be needed to deal with these complications?
- Can adequate angiographic runs be performed when single or multiple devices are inside it? i.e., to what degree will the inner lumen of the catheter be obturated?

Guide Catheter Types

Standard Guide Catheters (Guider, Envoy)

- Designed only to be positioned in the extracranial neck vessels
- Typically 5–8 F
- Angled or straight tip commonly used
- Delivered through an appropriately sized sheath in the groin
- Typically come in lengths of between 90 and 110 cm, with longer lengths for taller patients
- Common choice for simpler procedures (e.g., unassisted aneurysm coil embolization, embolization of intracranial AV shunt, or tumor)

Long Sheaths (e.g., Cook Shuttle)

- Designed only to be positioned in the extracranial neck vessels
- Typically 5–7 F (denotes internal capacity, not outer diameter)
- Straight tip – more complex to position using an exchange technique or as a single step using dedicated tip-shaped inner coaxial catheters sold as part of the system
- Kink resistant and very stable – can often be used to straighten tortuous proximal anatomy, providing greater stability with reduced chance of catheter prolapse
- Relatively large inner lumen – for simultaneous passage of multiple devices
- Common choice for complex procedures e.g., balloon-assisted aneurysm coil embolization or stent procedures requiring a large capacity guide

Intracranial Access (e.g., Neuron, Distal Access Catheters)

- Designed to be positioned more distally than standard guide catheters, e.g., in the petrous or cavernous portions of the internal carotid artery or around the C2 and C1 loops of the vertebral artery
- 6 F proximally and either 6 F distally or tapering to 5 F (relatively small lumen may be a weakness)
- Can be positioned using proprietary 3 or 5 F select catheters with a range of different shaped tips, or exchanged for a diagnostic catheter into the neck, then tracked more distally over a microcatheter/microwire
- Potential for greater stability in some circumstances, but only if truly positioned within the proximal intracranial vessels. Can be combined coaxially within long sheath devices when "extreme stability" is required
  - Useful for overcoming tortuous distal neck or proximal intracranial anatomy, particularly when trying to track balloons and stents to the intracranial circulation, e.g., around tonsillar loops in the cervical carotid artery
- Adopted by some operators first choice guide catheter for most intracranial embolizations, regardless of anatomy

Balloon Guide Catheters

- Designed to be positioned in the extracranial neck vessels (CCA/ICA).
- Typically 8 F.
- Straight tips.
- Reasonably small inner lumen relative to large outer diameter.
- The author reserves the use of these catheters for use in mechanical thrombectomy in acute stroke cases, where inflation of the balloon allows flow arrest/reversal and more effective aspiration.

Some Commonly Used Guide Catheters and Their Properties

Guider Softip (Boston Scientific)

- Typical sizes used: 6 and 7 F (5, 8, and 9 F also available).
- Respective internal diameters: 0.064 in and 0.073 in.
- Available lengths: 90 and 100 cm.
- Advantages: As the name suggests, it has a soft tip. Seven centimeter flexible distal segment. Relatively atraumatic and less likely to cause spasm. Easy to torque – good for direct selection of vessels from the arch (with or without a wire) in young patients.
- Disadvantages: 6 F version has a relatively small inner lumen compared to other 6 F guides. Less rigid/stable than some guide catheters, with a tendency to back out towards the aorta when negotiating inner microcatheters/devices etc. through tortuous distal anatomy.

5 F or 6 F Envoy (Codman Neurovascular)

- Typical sizes used: 5 and 6 F (only these sizes available).
- Respective internal diameters: 0.056 in (1.4 mm) and 0.070 in (1.8 mm).
- Available lengths: 90 and 100 cm.
- Advantages: Large inner lumen. Relatively rigid, often giving a stable position even in tortuous anatomy.
- Disadvantages: As in all cases, the trade-off for the rigidity is greater potential for trauma. The tip is also not as "vessel friendly" as the Guider Softip – it has quite a sharp lip. May "soften" during a procedure and lose its stability or rigidity.

5, 6, and 7 F Shuttle (Cook)

- Typical sizes used: 5, 6, and 7 F (8 F also available for carotid access).
- Respective internal diameters: 0.074, 0.087, and 0.100 in.
- Available lengths: 80 and 90 cm.
- Advantages: Very large inner lumen. Extremely stable. Track well over selective catheters. Straighten out tortuous aortoiliac anatomy. Good kink-resistance.

- Disadvantages: Large inner lumen can empty a flush bag in seconds if not closely monitored, with risk of gas embolus. Large lumen also forms large clots quickly –need to actively manage blood reflux. Again, stiff catheter is more spasm prone and has greater potential for dissection.
- Tip: if exchanging rather than using select catheters, be sure to use the inner obturator provided; this will help minimize vessel trauma.

Cello Balloon Guide (EV3 C3ovidien)

- Typical sizes used: 8 F only.
- Respective internal diameters: 0.075 in (1.9 mm).
- Available lengths: 95 cm effective length.
- Advantages: Soft atraumatic hydrophilic tip. Balloon inflation can achieve ICA flow arrest in mechanical thrombectomy cases and may allow for more effective aspiration during device/thrombus retrieval.
- Disadvantages: Relatively small inner lumen when compared to outer diameter. Like most balloons, need to carefully purge balloon of gas during preparation.
- Tip: a 125 cm 5.5 F SIM-2 Shuttle Select catheter inside this catheter provides a formidable access tool when used for mechanical thrombectomy in acute stroke patients (who often have challenging aortic arch and neck vessel anatomy).

Chaperon (Microvention)

- Typical sizes used: 5 and 6 F.
- Respective internal diameters: 0.059 and 0.071 in.
- Available lengths: 95 cm.
- Advantages: Thin wall profile, so 6 F version has slightly larger inner lumen than some of the other 6 F competitors. Good torque control. Comes with dedicated "inner" selective catheters for coaxial method.
- Disadvantages: While it offers a relatively stable position, it is not as stable as some of its competitors.

Neuron (Penumbra Inc.)

- Typical sizes used: 6 F.
- Respective internal diameters: 0.053 and 0.070 in (053 tapers to 5 F distally, both are 6 F proximally).
- Available lengths (working): 053 = 105 cm and 115 cm; 070 = 95 cm and 105 cm.
- Advantages: Can be positioned in petrous (070) and cavernous (053) ICA or the more distal vertebral arteries – assists in overcoming tortuous anatomy. Can allow for easier tracking of large/stiff kit such as balloons and stents. 5 F Select catheters for use in the 070 versions are useful for vessel selection.

- Disadvantages: Unless positioned distally as per the design intention, they can be less stable than ordinary guides – so either put it distally or choose another catheter. May require the additional support of a long sheath otherwise (but be careful to calculate the usable length of neuron at the distal end in advance).

Guide Catheter Positioning

Guide catheters can be positioned in the following ways:

- Direct selection of a vessel from the aorta, usually using a suitable guidewire
- Using a coaxial technique with a smaller and pre-shaped inner "select" catheter
- Exchanging over a wire having accessed the vessel using a smaller tip-shaped (diagnostic angiography) catheter

Direct Selection

- Direct selection of a vessel without a wire, but with intermittent "puffing" of contrast upon catheter advancement, should probably be reserved for relatively young patients in whom diseased neck vessels is not anticipated.
- Using this method in tortuous or grossly diseased vessels is likely to result in a higher incidence of vessel dissection and vasospasm.
- Puffing of contrast helps keep the catheter tip away from the vessel wall, allowing for prompt identification of any impediments to passage and dissections.
- If wire is used, an RHV and flush bag should always be attached to the guide catheter to prevent blood reflux around the wire and intraluminal thrombus formation, leading to subsequent thromboembolic complications.

Coaxial Technique

- Smaller catheter with a shaped tip.
- Loaded into the inner lumen of the guide catheter to select the desired vessel.
- Once the smaller inner catheter is advanced into the vessel over a wire, the external guide catheter can be advanced smoothly over the inner catheter.
- Helps minimize trauma to the vessel wall and likely reduces embolic events arising from an atheromatous aortic arch.
- Some guide catheters have accompanying proprietary inner catheters in a range of different shapes for the express purpose of coaxial catheter placement. *Examples*:
  - Shuttle long sheath (Cook)
  - Chaperon (Microvention)
  - Neuron (Penumbra Inc)
- Advantages: forming a snug fit within the guide catheter minimizing blood reflux and presenting a much smoother transition profile to the vessel on advancing.

Exchange Technique

- Inherently more dangerous than direct selection techniques
- Higher thromboembolic risk
- Exchange technique reserved (by authors) for tortuous or otherwise difficult anatomy and when either of the above two methods fail.
- If unavoidable, it is generally advisable to employ systemic heparinization prior to exchanging wherever possible.

Managing Guide Catheter Related Problems

Spasm and Flow Limitation

- Failure to observe and promptly correct limited or absent flow caused by a guide catheter can lead:
  - Thromboembolic
  - Hemodynamic ischemic stroke
- If flow is borderline, reduce the risk of thrombus formation by:
  - Higher flush rates.
  - Judicious use of systemic heparinization (to achieve an ACT of 2–3× baseline).
  - Does not eliminate the risk completely.
- With evidence of limited washout of contrast, but no obvious spasm or dissection:
  - Selected guide catheter may simply be too large for the vessel.
  - Downsizing the catheter or selecting a more proximal guide catheter position may be the only safe solution.
- Where spasm is seen at the tip of the guide catheter immediately after placement, with unacceptable impediment to distal flow:
  - Incrementally pulling the guide catheter back, short distances will usually restore acceptable flow.
  - Guide catheter can often be repositioned more distally later in the procedure (often over the microcatheter) once initial vasospasm has settled.
- Antispasmodic agents such a nimodipine and GTN may help relieve spasm and allow for a distal catheter placement with preserved flow.
- Some interventionists use GTN for catheter-induced spasm, reserving nimodipine for the treatment of spasm related to subarachnoid hemorrhage. Others use nimodipine for both causes of spasm.
- Nimodipine 1–2 mg boluses can be given slowly through the guide catheter until the desired effect is achieved.
- Caution: Inform the anesthetist before injecting, as there may be profound effects on systemic blood pressure.
- Nimodipine can also be added to flush bags, and some operators do this for every case. GTN may be given in small 30 µg aliquots – *again warn the anesthetist first.*

Arterial Dissection

- Much-feared problem in neurointervention, whether in the extra- or intracranial vessels.
- Potential complications: vessel occlusion or distal thromboembolism.
- Clinical situation will often determine the appropriate course of remedial action, if any.
- Limited flow but patent vessel lumen:
  - Consider balloon angioplasty or stent placement across the dissected segment.
  - Stent placement will usually require dual antiplatelet therapy: risk/benefit should be carefully considered. (Discussion with a colleague often helps.)
- No flow limitation:
  - Case is elective.
  - In its early phases, may be appropriate to defer the procedure and place the patient on anticoagulants/antiaggregants.
  - Decision making becomes more challenging in the emergency setting (e.g., acute subarachnoid hemorrhage) where it is necessary to cross the dissected segment to protect a lesion downstream.

The "Bouncing" Guide Catheter

- In patients with hypertension and/or tortuous access, guide catheter may "see-saw" back and forth along the axis of the vessel with each cardiac pulsation.
- The bouncing motion is often then transmitted to microcatheters, and this can be very disconcerting (and dangerous), particularly while trying to access fragile structures such as recently ruptured intracranial aneurysms.
- Allowing for anatomy, advancing the guide catheter to a more distal position (almost invariably, a more proximal position will only worsen the problem) may be attempted.
- Alternative strategies include:
  - Place a stiff "buddy" microwire alongside the microcatheter with its tip in the guide catheter to provide additional support without traumatizing the vessel (e.g., Platinum plus 014, Boston Scientific).
  - Change to a stiffer guide catheter or a long sheath.

Arterial Embolus

- Guide catheter related embolus is always avoidable by:
  - Meticulous catheter techniques
  - Judicious use of pressurized heparinized saline flush bags
  - Systematic organization of the angiography environment
  - Careful training of angiography staff
- One must be on high alert for embolic complications at all times and be prepared to act swiftly once recognized.

Emboli can occur in a number of ways:

Atherosclerotic Plaque Disruption: From Aortic Arch/Extracranial Arteries

- Appearance: Varying size emboli – often calcified/fatty fragments on CT.
- Prevention: These are predictable and can be avoided by vigilance in recognition of plaque on access imaging and appropriate modification of technique.
- Treatment: Difficult to treat as often small, distal, and unresponsive to drug therapies.

Fresh Thrombus: Stationary Blood-Forming Clot in Guide Catheter Lumen and Then Being Flushed Out or Clot Forming on Exposed Wires During Exchange Technique

- Appearance: long strings of clot or casts of the catheter lumen on angiography (red thrombus)
- Prevention: Scrupulous guide catheter flush management and avoidance of exchange techniques. Recognizing patient factors predisposing to thrombosis, e.g., sepsis, malignancy, clotting disorders. Early heparin administration
- Treatment: Consider thrombus retrieval for large proximal emboli or drug therapies such as IV tPA or antiplatelet therapies: abciximab > clopidogrel > aspirin

Arterial Gas Embolus: Gas Bubbles Entering via Flush Line or Directly Injected with Contrast

- Appearance: Showers of small distal emboli – gas locules often visible on post-procedure CT.
- Prevention: There are many potential initiatives including sealed contrast systems// meticulous handling of contrast syringes. Low volume alarms on flush bags etc.
- Treatment: anecdotal experience has found increasing patient's inspired oxygen concentration to maximum for duration of case promotes resorption of intravascular gas bubbles and minimizing deficit (no cost in doing this even if it doesn't work!).

Device Compatibility: French, Gauge and Inches Made Easy

- No single standardized method for communicating sizes of the wide range of equipment used in neurointervention.
- The following outlines the commonly used sizing systems in neurointervention, with an easy guide to conversion between these systems.
- Two reference tables are provided for everyday use.

French (Charrière) Gauge System

- Named after Joseph-Frédéric-Benoît Charrière, a nineteenth century Parisian cutler.
- Symbols: F, Ch, and CH.
- 1 F = 0.33 mm.

Table 1 Examples of size compatibility[a]

Procedure	Example equipment	Individual OD sizes (F/in)	Minimum inner guide lumen (F/in)	Usable guide catheters
Stent-assisted aneurysm coiling (jailing technique)	4 mm Solitaire stent delivery catheter (021 class)	2.8/0.037	5.2/0.069	6 F Envoy
	014 class microcatheter	2.4/0.032		6 F Chaperon
	Enterprise stent delivery catheter (021 class)	2.8/0.037	5.2/0.069	7 F Guider Softip
	014 class microcatheter	2.4/0.032		6 F Neuron
				5 F Shuttle
Balloon-assisted aneurysm coiling	Hyperglide/Hyperform balloon	2.8/0.037	5.2/0.069	
	014 class microcatheter	2.4/0.032		
Extracranial carotid stenting	Carotid Wallstent (8 mm)	5/0.066	6.1/0.080	6 F Shuttle
	Platinum Plus 014 "buddy" wire	1.1/0.014		8 F Guider Softip

[a]This type of table is easily modified and extended for individual practice and can prove to be an invaluable reference on the wall of a lab/angiography suite

F/3 = external diameter of a catheter in mm.

- Usage: Commonly used to refer to the OUTER DIAMETER (OD) of a catheter.
- However, confusingly, when describing a sheath size, it refers to the largest-sized catheter that will fit inside the sheath, i e., the INNER DIAMETER (ID) not the OD of the sheath itself. Example: a 6 F Shuttle (Cook) long sheath will accept a 6 F catheter inside it, and itself has an OD of 7.8 F (0.104 in).
- Unfortunately, catheter size in F does not reliably define the internal diameter of the catheter; this is also determined by catheter wall thickness. However, most catheters of a given F will have inner lumen that falls within a fairly narrow range (see Table 1).

Stubs Iron Wire Gauge System

- Developed by the Stubs Iron Works in the mid nineteenth century.
- Symbols: G, Ga, Gg, and g.
- Usage: needles and venous/arterial access catheters.
- Designated as the number of a particular device that can fit inside a circular orifice of standard diameter.

Table 2 Converting units

F	in	mm	G[a]
0.6	0.008	0.20	33
0.8	0.010	0.25	31
0.9	0.012	0.30	30
1.1	0.014	0.36	28
1.2	0.016	0.41	27
1.4	0.018	0.46	26
2.6	0.035	0.89	20
2.9	0.038	0.96	19
4	0.053	1.35	17
5	0.066	1.67	16
6	0.079	2.0	14
7	0.092	2.3	13
8	0.105	2.7	12
9	0.118	3.0	11

[a]The gauge sizing listed is an approximation to the nearest measurement in inches. Where a given G size is roughly equidistant between two sizes in inches, the larger G size has been listed

- Inverse and nonlinear scale: the larger the number, the smaller the caliber.
- It is sometimes useful to be able to convert F (Ch) to gauge e.g., when choosing an appropriately sized (same size or slightly larger) arterial or venous access catheter for exchange with the sheath at the end of a procedure.

Inch

- Imperial system unit of length.
- Symbol: in.
- 1 in = 25.4 mm.
- Usage: the internal diameter of a guide catheter is commonly measured in inches and class of microcatheter commonly referred to in terms of fractions of inches. In the latter case, this is not the true internal diameter of the microcatheter, but rather the maximum external diameter microwire that can be accommodated within it. Microwire diameters are entirely referred to in fractions of inches.
- To convert F to inches: F/76.2 = in (Table 2).

Key Points

> The neurointerventionalist requires a clear understanding of the following:
> — Principles of guide catheter design, selection, and usage
> — Guide catheter related complications – minimizing incidence and mitigating their effects
> — Complexities of device sizing and conversion between sizing systems
> Give careful thought to guide catheter selection in every case. Ask yourself in advance: what could go wrong, what equipment might be needed to fix the problem, and will the guide catheter be up to the task?
> Guide catheters can be navigated into the neck vessels in a number of ways. Choice of method depends on a number of factors including personal experience, patient age, and vessel tortuosity/disease. Avoid the exchange technique where possible, but if necessary, ensure the patient is heparinized.
> For catheter-induced spasm, first try slowly withdrawing the catheter until adequate flow is restored. Either GTN or nimodipine can be given slowly in small aliquots via the guide catheter. Warn the anesthetist regarding potential drops in blood pressure before giving either of these drugs.
> Keeping a chart of size-compatible equipment on the wall of the lab/angio suite is useful as an aide memoir and can prevent procedural delays and wastage by helping to choose the appropriate kit first time.

Suggested Reading

1. Ahn W, Bahk JH, Lim YJ. The "gauge" system for medical use. Anesth Analg. 2002;95(4):1125.
2. Iserson KV. J.- F.- B. Charrière: the man behind the "French" gauge. J Emerg Med. 1987a;5:545–8.
3. Iserson KV. The origins of the gauge system for medical equipment. J Emerg Med. 1987b;5:45–8.
4. ISO 10555–1: Sterile, single-use intravascular catheters – part 1: general requirements. 1st ed. Geneva: International Organization for Standardization; 1995. p. 1–3.
5. ISO 10555–2: Sterile, single-use intravascular catheters – part 2: angiographic catheters. 1st ed. Geneva: International Organization for Standardization; 1996. p. 1–3.

Part II

Aneurysm Treatment

Basic Principles and Simple Techniques

Rufus Corkill

Abstract

The incidence of spontaneous aneurismal subarachnoid hemorrhage is 6–10 per 100,000 patients per year, and the prevalence of intracranial aneurysms is between 1 and 5 % of the population. This suggests that 0.2–1 in 100 aneurysms rupture each year. One third of patients who have a subarachnoid hemorrhage will die before they get to a hospital, and another third will die within a month as a result of the damage done at the time of the bleed. Aneurismal rebleeding is the greatest risk to life. This has two peaks of increased risk: in the early and subacute phases within 24 h and at 7–10 days. If left unsecured, about 25 % will rebleed in the first 2 weeks and two-thirds within the first 2 months. Treatment options include supportive resuscitation, neurosurgical clipping, and endovascular therapy.

Keywords

Spontaneous aneurismal subarachnoid hemorrhage • Intracranial aneurysm • Rupture • Mortality • Bleeding • Aneurismal rebleeding • Subacute phase • Early phase • Supportive resuscitation • Neurosurgical clipping • Endovascular therapy • Treatment

Introduction

The incidence of spontaneous aneurismal subarachnoid hemorrhage (SAH) is 6–10 per 100,000 patients per year, and the prevalence of intracranial aneurysms is between 1 and 5 % of the population. This suggests that 0.2–1 in 100 aneurysms rupture each year.

R. Corkill, MBBS, BSc, FRCS, FRCR, MSc
Department of Neuroradiology, Level 1, John Radcliffe Hospital, Oxford, UK
e-mail: rufus.corkill@orh.nhs.uk

K. Murphy, F. Robertson (eds.), *Interventional Neuroradiology,*
Techniques in Interventional Radiology,
DOI 10.1007/978-1-4471-4582-0_4, © Springer-Verlag London 2014

One-third of patients who have a subarachnoid hemorrhage will die before they get to a hospital, and another third will die within a month as a result of the damage done at the time of the bleed. Aneurismal rebleeding is the greatest risk to life. This has two peaks of increased risk: in the *early* and *subacute* phases within 24 h and at 7–10 days. Overall, if left unsecured about 25 % will rebleed in the first 2 weeks and two-thirds within the first 2 months.

Treatment Options

Treatment options include:

Supportive Resuscitation

Supportive resuscitation should aim to maintain normotension until the aneurysm is secured, vasospasm prophylactic therapy with nimodipine and consideration for cerebrospinal fluid (CSF) drainage procedures. This is used on all patients while waiting for definitive treatment and those who are too unwell to undergo treatment and the nimodipine is continued for 21 days.

Neurosurgical Clipping

Neurosurgery has been available since the 1950s and has improved with the advent of the operating microscope and well-designed clips.

Endovascular

Endovascular therapy has been available since the early 1990s and offers a minimally invasive alternative to craniotomy and clipping.

Clinical Presentation

The most common cause of SAH is trauma. Usually there is a good history of the preceding traumatic event. When the history is not clear and it is not possible to exclude a sudden onset of a severe headache as the cause of the trauma, the distribution of the blood on the

Fig. 1 CT head showing traumatic SAH

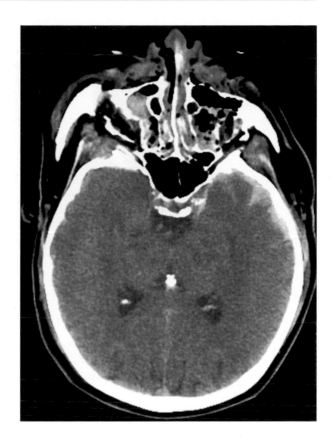

computed tomography (CT) scan can be helpful. Characteristically the SAH is peripheral in trauma (Fig. 1) and central in and around the suprasellar cistern in aneurismal SAH (Fig. 2).

Spontaneous SAH is most often (85 %) caused by a ruptured aneurysm. More rare causes include ruptured arteriovenous malformations at about 8 % and dural arteriovenous fistula at less than 1 %. This leaves about 5–10 % of cases in which no cause is found, and a venous rupture causing a perimesencephalic bleed is suspected. The importance of this latter group is that their risk of rebleeding is low and no definitive treatment is required. Due to the high rebleed rate in aneurismal SAH, urgent investigation and treatment has become the routine following the publication of the International Study of Aneurysm Treatment (ISAT), and this has led to the subsequent development of interventional neuroradiology and endovascular neurosurgery. Aneurysms can present with mass effect (Fig. 3a, b) or rarely with thromboembolic complication of the intraluminal thrombus.

Fig. 2 Unenhanced axial CT
brain showing central
aneurismal SAH

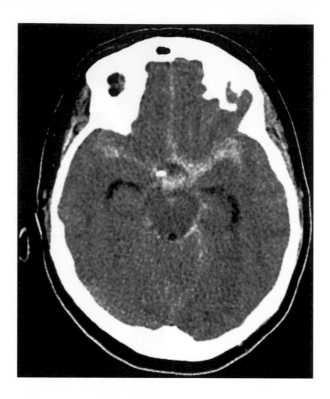

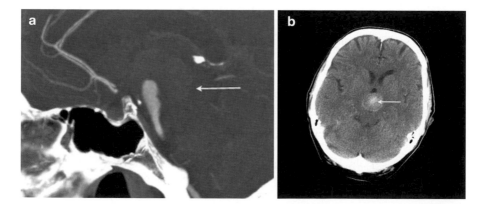

Fig. 3 (a) Sagittal maximum intensity projection (MIP) of a contrast-enhanced CT angiogram
showing the mass effect of a giant basilar tip aneurysm that is substantially thrombosed. (b)
Unenhanced axial CT brain showing the same aneurysm with high attenuation thrombus demonstrated near the aneurysm dome (*arrow*)

Risk Factors

- Smoking
- Hypertension
- Alcohol abuse
- Positive family history
- Collagen dysfunction diseases
- Female predominance over 30 years of age

Investigations

CT to Show SAH

- Sensitivity for SAH at 24 h = 98 %
- Sensitivity for SAH at 5 days = 70 %
- Sensitivity for SAH at 7 days = 50 %

Lumbar Puncture (LP) to Show SAH in CT-Negative Cases and Delayed Presentation

- Must be processed (spun down) by the lab immediately to decrease the false positive rate
- 98–100 % sensitive from 9 h to 2 weeks
- 70 % sensitive at 3 weeks
- 40 % sensitive at 4 weeks

Magnetic Resonance Imaging (MRI)

- T1, FLAIR, and gradient echo-/susceptibility-weighted imaging (SWI) sequences to look for blood

Computed Tomographic Angiography (CTA)

- May miss small aneurysms at the skull base

Digital Subtraction Angiography (DSA)

- Gold Standard with the best spatial and temporal resolution but comes at a cost of 1/2000 permanent neurological deficit

Endovascular Aneurysm Treatment (EVT)

- *Consent* is the cornerstone of the patient–doctor relationship. It is important to cover:

Indications

- Primary objective is to reduce the risk of rebleeding from 2 % per day to 0.2 % per year.
- Secondary objectives are to allow aggressive hypertensive treatment for delayed cerebral ischemia.
- Prevent recurrence.

Risks

- 5 % groin hematoma
- 2–4 % new neurological deficit (local data/ISAT)

Alternatives

- Neurosurgical clipping
- Conservative treatment
- Special techniques

Preoperative Medication

- Dual antiplatelet medication, used in the setting of unruptured aneurysms

World Health Organization (WHO) Checklist

- Confirmation of the correct patient and procedure
- Allergies
- Risk factors for bleeding
- Any special requirements
- Review previous imaging
- Performed under general anesthesia

Groin Puncture: Right, Left, or Both

- Right normally, as close to the operator.
- Left if indwelling lines already in the right or difficult access due to previously deployed stent, scar tissue, peripheral vascular disease, or bypass.

Fig. 4 (a, b) Shows dual ICA cannulation to allow contra lateral ACA control while coiling proceeds

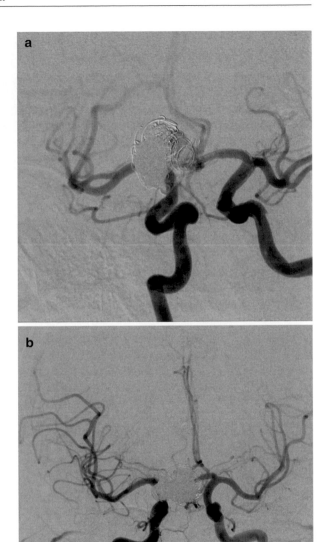

- Both, check if angiography of both internal carotid artery (ICA) is needed e.g. while treating an anterior communicating artery complex aneurysm (Fig. 4a, b).

Diagnostic Angiography

- Target aneurysm harboring vessel first with an AP and lateral whole head with which to compare the pre- and post-embolization images looking for distal embolic events followed by a 3-dimensional (3-D) rotational angiogram (Fig. 5a–d) for the selection of working projections and measurement of the aneurysm neck and dome. The remaining vessels can then be interrogated while processing and manipulating the volume data.

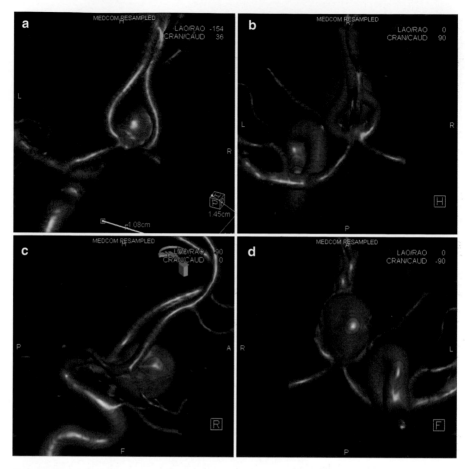

Fig. 5 (a–d) Showing a 3-D rotational angiogram of an ACom aneurysm viewed from behind, above, laterally, and below, respectively

Guide Catheter

- Stable safe position just below the skull base in the majority of cases on a heparin containing flush bag.

Intra-procedure Medication

- *Heparin in the bag*
  — 2,500 IU in the flush bag 500 ml of warmed normal saline
- *Systemic heparin*
  — 5,000 IU given at the time of coiling. The timing of this depends on the risk of on-table rupture and if the aneurysm is very small may not be given at all. If the

aneurysm is small, the first coil can be deployed before the heparin is given. In most cases the heparin is given once the guide catheter is in place.

- *Nimodipine in the bag or IA bolus*
  — If angiographic vasospasm is detected and is severe enough to impede the cannulation of the aneurysm, Nimodipine can be given as a bolus and the effect maintained with an infusion. Dose 2 mg per territory usually split into 1 mg IA bolus and 1 mg injected into the flush bag to irrigate slowly over the time of the procedure.
- *IV aspirin*
  — Given after stent insertion in an acute case or post procedure if there is a wide neck with a large surface area of coil in contact with the blood flow in the parent vessel. Proud coil loops in the parent vessel are another indication. Consider the risk of hydrocephalus requiring an External Ventricular Drain (EVD) and if thought to be of higher risk than that of thrombosis, omit Aspirin.
- *Nasogastric (NG) tube clopidogrel*
  — This can be given at the time of stent placement in the acute case but more commonly this is given after the case.
- *Contrast*
  — Iodinated contrast should be kept to a safe minimum allowing visualization of the EVT. Especially relevant to pediatric cases.

Microcatheter and Microwire

- *Microcatheter: Braided or not?*
  — Stability versus stiffness. Consider using a stiffer microcatheter in those proximal aneurysms where the catheter stability is a problem and a more delicate catheter for small distal aneurysms where the risk of on-table rupture is greater.
- *Micro wire: Hydrophilic or not?*
  — This is a personal decision based on the individual case weighing the risks of wire stiffness and torquability to achieve safe aneurysm cannulation.

Framing Coils

- *Diameter*
  — This should be close to the mean diameter of the aneurysm sac with an underestimate in ruptured aneurysms and an overestimate in unruptured aneurysms. Remember that if the first coil is too small (still tumbling in the aneurysm despite half to two-thirds of the length being deployed), it can be removed and used as the second coil. If the first coil is too large, then it will be discarded or put the patient at risk of on-table rupture.
- *Length*
  — The length of the first coil needs to be enough to give a stable peripheral configuration and cover the aneurysm neck with sufficient metal to prevent subsequent coil prolapse into the parent vessel. If too long there is a risk of compartmentalization of

the aneurysm lumen potentially leading to under packing or the need to reposition the microcatheter.

- *Number*
  - Several framing coils can be used in a concentric sphere fashion before moving on to filling coils.

Filling Coils

- Coating and biologically active fillings, stretch resistance.

Finishing Coils

- Soft fillers that find the gaps and reposition the catheter into the remaining space.

Coil Detachment and Pusher Removal

- Forward pressure on the microcatheter, is often necessary while deploying coils, in order to maintain microcatheter position in the aneurysm and overcome the coil pushing the microcatheter out of the aneurysm. This pressure will be released when the coil is detached and should be balanced to result in central intra-aneurysmal position on detachment. When the coil pusher is withdrawn, it should be done carefully under direct vision as it is possible for detachment to fail or to pull a coil tip into the microcatheter.

Catheter Withdrawal

- Carefully remove the microcatheter over the microwire or coil pusher to avoid displacing any of the previously deployed coils from the aneurysm neck.

Post-procedure Diagnostic Angiogram to Assess

- *Complications*
  - Parent vessel thromboembolic
- *Grade of occlusion*
  - Different scoring systems but share the concept of occlusion, residual aneurysm or neck filling.
- *Contraindications to groin closure device*

Arteriotomy Closure

- *Closure devices*
  - Numerous devices can be used as the patient may be systemically heparinized and on antiplatelets (see Chap. 1).
  - Alternatively consider reversal of the systemic heparinization and manual compression or delayed catheter removal.

Complications

- *Local acute*
  - Groin hematoma 5 %
- *Local delayed*
  - Pseudoaneurysm
  - Arteriovenous fistula (AVF)
- *Distal acute*
  - On-table rupture 2 %
  - Dissection
  - Distal embolic
  - Thromboembolic
- *Distal delayed*
  - Rebleed rate of 0.2 % a year
  - Recurrence requiring re-treatment
  - Recurrences requiring follow-up

Post-procedure Medication

- Heparinization
- Antiplatelets

Recovery: Daily Ward Rounds to Assess for

- *Headache*
  - Often this is significantly better for the next 24–72 h due to the delayed excretion of the anesthetic materials, and a recurrence of the patient's headache should be anticipated after this time and is not necessarily a sign of a rebleed or hydrocephalus. If the headache is persistent and so severe, it is not alleviated with regular analgesia, or lumbar puncture should be considered as hydrocephalus may be the cause and can give dramatic relief.

- *Hydrocephalus*
  - — Diagnosed clinically and confirmed on CT head. Treatment ranges from LPs to EVD/lumbar drain to permanent shunt placement
- *Delayed cerebral ischemia* (DCI, previously vasospasm)
  - — Optimize heart and lung function and consider intra-arterial treatment.
- *Electrolytes, Mg++*
  - — Monitor and replace.
- *Nimodipine*
  - — Until day 21
- *Blood pressure*
  - — Once the aneurysm is secured, the MAP can be elevated to prevent delayed cerebral ischemia (DCI).
- *Fluids*
  - — 3 1/24 h orally or topped up IVI
- *Pronator drift*
  - — Is an early clinical sign of DCI
- *Visual saccades*
  - — May be more sensitive
- *Decreased neurocognition*
  - — Suggests DCI

Follow-Up

- *MRI* at 6 months with neurovascular multidisciplinary discussion
  - — TOF-MRA (time-of-flight magnetic resonance angiography) of the Circle of Willis (COW) for most aneurysms.
  - — CEMRA in cases of stent remodeling or large aneurysms where a post contrast assessment of the aneurysm wall is required.
  - — CTA (computed tomography angiography) can be used to assess coincidental aneurysms in distant locations if there is a contraindication to MRI but is usually not good enough to look at the coiled or clipped aneurysm.
  - — DSA is used for clipped aneurysms.
  - — Outcome is for re-treatment or further follow-up at 2 years or before if there is evidence of instability but no indication for treatment.

Two Years from EVT

- Outcome is for discharge, re-treatment, or further follow-up even if stable and occluded aneurysm in at-risk groups such as young female smokers.

Five Years from EVT

- Retreat or discharge

Key Points

> Consent.
> Objective is to reduce the risk of rebleed with early effective treatment.
> Secondary objective is to allow aggressive hypertensive treatment of delayed cerebral ischemia (DCI) and prevent recurrence.

Suggested Reading

1. Adams Jr HP, Kassell NF, Torner JC, Sahs AL. CT and clinical correlations in recent aneurysmal subarachnoid hemorrhage: a preliminary report of the Cooperative Aneurysm Study. Neurology. 1983;33(8):981–8.
2. Brisman JL, Song JK, Newell DW. Cerebral aneurysms. N Engl J Med. 2006;355(9): 928–39.
3. de Rooij NK, Linn FHH, van der Plas JA, Algra A, Rinkle GJE. Incidence of subarachnoid haemorrhage: a systematic review with emphasis on region, age, gender and time trends. J Neurol Neurosurg Psychiatry. 2007;78(12):1365–72.
4. Flaherty ML, Haverbusch M, Kissela B, Kleindorfer D, Schneider A, Sekar P, Moomaw CJ, Sauerbeck L, Broderick JP, Woo D. Perimesencephalic subarachnoid hemorrhage: incidence, risk factors, and outcome. J Stroke Cerebrovasc Dis. 2005;14(6):267–71.
5. Graf CJ, Nibbelink DW. Cooperative study of intracranial aneurysms and subarachnoid hemorrhage. Report on a randomized treatment study. III. Intracranial surgery. Stroke. 1974;5:559–601.
6. Jeon TY, Jeon P, Kim KH. Prevalence of unruptured intracranial aneurysm on MR angiography. Korean J Radiol. 2011;12(5):547–53.
7. Molyneux AJ, Kerr RS, Yu LM, Clarke M, Sneade M, Yarnold JA, Sandercock P, International Subarachnoid Aneurysm Trial (ISAT) Collaborative Group. International subarachnoid aneurysm trial (ISAT) of neurosurgical clipping versus endovascular coiling in 2143 patients with ruptured intracranial aneurysms: a randomised comparison of effects on survival, dependency, seizures, rebleeding, subgroups, and aneurysm occlusion. Lancet. 2005;366(9488):809–17.
8. Vermeulen M, Hasan D, Blijenberg BG, Hijdra A, van Gijn J. Xanthochromia after subarachnoid haemorrhage needs no revisitation. J Neurol Neurosurg Psychiatry. 1989;52(7):826–8.

Balloon Remodeling

Prem S. Rangi

Abstract

There has been a progressive incremental paradigm shift for treating intracranial aneurysms, both ruptured and unruptured, via endovascular techniques. The appeal of endovascular techniques for patients is in its minimally invasive approach and reduced recovery periods. Several trials have shown efficacy of endovascular treatment against traditional neurosurgical techniques for both ruptured and elective cases. The major challenge for endovascular management of intracranial aneurysms is twofold, endovascular results need to be durable and endovascular techniques need to able to manage complex aneurysms, including large, wide necked, and branches arising from the aneurysm sac. The treatment of complex aneurysms has been advanced by utilization of hypercompliant microballoons, particularly in acutely ruptured aneurysms, where the permanent deployment of a device, such as a stent, as an adjuvant device is prohibited, largely due to increased complications.

Keywords

Complex aneurysms • Remodeling • Hypercompliant microballoons • Acutely ruptured aneurysms • Complex aneurysms • Coil assistance • Stent assistance • Intra-procedural rupture

P.S. Rangi, MB, ChB
Department of Radiology, The Royal Free Hospital, London, UK
e-mail: prem.rangi@nhs.net

K. Murphy, F. Robertson (eds.), *Interventional Neuroradiology,*
Techniques in Interventional Radiology,
DOI 10.1007/978-1-4471-4582-0_5, © Springer-Verlag London 2014

Indications

- Balloon remodeling technique or balloon-assisted coiling (BAC) first described in 1997 by Jacques Moret.
- Since its inception, its initial remit has been surpassed, allowing the treatment of an increasing complexity of aneurysm morphologies.
- The indications for using microballoons for remodeling are
  1. Broad-necked sidewall aneurysms
  2. Small aneurysms with branches arising from the sac
  3. Broad aneurysms with one or two branches arising at the neck or sac (typically MCA bifurcation, basilar tip) (Fig. 1)
- Additional adjuvant uses of microballoons include
  1. Rescue treatment of prolapsed coils
  2. Treating local thrombus formation

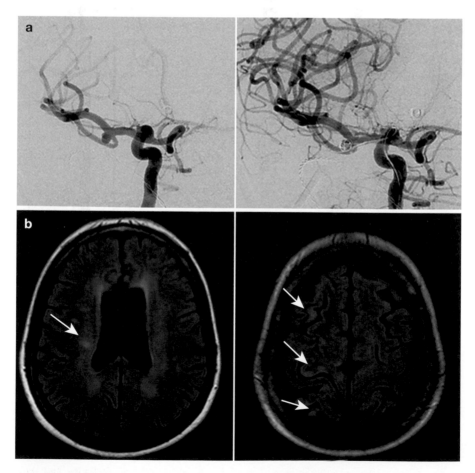

Fig. 1 Watershed ischemia post-balloon remodeling of right MCA aneurysm. (**a**) Pre- and post-angiograms using remodeling technique. MRI study post-embolization of right MCA aneurysm using remodeling technique. (**b**) FLAIR; (**b**) DWI; (**c**) ADC; (**d**) Maps show area of deep (*left*) and superficial (*right*) MCA watershed ischemia – *white arrows* show infarction

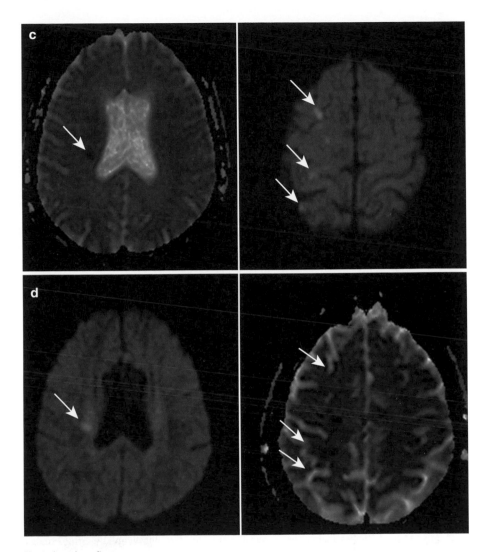

Fig. 1 (continued)

3. Concomitant angioplasty
4. Managing intra-procedural ruptures, whether at the time of microcatheter/coil placement or during intubation

Balloon Configuration

- Prior to incorporating microballoons within the repertoire of endovascular techniques, one must have an understanding of the basic subtypes of microballoons and their advantages and disadvantages.
- Until recently, balloons had two basic geometric shapes (with some minor variation in size to extend the range of aneurysms that can be managed):

- Sausage configuration.
  - Most widely utilized balloon: sausage configuration, oblong shaped.
  - One such balloon of this type is the HyperGlide™, ev3 (Covidien).
  - 3–6 mm diameter size and lengths from 10–30 mm.
  - Most commonly used: the 4×10–15 mm length.
- Rugby or football configuration (when unconstrained).
  - Typically more compliant than sausage configuration
  - One example: HyperForm™, eV3 (Covidien, Plymouth, MN, USA)
  - Available in two sizes: 4×7 mm and 7×7 mm

Hyperglide-Type Balloon

- Typically less compliant, which tends to determine its use for selective catheterization of branches arising at or within the proximal sac, in order to protect.
- Generally more predictable during placement and sequential inflation.
- During inflation, usually just prior to vessel occlusion, this balloon type has a tendency to move forward. With practice this can be anticipated for and compensated for by a small pull of the balloon just prior to vessel occlusion.
- The converse is equally true: the balloon tends to jockey proximally upon deflation.
  - For the most part, this motion is manageable and of little impact upon the subjacent microcatheter.
  - Can be extreme in some patients.
  - Extra care needs to be taken particularly with very small aneurysms where this movement can potentially propel the microcatheter through the aneurysm sac.

Microballoon Preparation (Fig. 2)

- Preparation of the microballoon is of utmost importance, with avoidance of introducing microbubbles within the system a prerequisite.
- Preparation is best undertaken within a designated area.
- Using a separate trolley makes for a natural "zone" to work within and by virtue creates "safe zone" to avoid contamination of the contrast-saline mixture.

There are several key stages:

Stage 1

Contrast-Saline Mixture

- A small gally pot is used to make the desired mixture by first placing 20 ml of saline, followed by 20 ml of 300 omnipaque contrast.
- The gally pot could be labeled for additional safety.

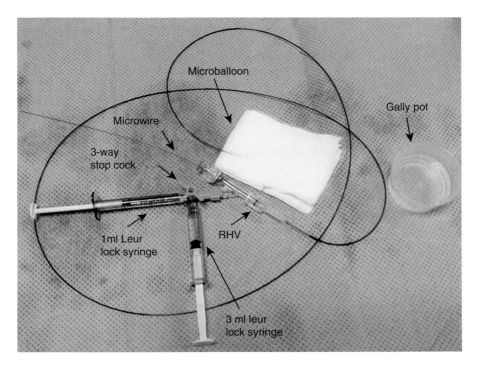

Fig. 2 Pictorial representation of microballoon configuration

- The importance of identifying the correct contrast-saline mixture cannot be overemphasized, to avoid inflating a balloon with clear saline and the inherent risk of overinflation and vessel rupture.
- Using neat contrast makes deflation of the balloon protracted, potentially necessitating microwire withdrawal to achieve deflation of the balloon.
- May potentially contaminate the microballoon with blood, making subsequent inflation difficult, reduce visibility, and make subsequent deflation impossible, even once the microwire has been completely withdrawn.

Stage 2

Preparing the Microballoon

- A 1 ml Luer-Lok syringe is filled with the contrast-saline mixture and attached to a 3-way stopcock, which in turn is attached to a RHV (rotating hemostatic value), without introducing any bubbles. This then is attached to the microballoon, which is subsequently flushed. This ensures the microballoon "system" is flushed with the desired contrast-saline mixture and free of microbubbles.
- A 3 ml Luer-Lok syringe is attached, again flushed with the contrast-saline mixture, to the vacant hub of the 3-way tap.

Stage 3

- The Luer-Lok is opened sufficiently to introduce the appropriate microwire for the balloon and advanced into the balloon microcatheter system, but avoiding occluding the balloon.
- Once the wire is sufficiently advanced, the 3 ml syringe is used to flush the hub of the RHV in a retrograde fashion, to ensure no bubbles have been inadvertently introduced into the system.
- Wire is advanced across the balloon and little beyond to seal the system, and a test inflation and deflation performed.
- The wire should be withdrawn to just protrude out of the microballoon; catheter tip; this will ensure no air or blood entry into the balloon.

Safety and Efficacy

- Use of balloons in treating intracranial aneurysms has come under considerable scrutiny.
- Initial experience was associated with higher thromboembolic sequelae. More contemporary published literature (some in the form of randomized multicenter trials) shows no increased complication rates but infers safer procedural rates, with reduced embolic phenomena, reduced rupture rates, and better packing density. The latter feature of the remodeling technique is being associated with reduced early re-hemorrhage and recurrence.
- Increasingly recognized safety profile of the balloon remodeling technique compared to unassisted coil embolization likely reflects increased practitioner experience, improved technology, and use of anticoagulation and antiplatelet regimes.
- One should be cognizant that more complex aneurysms tend to be treated with microballoon/multicatheter techniques.

Principle of Balloon Remodeling Technique

- Principle: Place a nondetachable balloon across the aneurysm neck.
- Balloon is temporarily inflated using a prepared mixture of contrast and saline, to a maximum volume predetermined by the particular balloon manufacturer.
- Balloon inflation is controlled under fluoroscopic guidance and maintained during coil placement.
- Once a coil is successfully placed within the aneurysm sac, the balloon is totally deflated.

- Subsequent coil placement is performed with the balloon reinflated.
- Process is repeated until a dense coil packing is achieved.
- Duration of balloon inflation should be minimized, avoiding extended times of inflation, beyond 2 min.

Aneurysm Morphology and Remodeling Technique

Type 1: Sidewall Aneurysm (Fig. 3)

- Basic utilization of the remodeling technique first described for managing sidewall aneurysms.
- Temporary inflation of a microballoon within the parent vessel artificially reduces the neck size, consequently improving the neck-to-dome ratio, allowing safe coil placement within the aneurysm sac.
- This mitigates for coil migration or coil prolapse into the parent vessel in wide-necked aneurysms.

Type 2: Broad-Necked Aneurysm, with Branches at the Neck, Single Balloon (Fig. 4)

- A single balloon is placed across the neck of the aneurysm, with protrusion of balloon such that it protects the second unengaged vessel.
- Either hyperglide- or hyperform-type balloons can be used.

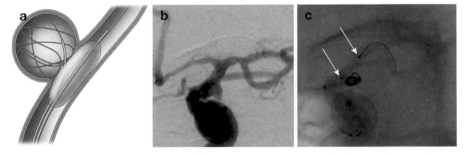

Fig. 3 Treatment of sidewall aneurysm using remodeling technique. (**a**) Schematic – showing sidewall aneurysm and balloon placement bridging the neck. (**b**) Angiogram of wide-necked left PCOM-origin aneurysm. (**c**) Balloon placed across left PCOM aneurysm, tips of which are delineated by *white arrows*

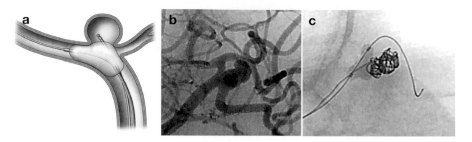

Fig. 4 Treatment of wide-necked aneurysm, with vessel incorporation using a single balloon: (**a**) Schematic – showing left MCA wide-necked aneurysm, with inflated balloon crossing the neck and protecting the second unengaged branch. (**b**) Broad-necked left MCA bifurcation aneurysm. (**c**) Single hyperform-type balloon, shown inflated protecting both the catheterized and the non-engaged MCA branches with the balloon

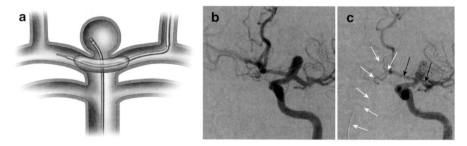

Fig. 5 (**a**) Schematic of parallel balloon placement utilizing Integraty of the Circle of Willis. (**b**) Left carotid "T" bifurcation aneurysm, with wide neck and a widely competent ACOM complex anastomotic channel. (**c**) Balloon placed parallel across aneurysm sac (*black arrows* marking balloon position), via contralateral right ICA-ACOM complex (*white arrows* demark the path of the balloon via the right ICA, ACA, ACOM, left A1 segment)

Type 3: Figure 3. Broad-Necked Aneurysm, Balloon Placed Parallel to Neck via Circle of Willis (Fig. 5)

- Greater coverage of the neck can be achieved by placing a balloon parallel to the neck of the aneurysm, such as:
  - A basilar or carotid "T" bifurcation aneurysm, via PCOM (posterior communication)
  - ACOM (anterior communication) anastomotic channels the Circle of Willis, respectively

Type 4: Broad-Necked Aneurysm, with Branches Arising at Neck/Proximal Sac, Double Balloon (Fig. 6)

- Tackling more complex aneurysm morphologies should only be considered once sidewall aneurysms have been treated successfully using microballoons.
- Appreciating the interaction (interplay) between microcatheter(s) and microballoon(s) is paramount when approaching such cases.

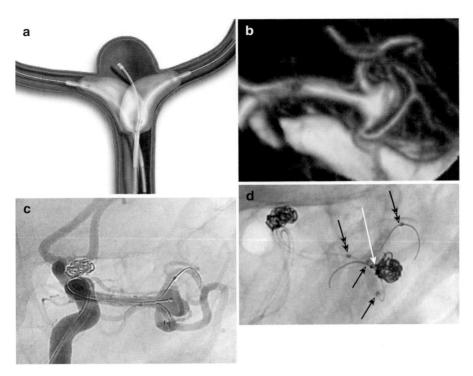

Fig. 6 (**a**) Schematic showing placement of two balloons across the broad aneurysm neck, with selective branch catheterization of the branches. (**b**) CTA showing complex left MCA morphology, with superior branch incorporated with the proximal sac and inferior branch an integral part of the neck/sac interface. (**c**) Corresponding angiographic run of left MCA aneurysm shown in CTA. Balloons and microcatheter in situ, bridging the broad aneurysm neck. (**d**) Balloons inflated with several coils deployed within aneurysm sac, showing successful remodeling, formation of a new parent vessel-sac interface (*white arrow*). Superior balloon markers show as double black arrows and inferior as single *black arrows*

- Not infrequently, beyond wide-necked aneurysms, complex aneurysms have a variable configuration of branches at the aneurysm neck/sac, with each branch needing to be preserved.
- A typical aneurysm incorporating more than one branch at the neck or proximal sac is a MCA bi/trifurcation aneurysm.
- Selectively the order of branch catheterization needs planning, with preference for the more difficult branch first. Although, one must be prepared to change strategy, and thus an alternative must be contemplated in advance.

Type 5: Small Aneurysm, with Branch Arising from Sac, Single Balloon/Multicatheters (Fig. 7)

- Small aneurysms associated with branches from the neck or proximal sac comprise a group of aneurysms that are difficult to treat.
- A balloon or a microcatheter can be positioned into the origin and proximal segment of the vessel needed to be "protected."

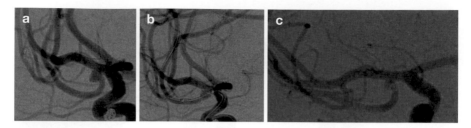

Fig. 7 Balloon utilization to protect a small branch arising from aneurysm sac. The vessel could alternatively be protected with a large microcatheter (0.21″): (**a**) Angiogram, showing a small 2 mm aneurysm arising from a right anterior temporal branch, which is incorporated within the aneurysm sac. (**b**) Balloon place within the anterior temporal branch, with accompanying anatomical distortion. (**c**) Post-embolization with anatomical restoration, occlusion of the aneurysm with preserved flow within the temporal branch

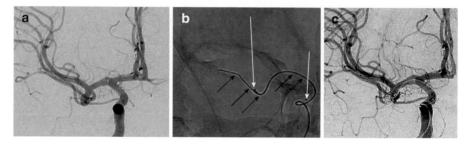

Fig. 8 Multicatheter technique. (**a**) Angiogram, showing right MCA bifurcation aneurysm, with inferior branch incorporated in neck. (**b**) First microcatheter positioned within aneurysm sac, distal tip show with *white arrow*. Second, larger microcatheter course shows with *black arrows*. (**c**) Angiogram, after second coil placement, showing dual catheter placement, with preservation of local anatomy

- Care is needed with subsequent microcatheter placement.
- Alternatively, the balloon can be further advanced into the more distal portion of the vessel, allowing the microcatheter to be positioned. However, withdrawing the balloon can displace the microcatheter and may require controlled forward pressure on the microcatheter during maneuvering of the balloon.
- An alternative to using a balloon to protect a branch is to use a microcatheter, such as a PROWLER®SELECT™ Plus (Cordis Neurovascular, Inc., Miami Lakes, FL, USA) with a large caliber, 0.021″. This will afford protection to the branch, without local anatomical distortion. The degree of protection is often less than with a balloon, and one must be prepared to rescue the branch with stent placement if necessary, a further reason for selecting a large microcatheter (Fig. 8).

Key Points

> There has been a progressive incremental paradigm shift for treating intracranial aneurysms, both ruptured and unruptured, via endovascular techniques.

> The appeal of endovascular techniques for patients is in its minimally invasive approach and reduced recovery periods.

> Several trials have shown efficacy of endovascular treatment against traditional neurosurgical techniques for both ruptured and elective cases.

> The major challenge for endovascular management of intracranial aneurysms is twofold:
>
> — Endovascular results need to be durable.
> — Endovascular techniques need to able to manage complex aneurysms, including large, wide necked, and branches arising from the aneurysm sac.

> Treatment of complex aneurysms has been advanced by utilization of hypercompliant microballoons, particularly in acutely ruptured aneurysms, where the permanent deployment of a device, such as a stent, as an adjuvant device is prohibited, largely due to increased complications.

Suggested Reading

1. Cekirge HS, Yavuz K, Geyik S, Saatci I. HyperForm balloon remodeling in the endovascular treatment of anterior cerebral, middle cerebral, and anterior communicating artery aneurysms: clinical and angiographic follow-up results in 800 consecutive patients. J Neurosurg. 2011;114(4):944–53. Epub 2010 May 14.
2. Moret J, Cognard C, Weill A, et al. Reconstruction technique in the treatment of wide-neck intracranial aneurysms: long-term angiographic and clinical results apropos of 56 cases. J Neuroradiol. 1997;24:30–44.

Flow-Diverting Stents in the Treatment of Intracranial Aneurysms

David Fiorella, Peter Kim Nelson, and Lissa Peeling

Abstract

Aneurysms are regarded as "complex" when they are challenging to treat using conventional surgical or endovascular approaches. Complexity is typically associated with very large or giant size, dysplastic or fusiform morphology, recurrence after prior surgical or endovascular treatment, and other anatomical features making conventional surgical or endovascular treatment challenging or impossible. Flow-diverting stents may allow a constructive, technically feasible, definitive, and durable treatment option in many of these cases that were previously deemed "complex" or "untreatable" in the past.

Keywords

Flow diversion • Giant skull base aneurysm • Coil compaction

Introduction

- Aneurysms are regarded as "complex" when they are challenging to treat using conventional surgical or endovascular approaches.
- Complexity is typically associated with any of the following characteristics (Fig. 1):

D. Fiorella, PhD, MD (✉) • L. Peeling, MD
Department of Neurosurgery, Cerebrovascular Center,
Stony Brook University Medical Center, Stony Brook, NY, USA
e-mail: dfiorella@notes.cc.sunysb.edu

P.K. Nelson, MD
Department of Radiology and Neurosurgery, NYU: Langone Medical Center,
New York, NY, USA

K. Murphy, F. Robertson (eds.), *Interventional Neuroradiology,*
Techniques in Interventional Radiology,
DOI 10.1007/978-1-4471-4582-0_6, © Springer-Verlag London 2014

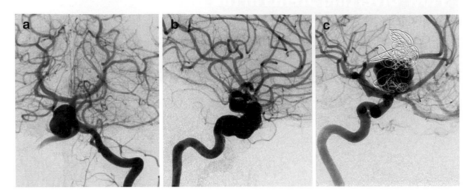

Fig. 1 Complex aneurysms which are suboptimally addressed by conventional endovascular techniques. (**a**) Very large, wide-necked basilar trunk aneurysm. (**b**) Long segment fusiform, circumferential aneurysm of the internal carotid artery. (**c**) Giant recurrence of an aneurysm after conventional coil embolization. All three of these lesions are potentially amenable to reconstruction with flow-diverting constructs

1. Very large or giant size
2. Dysplastic or fusiform morphology
3. Recurrence after prior surgical or endovascular treatment
4. Other anatomical feature(s) making conventional surgical or endovascular treatment challenging or impossible

- Flow-diverting stents may allow a constructive, technically feasible, definitive, and durable treatment option in many of these cases that were previously deemed "complex" or "untreatable" in the past.

Theoretical Background for Flow Diversion

Clinical Need for Flow Diverters

Aneurysms Amenable to Conventional Endovascular Treatment

Amenable Lesions

- Small (<10 mm) cerebral aneurysms with (<4 mm) narrow necks are typically optimal for endovascular therapy.
- Account for the majority of ruptured and many of the unruptured aneurysms encountered in clinical practice.

Conventional Endovascular (Endosaccular) Therapy

- Endovascular treatment of aneurysms has been predicated upon filling the aneurysm sac with embolic material: most commonly platinum coils.

Clinical Evidence: Endovascular Coil

- *Embolization* has been demonstrated to lead to favorable clinical outcomes for the majority of cerebral aneurysms.
- When compared directly, outcomes with endovascular therapy are as good, if not better than surgery, for the majority of the ruptured and unruptured aneurysms that are encountered in clinical practice.

Complex Aneurysms: Often Difficult or Impossible to Treat with Conventional Endovascular Approaches

Large and Giant Aneurysms

- Very high levels of incomplete occlusion (with estimates ranging between 50 and 85 %) and recurrence (40–70 %) and frequently require multiple treatments and re-treatments.
- Treatments and re-treatments, potentially along with the progressive aneurysm growth, may result in significant cumulative morbidity and mortality. Jahromi et al. calculated rates of per treatment mortality and morbidity of 8 and 20 %, respectively, with an overall cumulative morbidity and mortality of 55 % for the endovascular treatment of giant aneurysms.

Failed Prior Treatment: Aneurysms Which Fail Initial Endovascular Treatment, Regardless of Size, Also Represent a Challenging Subtype of Lesions

- Approximately 50 % of re-treated aneurysms demonstrate another recurrence after re-treatment.

Fusiform, Circumferential, and Very Wide-Necked Aneurysms

- Occurrence: Rare and highly variable group of lesions. b. Treatment: Conventional treatment of these lesions is associated with a relatively high rate of periprocedural and intra-procedural complications, particularly when a reconstructive approach (rather than a vessel occlusion) is required. Oftentimes, when a conventional constructive approach is taken, the result is temporary, and the lesions continue to recur locally and enlarge.

Complex Aneurysms: Reasons for Failure with Conventional Endovascular Therapy

- These complex aneurysms often fail conventional endovascular treatment for two main reasons:

Low Packing Density

- For small, narrow-necked aneurysms, packing densities in the range of 40 % are possible, and at this level of aneurysm occlusion, recanalization is uncommon.

- For larger and giant aneurysms, packing densities are more commonly in the range of 20 %, which may not provide the structural integrity to support a durable aneurysm occlusion.
- This is a particular problem if the aneurysm contains a large volume of soft, intraluminal thrombus, as with time, the coil mass can become compacted into the thrombus, leading to relatively rapid and large recanalizations (Fig. 1).

Inadequate Reconstruction of the Aneurysm-Parent Vessel Interface

- When the aneurysm neck comprises a significant length and circumference of the parent artery, it is very difficult to reconstruct a homogenous, smooth, and continuous surface by packing the aneurysm with embolization coils (even with the use of an adjunctive device such as a balloon or conventional coil-assist stent).
- The interface is usually irregular with large interstices between coil loops in the region of the aneurysm neck.
- These gaps allow continued flow into the aneurysm.
- This incomplete neck reconstruction leaves the aneurysm susceptible to recanalization.

Flow Diversion: Mechanistic Basis

Concept

- Flow diversion differs from conventional endovascular, endosaccular aneurysm treatment.
- In contrast to endosaccular treatment, flow diversion is a primarily endoluminal approach to aneurysm treatment.

Device Characteristics

- Flow diverters are typically braided stent-like constructs with low pore density and high metal surface area (Fig. 2).
- The devices are deployed through a microcatheter and positioned to completely bridge the aneurysm neck, spanning from normal vessel proximally to normal vessel distally.
- While aneurysms fill solely due to the trajectory of inflow and outflow vectors, regional branches fill on the basis of an arterial to venous pressure drop.
- Pressure gradients drive flow through the branches and support their patency despite substantial degrees of metal coverage over their ostia.

Fig. 2 Pipeline Embolization Device (PED): The PED is a flexible, braided, self-expanding microstent, which is delivered through a microcatheter with a 0.027″ internal diameter. When deployed, the device provides approximately 30–35 % metal surface area coverage over the reconstructed segment

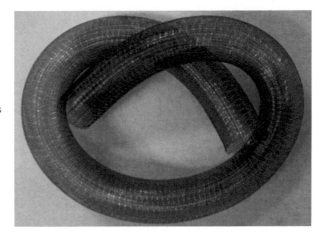

- Optimally designed flow-diverting constructs are of a porosity that efficiently induces aneurysm occlusion while at the same time reliably allowing the continued patency of regional eloquent branches which are also covered by the construct.
- The operator to some degree can customize the degree of metal surface area coverage during the procedure by applying variable load to the microcatheter during deployment, compressing the braid over segments of the parent artery.

Process of Reconstruction

- Reconstruction of the parent artery with aneurysm occlusion occurs over a period of days to months through the following sequence:

Mechanical: Flow Disruption (Immediate)

- The construct disrupts both the inflow and outflow of blood within the aneurysm, redirecting the primary vector of blood flow along the course of the anatomically reformed parent artery.
- While the aneurysm may still fill with contrast, the intra-aneurysmal flow is disrupted and shear forces upon the aneurysm wall are reduced (Fig. 3).

Physiological: Aneurysm Thrombosis (Days to Weeks)

- The intra-aneurysmal flow disruption creates an environment conducive to progressive thrombosis.

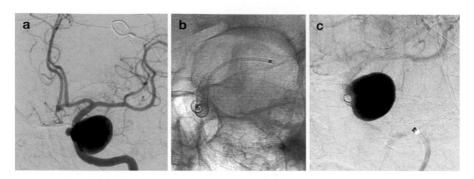

Fig. 3 Progression of curative reconstruction after successful flow diversion: mechanical reconstruction. Subtracted angiogram in the PA projection demonstrates a giant aneurysm involving the cavernous segment of the left internal carotid artery (**a**). Native image in the same projection depicts a construct composed of three pipeline devices reconstructing the left internal carotid artery (**b**). Subtracted image in the capillary phase of angiography demonstrating the hemodynamic effects of mechanical reconstruction with persistent stasis of contrast within the aneurysm (**c**)

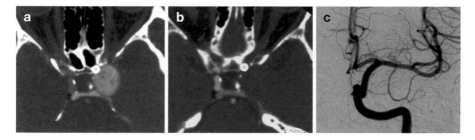

Fig. 4 Progression of curative reconstruction after successful flow diversion: physiological reconstruction. Computed tomographic angiographic image in the axial plane 24 h after reconstruction of the aneurysm depicted in Fig. 2 demonstrates the construct in position with continued filling of the aneurysm with contrast (**a**). Follow-up CTA 2 weeks later demonstrates complete thrombosis of the aneurysm (**b**). Angiographic follow-up performed 6 months after treatment confirms complete occlusion of the aneurysm with anatomical remodeling of the parent artery (**c**)

- When this process is complete, angiographic imaging demonstrates complete occlusion.
- Cross-sectional imaging demonstrates a thrombus mass within the aneurysm.
- The rate of this thrombosis seems to vary significantly with aneurysm size, location, and the degree of neck coverage.
- Clinically, local mass effect and/or transmural inflammatory changes secondary to the thrombosis may result in an exacerbation of the originally present clinical symptoms or, in some cases, new symptoms (e.g., headache or cranial neuropathy).
- In some cases, these new symptoms can be treated with steroids (Fig. 4).

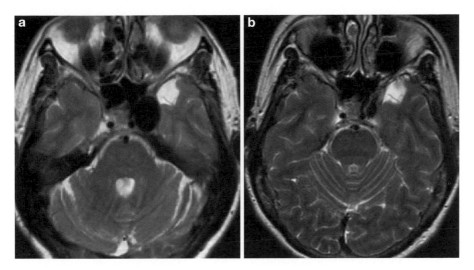

Fig. 5 Progression of curative reconstruction after successful flow diversion: anatomical restoration. Long TR-weighted sequence in the axial plane demonstrates the left cavernous segment aneurysm as a hypointense mass with some regional mass effect (**a**). Follow-up MR performed at 6 months demonstrates near-complete resolution of mass effect after curative reconstruction and resorption of the intra-aneurysmal thrombus mass (**b**)

Biological: Construct Endothelialization and Thrombus Resorption (Months)

- When the aneurysm is completely occluded, the construct may become endothelialized.
- This forms a permanent biological seal across the aneurysm-parent artery interface, to functionally bridge the normal proximal and distal parent arterial segments.
- When the aneurysm is completely excluded from the circulation, the intra-aneurysmal thrombus begins to resorb and the entire aneurysm mass collapses around the periphery of the construct (Fig. 5).
- Symptoms related to aneurysm mass effect or pulsation may resolve at this point (to the extent that they are reversible).

Clinical Applications of the Pipeline Embolization Device: Available Data

Available Devices

Pipeline Embolization Device (PED; Covidien/ev3, Mansfield, MA, USA)

- The PED is the only flow diverter that has been cleared by the US Food and Drug Administration and has CE Mark.
- Commercially available in the USA and worldwide.

Silk+ (Balt Extrusion, Montmorency, France)

- CE Mark in Europe with clinical application outside of the USA

Surpass (Surpass Medical Ltd., Tel-Aviv, Israel)

- CE Mark in Europe with clinical application outside of the USA

Pipeline Embolization Device: Clinical Experience

Compassionate Use

- Initial cases performed with the PED predated its regulatory approval.
- Cases most often performed within the context of "compassionate use": Case-specific permission was obtained from regulatory bodies for patients with aneurysms not treatable with conventional surgical or endovascular approaches.
- These cases provided the first "proof of concept" that flow diversion could be successfully and safely applied in cases which lacked other options.

Clinical Trials

Pipeline for the Intracranial Treatment of Aneurysms (PITA) Study

- Patients: 31 patients with 31 intracranial aneurysms.
- Aneurysms: Most arose (28 of 31) from the internal carotid artery.
- Aneurysms were large (average size 11.5 mm) with wide necks (average 5.8 mm).
- Technical success: 96.8 %.
- Angiographic results: Complete aneurysm occlusion at 6-month follow-up in 28 of 30 patients (93.3 %).
- Complications: 2 of 31 patients with major periprocedural stroke.

Pipeline for the Treatment of Uncoilable or Failed Aneurysms (PUFS)

- Patients: 108 patients with 108 target aneurysms.
- Aneurysms: Large (mean size of 18.2 mm) and wide necked (mean of 8.8 mm).
- Technical success: 97.7 %.
- Angiographic Results: Complete angiographic occlusion in 82 % at 6 months and 86 % at 1 year.
- Complications: Major ipsilateral stroke or neurological death occurred in 6 of 108 subjects (5.6 %) assessed at 180 days.

Practical Considerations for the Application of Flow Diversion

Patient Selection

Regulatory Aspects

- Pipeline Embolization Device labeled indications for use: PED has PMA clearance for the endovascular treatment of adults (≥22 years) with large or giant wide-necked intracranial aneurysms (IAs) from the petrous to the superior hypophyseal segments of the internal carotid artery.
- US physicians may elect to use the device outside of the labeled indications at their discretion. Similarly, outside of the USA, regulatory bodies have not placed specific anatomical restrictions upon the application of the PED. The discussion of patient selection should not be considered to represent an endorsement of off-label use in the USA but rather a summary of the available experience.

Proximal Carotid Aneurysms

- Proximal carotid aneurysms are defined as those arising from the petrous to the paraclinoid segment of the carotid artery.

Indications for Treatment

- Asymptomatic extradural aneurysms, regardless of size, pose little risk to the patient and are not typically appropriate candidates for treatment with flow diversion.
- Intractable pain or progressive optic neuropathy represents excellent indications for the treatment of cavernous aneurysms.

Patient Age

- Advanced patient age is often associated with more hostile cervical carotid anatomy and a greater burden of atherosclerotic vascular disease.
- Not only do these patients frequently pose more technical challenges to treatment, but they also are far less resilient and can be badly injured after even a minor periprocedural complication.

Carotid Anatomy

- Tortuous cervical and intracranial carotid anatomy frequently poses a considerable technical challenge to the delivery and accurate deployment of flow diverters.

- More flexible distal intracranial access guiding catheters (Neuron, Penumbra Inc., Alameda, CA; Reflex, Reverse Medical/Covidien) are important tools in overcoming such anatomical features.

Antiplatelet Medication Compatibility

- Patients treated with flow diverters require long-term dual antiplatelet medications.
- Operator should consider screening patients for:
  - Known bleeding disorders
  - Resistance to antiplatelet medications
  - Medication noncompliance
  - Any requirement for long-term anticoagulation (e.g., atrial fibrillation)
  - Any predictable future invasive procedures (e.g., dental reconstruction, orthopedic surgery) that may require the interruption of antiplatelet therapy

Non-proximal Carotid and Posterior Circulation Aneurysms

- Aneurysms located outside of the proximal carotid distribution, particularly those involving the posterior circulation, have been associated with higher rates of periprocedural complications and poor clinical outcomes.
- Several features of these more complex aneurysms seem anecdotally to be associated with poorer clinical outcomes:

Incorporated Branch Vessel(s)

- Posterior circulation aneurysms and more distal anterior circulation aneurysms often incorporate pial vessels or involve major bifurcations.
- In either circumstance, the incorporation of branches into the actual aneurysm has been associated with continued patency of the aneurysm, progressive growth, and occasionally delayed rupture.
- Any branches incorporated into the aneurysm at the time of PED treatment should be deconstructed with coils if possible to avoid continued intra-aneurysmal flow which preclude progression to complete occlusion.
- If these vessels cannot be safely deconstructed, flow diversion may represent a suboptimal treatment option.

Primary Ischemic Presentation

- Aneurysms arising from diffusely diseased, atherosclerotic vessels, particularly those presenting with primary ischemic symptoms related to progressive perforator interruption, have almost invariably had dismal outcomes after treatment with flow diversion.

Older Age

- While younger patients demonstrate remarkable vascular remodeling over long segments after flow diversion, older patients often times do not.
- Younger patients often have very normal appearing vascular segments proximal and distal to the aneurismal segment.
- Older patients are more likely to demonstrate diffusely diseased vessels.
- The regional perforator origins are more likely to be compromised to some extent by atheromatous disease and may be more likely to become occluded following flow diversion.

Patient Preparation: Antiplatelet Medications

- The high metal surface area coverage characteristic of these devices presents a large, thrombogenic interface to the parent artery after implantation.
- Adequate dual antiplatelet therapy is required to maintain device patency after treatment. Several pretreatment protocols have been successfully employed:
  - Daily clopidogrel (75 mg) for a minimum of 5–7 days and aspirin daily (81–325 mg) for a minimum of 48 h.
  - A 600 mg loading dose of clopidogrel represents an alternative to the 75 mg daily dose. The loading dose has been shown to have a faster onset of activity (a little as 2 h after administration) and more reliably induces a therapeutic inhibition of platelets.
  - Testing of platelet function after the administration of aspirin and clopidogrel remains a controversial area. However, neurointerventionists are performing these tests with greater frequency.
  - Clopidogrel-resistant patients may be reloaded and maintained on a higher dose (150 mg/day) to achieve responsivity.
  - Prasugrel may represent an effective and more reliable oral P2Y12 inhibitor for patients who do not respond to clopidogrel.

Procedural Considerations

Precise Delineation of the Angiographic Anatomy

- A clear understanding of the anatomy of the aneurysm is required to efficiently cross the lesion and build an effective flow-diverting construct.
- Rotational angiography and three-dimensional reconstruction allow the delineation of optimal working two-dimensional projections:
  - Initially these projections are selected to provide the operator with an accurate biplane localization of the aneurysm outlet. This is particularly important for very large and giant cavernous aneurysms, which are challenging to navigate beyond.
  - Working projections for deployment should be chosen to optimally depict the distal and proximal landing zones. An understanding of these landing zones is more important than a consistent visualization of the aneurysm-parent artery interface (in contrast to aneurysm coiling).

Distal Guiding Catheter Access

- Stable distal access is prerequisite for the precise delivery and deployment of the flow diverters:
  - Anterior circulation: A long (80 cm) 6 F guiding sheath can be positioned within the proximal cervical carotid artery (NeuronMax, Penumbra Inc., Alameda, CA). An internal 6 F distal access guiding catheter can then extend the platform into the cavernous segment of the intracranial carotid artery (Neuron, Penumbra Inc., Alameda CA; Reflex, Reverse Medical Corporation, Irvine, CA).
  - Posterior circulation: A 6 F long ArrowFlex sheath (Teleflex Medical, Research Triangle Park, NC) can be positioned within the subclavian artery, with a 6 F distal access guiding catheter positioned within the distal (preferably the proximal intracranial segment) vertebral artery.
  - Aggressive pretreatment of the target artery with an antispasmodic agent (e.g., verapamil or nicardipine) can be helpful in preventing vasospasm.

Intra-procedural Imaging

Intra-procedural Angiographic CT (e.g., Cone Beam Volume CT, dynaCT Siemens Medical Solutions, Erlangen, Germany)

- Essential to accurately define the configuration of flow diverters in situ.
- Conventional fluoroscopic imaging is often inadequate to allow the visualization of deployed devices, particularly within segments of vasculature which overlie the osseous skull base.

Imaging Verifications After Deployment

- Construct bridges the entire diseased segment and extends from normal vessel proximally to normal vessel distally.
- All component devices are fully opened and well apposed to the vessel wall.

Post-procedural Management

- The post-procedural management of patients after flow diversion is highly controversial, and there are few data to guide these decisions. The authors present their current management strategies, which are based upon personal experience and continuously evolving:

Antiplatelet Therapy

- The duration of dual antiplatelet therapy varies with the complexity of the aneurysm and the length of the reconstructed vessel.

Conventional Lesions

- When a relatively short segment of aneurysmal involvement separates normal vascular segments, we maintain dual antiplatelet therapy for 6 months.
- If angiography demonstrates complete aneurysm occlusion at 6 months, we maintain aspirin therapy at traditional doses and reduce the clopidogrel dose by one-half.
- After 12 months we discontinue both clopidogrel and aspirin or, alternatively, maintain aspirin therapy at an 81 mg dose for life (depending on the patient's age, anatomical considerations related to branch vessels covered by the construct, or other medical considerations).

Complex Aneurysms

- When long circumferentially diseased vascular segments are reconstructed with multiple devices, we maintain dual antiplatelet medications for 1 year.
- If angiography demonstrates complete aneurysm occlusion at 1 year, we maintain aspirin therapy and half-dose clopidogrel therapy for another year.
- After 2 years we discontinue clopidogrel and continue aspirin indefinitely at an 81 mg dose.

Incompletely Occluded Aneurysms at Follow-Up

- We do not recommend the discontinuation of clopidogrel in circumstances in which flow persists through the construct and into the aneurysm.
- In these cases, we typically either continue dual antiplatelet therapy (full- or half-dose clopidogrel depending on the extent of the remnant) and wait or place additional devices across the remaining entry remnant.
- This approach to the discontinuation of dual antiplatelet therapy is based upon the observation of the very late thrombosis of flow-diverting constructs, occurring 1 year or more after the initial treatment in cases where dual antiplatelet medications were discontinued to perpetuate the occlusion of neck remnants.

Blood Pressure Management

- Following the PED reconstruction of anterior circulation aneurysms, it is prudent to ensure normal blood pressure.
- Several case reports and small case series have described delayed spontaneous ipsilateral parenchymal hemorrhages after the reconstruction of anterior circulation aneurysms with flow diverters.
- The etiology of these hemorrhages is unknown. They have been documented to occur at intervals ranging between 1 day and nearly 3 weeks after the procedure.
- While the etiology is unclear, the avoidance of periprocedural hypertension may be helpful in reducing the incidence and/or the severity of these hemorrhages should they occur.

Steroids

- With the exception of individuals presenting with acutely symptomatic aneurysms, we do not routinely treat patients with steroids in the periprocedural period.
- We typically reserve steroid for patients who develop new or worsening symptoms of mass effect or peri-aneurysmal edema after treatment.

Imaging Follow-Up

Angiography

- We typically perform angiographic follow-up between 3 and 6 months and then between 9 and 15 months.
- If the second angiogram confirms complete angiographic occlusion of the aneurysm and no evidence of in-construct stenosis, no further angiography is performed.

MR (or CTA)

- For all large and giant aneurysms, we perform MR imaging at these same intervals to monitor the expected, progressive resolution of the aneurysm-thrombus mass.
- If complete angiographic occlusion is confirmed at the 1-year follow-up, in most cases further follow-up is performed only with cross-sectional imaging.

Complications Related to Flow Diversion

Procedural Complications

- Procedural complications related to flow diversion are similar to those associated with standard stent-assisted coiling and have been described in detail in prior publications.

Delayed Complications

- Delayed complications after flow diversion are more unique to the technology.
- These complications may be observed days to weeks after an initially uncomplicated procedure.

Mural Destabilization

- Several case reports and small case series have described the delayed growth and/or rupture of previously unruptured aneurysms after flow diversion.

Aneurysm Characteristics

- Limited to very large aneurysms (>15 mm)

Timing

- The ruptures have been documented to occur days to months after aneurysm treatment.

Imaging Characteristics

- In most all cases where imaging is available, the aneurysms have demonstrated a large volume of accumulating intra-aneurysmal thrombus at the time of rupture.

Etiology

- While still uncertain, delayed rupture has been ascribed to a destabilization of the aneurysm wall related to physical phenomena or the evolving intra-aneurysmal thrombus, which is induced by flow diversion.
- Acute thrombus may induce ischemic, inflammatory, and destructive changes in the adjacent aneurysm wall following treatment, leading to thinning and in some cases complete dissolution.
- A similar phenomenon has been observed in partially thrombosed abdominal aortic aneurysms, which grow more rapidly if they are partially thrombosed and typically grow and rupture from the portion of the wall adjacent to the thrombus.

Predisposing Factors

- Some investigators have proposed that branch vessels incorporated into the aneurysm may perpetuate continued blood flow through the construct and prevent or delay complete aneurysm occlusion.
- Others have noted that symptomatic aneurysms, or those which have demonstrated recent growth, may be particularly susceptible to rupture after flow diversion.

Delayed Non-aneurysmal Parenchymal Hemorrhage

Anatomical Location

- Delayed parenchymal hemorrhage has been described after the treatment of anterior circulation aneurysms with flow diverters.

Associated Factors

- Timing: The hemorrhages have occurred between 24 h and 3 weeks after either complicated or uncomplicated procedures.
- Distribution: The hemorrhages have been primarily ipsilateral, in the vascular distribution of the treated aneurysm, but anatomically remote from the lesion itself. The distribution of hemorrhage has been either exclusively or predominantly intraparenchymal.
- Other aneurysm characteristics: These events seem to be independent of the size, morphology, or preoperative symptomatic status of the aneurysm.

Proposed Etiologies

- Reperfusion bleeds into small, clinically silent procedure-associated infarcts.
- Foreign body emboli produced during the flow diverter placement.
- Deleterious hemodynamic phenomena resulting from exclusion of a high-volume, large-capacitance aneurysm from the vascular circuit or the induction of a change in vascular compliance over the reconstructed segment, resulting in a loss of the Windkessel effect and the transmission of a less dampened arterial wave form to the cerebral vasculature.
- Clinical presentation: Presentations have ranged in severity from minor neurological impairment to death.
- Management: Challenging in the recent periprocedural period, given the difficulties involved in reversing antiplatelet medications to control hemorrhage progression or facilitate surgical evacuation of the hematoma in a patient with a newly implanted (thrombogenic) flow diverter construct. Decisions must be made on a situational- and patient-specific basis.

In-Construct Stenosis or Thrombosis

In-Stent Stenosis or Thrombosis at 6–12-Month Follow-Up

- The rate of in-construct stenosis or occlusion of flow diverters at 6–12-month follow-up is similar (~5 %) to what has been described for other intracranial aneurysm stents.
- In PUFS, 6 of 91 patients (6.6 %) with angiographic follow-up had in-stent stenosis ($n=2$) or construct thrombosis ($n=4$) at follow-up. Only two of these patients (2.2 %) were symptomatic.

Very Late Thrombosis (>1 Year)

- There are three reported cases of very late thrombosis of flow-diverting constructs 1 year or more after their implantation.

- Etiology: In two of three cases, the discontinuation of clopidogrel in response to the observation of a small amount of residual aneurysm filling at 1 year follow-up was followed by construct occlusion.
- For this reason, we typically maintain dual antiplatelet medications until complete aneurysm occlusion is documented on angiography (as discussed above).
- If a persistent entry remnant is identified, we often will place additional flow diverters over the involved segment as needed to augment the surface coverage and encourage the progression to complete occlusion.

Key Points

> Flow-diverting stents allow effective treatment of aneurysms considered unsuitable for "conventional" endovascular treatments.
> A theoretical appreciation of each device's physical properties, delivery, mechanism of action, and side effect profile is vital for appropriate and safe use.
> Appropriate patent selection is critical.
> Patient preparation, peri- and post-procedural care, in particular management of antiplatelet medication, is crucial for safety and success.
> The devices can be technically challenging to deploy and experienced proctor support in each operator's early cases is strongly recommended.

Suggested Reading

1. Cruz JP, Chow M, O'Kelly C, et al. Delayed ipsilateral parenchymal hemorrhage following flow diversion for the treatment of anterior circulation aneurysms. AJNR Am J Neuroradiol. 2012;33(4):603–8.
2. Devulapalli KK, Chowdhry SA, Bambakidis NC, Selman W, Hsu DP. Endovascular treatment of fusiform intracranial aneurysms. J Neurointerv Surg. 2013;5(2):110–6.
3. Fiorella D, Woo HH, Albuquerque FC, Nelson PK. Definitive reconstruction of circumferential, fusiform intracranial aneurysms with the pipeline embolization device. Neurosurgery. 2008;62:1115–20; discussion 1120–1.
4. Fiorella D, Lylyk P, Szikora I, et al. Curative cerebrovascular reconstruction with the pipeline embolization device: the emergence of definitive endovascular therapy for intracranial aneurysms. J Neurointerv Surg. 2009;1:56–65.
5. Fiorella D, Albuquerque F, Gonzalez F, McDougall CG, Nelson PK. Reconstruction of the right anterior circulation with the pipeline embolization device to achieve treatment of a progressively symptomatic, large carotid aneurysm. J Neurointerv Surg. 2010a;2:31–7.
6. Fiorella D, Hsu D, Woo HH, Tarr RW, Nelson PK. Very late thrombosis of a pipeline embolization device construct: case report. Neurosurgery. 2010b;67:E313–4; discussion E314.
7. Hampton T, Walsh D, Tolias C, Fiorella D. Mural destabilization after aneurysm treatment with a flow-diverting device: a report of two cases. J Neurointerv Surg. 2011;3:167–71.

8. Klisch J, Turk A, Turner R, Woo HH, Fiorella D. Very late thrombosis of flow-diverting constructs after the treatment of large fusiform posterior circulation aneurysms. AJNR Am J Neuroradiol. 2011;32:627–32.
9. Kulcsar Z, Houdart E, Bonafe A, et al. Intra-aneurysmal thrombosis as a possible cause of delayed aneurysm rupture after flow-diversion treatment. AJNR Am J Neuroradiol. 2011;32:20–5.
10. Lylyk P, Miranda C, Ceratto R, et al. Curative endovascular reconstruction of cerebral aneurysms with the pipeline embolization device: the Buenos Aires experience. Neurosurgery. 2009;64:632–42; discussion 642–3; quiz N636.
11. Nelson PK, Lylyk P, Szikora I, Wetzel SG, Wanke I, Fiorella D. The pipeline embolization device for the intracranial treatment of aneurysms trial. AJNR Am J Neuroradiol. 2011;32: 34–40.
12. Siddiqui AH, Abla AA, Kan P, et al. Panacea or problem: flow diverters in the treatment of symptomatic large or giant fusiform vertebrobasilar aneurysms. J Neurosurg. 2012;116(6):1258–66.
13. Turowski B, Macht S, Kulcsar Z, Hanggi D, Stummer W. Early fatal hemorrhage after endovascular cerebral aneurysm treatment with a flow diverter (SILK-stent): do we need to rethink our concepts? Neuroradiology. 2011;53:37–41.
14. Velat GJ, Fargen KM, Lawson MF, Hoh BL, Fiorella D, Mocco J. Delayed intraparenchymal hemorrhage following pipeline embolization device treatment for a giant recanalized ophthalmic aneurysm. J Neurointerv Surg. 2012;4(5):e24.

Parent Artery Sacrifice

Fergus Robertson and Andy Platts

Abstract

The goal of treatment of cerebral aneurysms is complete, permanent aneurysmal occlusion with preservation of parent artery and its branches (constructive techniques). Developments in endovascular and neurosurgical techniques mean most aneurysms are treatable by constructive techniques. Constructive techniques remain inappropriate for a small number of aneurysms (i.e., fusiform, giant, or blister aneurysms). Parent artery occlusion or trapping aneurysmal segment (deconstructive) techniques remain the safest option in some settings.

Keywords

Cerebral aneurysm • Permanent occlusion • Preservation • Parent artery sacrifice • Occlusion • Constructive technique • High risk • Giant aneurysm • Blister aneurysm • Trapping aneurysmal segment • Deconstructive technique • Arteriovenous malformation • Bleeding

F. Robertson, MA, MBBS, MRCP, FRCR (✉)
Department of Neuroradiology, National Hospital for Neuroradiology and Neurosurgery, Queen Square, London, UK
e-mail: fergusrobertson@nhs.net, fergus.robertson@uclh.nhs.uk

A. Platts, MBBS, FRCS, FRCR
Department of Radiology, Royal Free Hospital, London, UK
e-mail: andrew.platts@nhs.net

K. Murphy, F. Robertson (eds.), *Interventional Neuroradiology,*
Techniques in Interventional Radiology,
DOI 10.1007/978-1-4471-4582-0_7,© Springer-Verlag London 2014

Introduction

- The goal of treatment of cerebral aneurysms is complete, permanent aneurysm occlusion with preservation of parent artery and its branches (constructive techniques).
- Developments in endovascular and neurosurgical techniques mean most aneurysms are treatable by constructive techniques. Constructive techniques remain inappropriate for a small number of aneurysms (i.e., fusiform, giant, or blister aneurysms).
- Parent artery occlusion or trapping aneurysmal segment (deconstructive) techniques remain safest option in some settings.
- Technique also useful in other clinical settings, e.g., as an adjunct to tumor resection or in management of traumatic/iatrogenic major vessel injury.
- Rigorous assessment of arterial collateral pathways including balloon test occlusion is essential to assess likelihood of subsequent ischemic injury.
- May occasionally be combined with surgical vascular bypass procedure where native collateral circulation is demonstrated to be inadequate.
- Historically achieved by surgical parent artery ligation, more commonly now achieved by endovascular occlusion.

Diagnostic Evaluation

Clinical

Comprehensive medical, neurological, cognitive, and radiological assessment.

Laboratory

Basic screening bloods including full blood count, urea and electrolytes, coagulation profiles and blood group and save ECG, etc., as required.

Imaging

MRI and/or CT

Vital to establish location/anatomy of target lesion and the level of occlusion necessary to achieve protection. Angiographic studies provide some information on collateral circulation and the presence of background parenchymal ischemic damage.

Cerebral Angiography

Is essential to evaluate arterial anatomy and is crucial for planning treatment: six-vessel angiography should always be considered.

Balloon Test Occlusion

Should be considered in all patients, except perhaps those with life-threatening major artery injury requiring immediate control, in young or noncompliant patients, or in very distal vessels. Balloon test occlusion techniques are beyond the scope of this chapter and are well documented in the literature.

Indications for Treatment

- *Cerebral aneurysm* in which constructive technique considered impossible, high risk, or unlikely to yield a robust treatment (i.e., fusiform, giant or blister-like aneurysms or in distal (mycotic) aneurysm)
- *Arteriovenous fistula* such as direct carotid cavernous fistula (see Chap. 11)
- *Adjunct to tumor surgery* prior to resection of tumor encasing vessel
- *Acute vessel injury* – trauma/iatrogenic following surgery

Contraindications

Absolute

Failure of balloon test occlusion – may still be possible in conjunction with distal neurosurgical vascular bypass.

Relative

- Other vascular lesions (i.e., contralateral aneurysm likely to be put under increased stress following occlusion or contralateral significant stenosis)
- Difficult access – including tortuous/occluded proximal arterial anatomy
- Iodinated contrast allergy
- Severe renal impairment

Anatomy

Thorough angiographic assessment should consider the following:

- Patency and caliber of all major brain-supplying arteries (exclusion of stenoses)
- Integrity of circle of Willis
- Presence of native external to internal carotid artery and pial-pial collateral pathways
- Nature of vessel segment where occlusion is contemplated
- Presence of other relevant vascular pathologies (i.e., aneurysms/arteriovenous shunts or vascular anomalies or stenoses)

Equipment

- Biplane angiography is desirable but not essential.
- Guide catheter of suitable caliber to allow safe passage of embolization device.
- Familiar embolization device (see below).

Embolization Techniques

- The aim is to cause rapid cessation of flow in the parent vessel (to prevent distal clot embolization).
  There are essentially two treatment goals, depending upon clinical setting:

Proximal occlusion: merely blocking the vessel proximal to the pathology – this may permit continued perfusion of the pathological segment via collateral circulation, albeit at a decreased pressure or with altered flow dynamics/shear stress. This is often enough to promote subsequent thrombosis of the pathological segment (i.e., giant cavernous carotid aneurysm causing cranial nerve compression). This technique does no guarantee occlusion of the aneurysmal segment as back filling may cause continued perfusion.

Segmental trapping: blocking the vessel proximal and distal to the pathological segment – eliminates the pathology from the circulation (i.e., dissecting arterial aneurysm, ruptured mycotic distal MCA aneurysm, or extracranial artery sacrifice prior to resection of skull base/cervical tumor resection).

A number of occlusion techniques/devices are available and may be used in combination tailored to the treatment goal.

Detachable Balloon Occlusion (Fig. 1)

- Goldballoon (Goldbal 1–5; Balt Medical, Montmorency, France)
- Commercially available in most countries (excluding USA)
- Range of sizes available: match to vessel lumen
- Technically challenging/fragile in unfamiliar hands

Tips on Preparation

- A minimum of two balloons should be prepared at the outset – prepare the first balloon and inflate with 50 % contrast/saline and leave inflated while preparing the second device. This will confirm integrity of the first balloon.
- Reinsert the mandrill into the delivery microcatheter (with tip just inside the deflated balloon taking care not to damage it). This will support its passage through the guide catheter.

Tips on Safe Deployment

- Always have a second balloon prepared and ready for deployment before introducing the first.
- Once in the parent artery, remove the mandrill. Attach a 1 mL syringe of contrast/saline mixture via a two-way tap to the microcatheter.
- Once fully clear of the guide catheter, partially inflate the balloon to ensure visualization and use flow guidance to navigate the balloon catheter to the desired position.

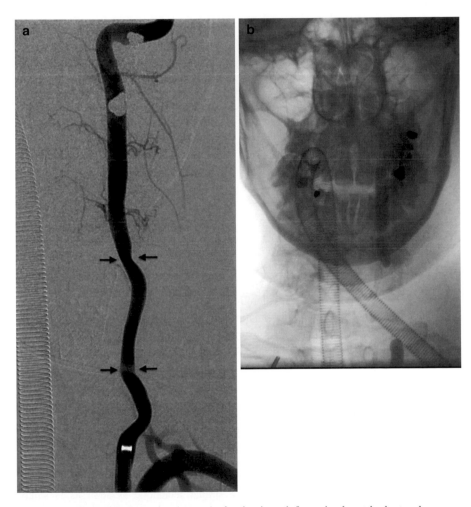

Fig. 1 (**a**) Angiographic narrowing (*arrows*) of codominant left proximal vertebral artery by encasing recurrent malignant cervical sarcoma. (**b**) Native image showing position of three detachable balloons which resulted in immediate/permanent vessel occlusion facilitating en bloc tumor resection 2 weeks later. (**c**) Preparation of the Goldballoon (With Permission from Balt Extrusion, Montmorency, France)

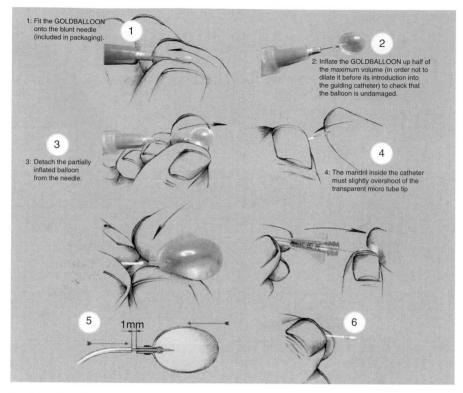

Fig. 1 (continued)

- Further inflate the balloon gently until it fills the lumen and begins to elongate along the long axis of the parent artery (maximum inflation volume should never be exceeded).
- It may be necessary to deflate and reinflate the balloon more than once while advancing/withdrawing the microcatheter to ensure appropriate positioning.
- Once adequately inflated, perform *gentle* guide catheter angiography to confirm parent vessel occlusion while avoiding washing the balloon from the microcatheter prematurely and risking distal balloon embolization.
- Once satisfied gently pull the microcatheter until the balloon detaches from the microcatheter tip – often requires considerable retraction force and may be assisted by advancing the guide catheter to abut the lower end of the balloon to hold in place; care must be taken not to allow the guide catheter to push the balloon forwards.
- This is the most dangerous stage and further angiography should be avoided until position secured with additional proximal balloon(s).
- Deploy a second proximal balloon using similar technique as soon as is safely possible.
- Consider a third balloon for security (should one of the first two subsequently fail).
- Final angiography is necessary to confirm occlusion and collateral flow and exclude complications.

Pros: Rapid occlusion, inexpensive

Cons: Fiddly to use, device fragile and may be damaged, risk of distal embolization of undersized balloon, risk of balloon deflation over time and recanalization of vessel, limited availability in some areas

Detachable Coil Occlusion (Fig. 2)

Coil occlusion involves familiar devices but occlusion of a "normal" vessel can be a difficult and lengthy procedure with two major challenges:

1. Getting first coil to form a stable platform in a tubular structure
2. Achieve sufficient packing density to establish rapid occlusion

May be assisted by:

- Start coil deployment at a bend, dilatation, narrowing, or branch in the parent vessel to engage the first coil and promote formation a complex structure.
- More rapid occlusion may be achieved by hydrogel coils which will swell inside the vessel or fibered coils which promote thrombosis.
- Two-catheter technique – holding the undetached first coil in place and deploying further coils against it via a second catheter.
- Proximal nondetachable to occlusion balloon to temporarily eliminate antegrade flow during coiling (especially dual lumen balloons such as Ascent (Micrus/Johnson & Johnson) and Sceptre (MicroVention) where coils can be deployed directly through balloon lumen).

Pros: Familiar devices, widely available

Cons: May be difficult to get coils to sit in tubular lumen

Usually slow, gradual occlusion – risk of distal embolization

Expensive – often needs many coils

Amplatzer Occlusion Device (Vascular Plug) (Fig. 3)

- Amplatzer occluder family of devices may be used to occlude extracranial vessels.
- The vascular occlusion plugs come in a range of sizes and configurations. All are delivered via a catheter or sheath and cause rapid, but not immediate vessel occlusion.
- The device is attached to a pusher wire and advanced from the delivery catheter, or operating sheath where it is to be deployed. If a satisfactory position is not achieved immediately, the device can be retrieved into the delivery system and removed or redeployed at a different site.

Fig. 2 (**a**) Recently ruptured right posterior inferior cerebellar artery (PICA) origin aneurysm in patient with poor grade subarachnoid hemorrhage. (**b**) Occlusion of aneurysm lumen and proximal PICA with detachable coils (no resulting attributable cerebellar or brainstem infarct in this case)

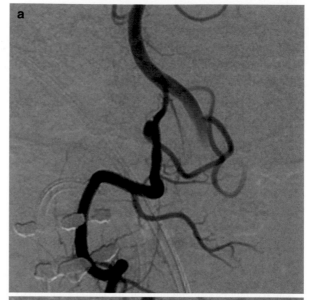

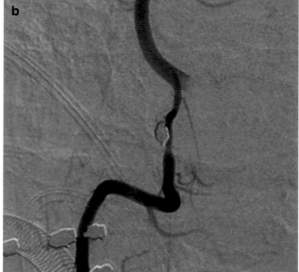

- When satisfactory placement has been achieved, the device is detached from the delivery wire by simply unscrewing it and the delivery wire is then removed.
- The device is selected to be oversized in the target vessel in the order of 20–50 %.

Each model of the device has advantages and disadvantages.

- *The Amplatzer 1* device uses a relatively low-profile delivery system and is generally easy to advance through the operating sheath or guiding catheter. It has only two membranes of nitinol mesh covering the vessel lumen and so vessel occlusion may be slow

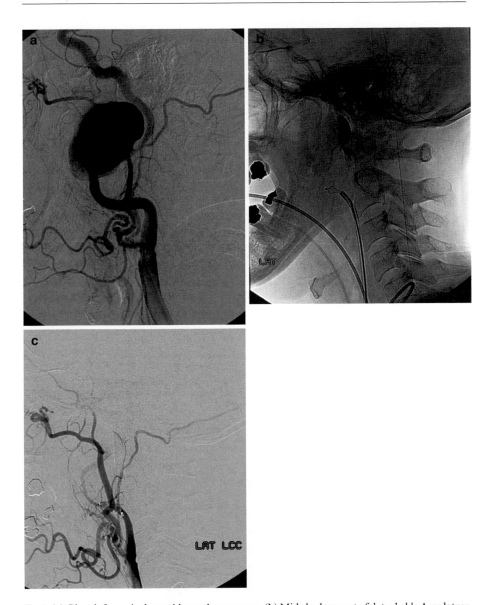

Fig. 3 (**a**) Giant left cervical carotid pseudoaneurysm. (**b**) Mid-deployment of detachable Amplatzer occlusion device (AOD). (**c**) Post-detachment of AOD with near occlusion of distal vessel

or may never occur particularly if the patient remains anticoagulated after the procedure.

- *The Amplatzer 2 device* is much longer than the Amplatzer 1 device when constrained within the delivery system and requires more effort to deliver through the operating sheath. It deploys within the vessel and results in six membranes of nitinol mesh across the lumen. Vessel occlusion is rapid and reliable but not immediate.

- *The Amplatzer 4 device* is very attractive in that it may be delivered through a simple 4 F angiographic catheter that has a 0.038″ lumen. Four membranes of nitinol mesh cover the lumen, but the wire is of thinner grade so occlusion is not as rapid as the Amplatzer 2 device and more than one device may be required to achieve occlusion.
- If any of the devices is to be used for extracranial arterial occlusion, then normal vigorous attention must be paid to prepare the operating sheath or guiding catheter to prevent air or thrombus resulting in intracranial embolus. The operating sheath should be continuously flushed with heparinized saline and the patient systemically heparinized before the deployment system is advanced into the vessel that is the target for occlusion.
- If after deployment vessel occlusion does not occur rapidly, then a second device may be used or a temporary occlusion balloon inflated proximally to encourage stasis and thrombosis.
- If the patient has been pretreated with antiplatelet agents and is anticoagulated, then rapid occlusion is unlikely to occur with a single device. Adding an additional vascular plug may be required or microcoils may be deployed proximally.

Liquid Embolic (Histoacryl) (Fig. 4)

- Reserved for distal embolization in a small artery where parent artery cannot be preserved and where focal occlusion is unlikely to cause major neurological deficit (test occlusion usually not practical/possible – e.g., in ruptured distal mycotic intracranial aneurysm).
- Considered by some to be a safer alternative to coil embolization, particularly where parent artery is small and there is inflamed friable aneurysm wall liable to rupture with coil placement.
- Challenge is to ensure occlusion of the diseased segment and the immediately proximal normal segment while preventing distal travel of embolic material to occlude cortical territories.
- A drop or two of concentrated (60–90 %) Histoacryl/Lipiodol injected via microcatheter with tip positioned at the proximal junction of the abnormal segment.

Pros: quick, cheap, low risk of rupture, permanent
Cons: difficult to control, risk of distal embolization

Pre-procedure Medications

- Formal loading with intravenous heparin appropriate in most settings should be performed after groin puncture using the operator's usual protocol. This should only be avoided where there is concern about ongoing extravasation, such as in iatrogenic arterial trauma.
- Antihypertensive medications should usually be discontinued prior to the procedure.
- Many advocate the use of antiplatelet agents with large vessel occlusion, but this practice is not consistent.
- Procedure is almost always performed under general anesthetic.

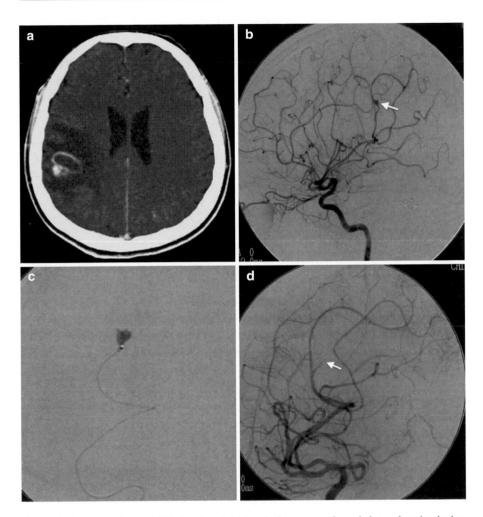

Fig. 4 (**a**) Contrast-enhanced CT showing right-hemisphere parenchymal ring enhancing lesion in a patient with bacterial endocarditis. (**b**) Lateral projection right carotid angiogram showing mycotic aneurysm in post-central middle cerebral artery branch (*arrow*). (**c**) Histoacryl/Lipiodol (glue) injection via microcatheter at aneurysm neck to occlude aneurysm and immediately proximal segment of parent artery. (**d**) Lateral projection of right carotid angiogram showing aneurysm occluded with stump of blocked vessel filling (*arrow*) with no clinical deficit resulting in this case

Post-procedural Care

Hydration

- Keep the patient well hydrated – 2 L, 0.9 % saline in 24 h in addition to oral fluids.

Close Monitoring

- Patient may be extubated immediately post-procedure; they optimally should be monitored in Neuro ITU or HDU for 24 h.

Blood Pressure Control

- Patient must not be allowed to become hypotensive – a period of relative hypertension should be tolerated and antihypertensive agents should only be used and reinstated later, gradually and after careful review.

Antithrombotics

- Large vessel occlusion (ICA or vertebral artery): uninterrupted therapeutic heparinization should continue for at least 48 h.
- The author converts from IV intraprocedural heparin to subcutaneous unfractionated heparin immediately post-procedure and for 48–72 h afterwards.
- Continued antiplatelet usage again is inconsistent and should be considered on a case-by-case basis.

Complications

- Main complication is distal cerebral ischemia – thromboembolic or hemodynamic occurring intra-procedurally or delayed.
- Risk is approximately 5 % of ICA occlusion (despite passing test occlusion), higher for distal intracranial artery occlusion and lower for vertebral artery occlusion.
- In the event of new neurological deficit, urgent MRI with diffusion-weighted imaging should be performed to identify lesion.
- Hemodynamic ischemia can be managed with fluid filling and blood pressure elevation in a monitored environment.
- Modification of antiplatelet/antithrombotic medication should be considered in thromboembolic complications.

Follow-Up

- Recanalization of large vessel occlusions is unusual if proper techniques employed.
- Noninvasive follow-up vascular imaging with CTA/MRA is often adequate for extradural vessel occlusion.
- Follow-up angiography in parent sacrifice for intradural aneurysm is usually considered desirable.

Alternative Treatments

- Technical improvements in stent graft and flow-diverting stent technology have increased the scope of reconstructive techniques for large vessel problems traditionally only suitable for "deconstruction."

Key Points

Large vessel:
> Test occlusion should be performed for all ICA occlusions and considered in other settings.
> Range of possible occlusion techniques, dependent on clinical setting and local experience.
> Ideal occlusion is rapid with occlusion proximal and distal to the diseased segment.
> Close post-procedural monitoring essential to mitigate delayed ischemic complications.

Small vessel:
> Coil occlusion/liquid embolic agent according to lesion and experience

Suggested Reading

1. Elhammady MS, Wolfe SQ, Farhat H, Ali Aziz-Sultan M, Heros RC. Carotid artery sacrifice for unclippable and uncoilable aneurysms: endovascular occlusion vs common carotid artery ligation. Neurosurgery. 2010;67(5):1431–6; discussion 1437.
2. Fox AJ, Viñuela F, Pelz DM, Peerless SJ, Ferguson GG, Drake CG, Debrun G. Use of detachable balloons for proximal artery occlusion in the treatment of unclippable cerebral aneurysms. J Neurosurg. 1987;66(1):40–6.
3. Lesley WS, Rangaswamy R. Balloon test occlusion and endosurgical parent artery sacrifice for the evaluation and management of complex intracranial aneurysmal disease. J Neurointerv Surg. 2009;1(2):112–20.
4. Ong CK, Lam DV, Ong MT, Power MA, Parkinson RJ, Wenderoth JD. Neuroapplication of amplatzer vascular plug for therapeutic sacrifice of major craniocerebral arteries: an initial clinical experience. Ann Acad Med Singapore. 2009;38(9):763–8.

Complications of Aneurysm Coiling

Mani Puthuran

Abstract

Endovascular coiling of intracranial aneurysm is an accepted treatment with good outcome and long-term efficacy. However like any interventional technique, it has procedural risks and complications. Large studies have shown a procedural complication rate leading to morbidity and mortality of around 5–6 %. Thromboembolic events followed by procedural rupture account for the majority of complications.

Keywords

Complication • Dissection hematoma • Retroperitoneal groin • Thrombosis • Clot • Stroke • Perforation aneurysm • Rupture • Coil prolapse

Every step of the procedure can cause a complication

Introduction

Endovascular coiling of intracranial aneurysm is an accepted treatment with good outcome and long-term efficacy. However like any interventional technique, it has procedural risks and complications. Large studies have shown a procedural complication rate leading to morbidity and mortality of around 5–6 %. Thromboembolic events and procedural rupture account for the majority of complications. The following is a brief summary of some of these complications.

M. Puthuran, MD, FRCR
Department of Neuroradiology, The Walton Centre for Neurology
and Neurosurgery NHS Trust, Liverpool, UK
e-mail: manipaul@hotmail.com

K. Murphy, F. Robertson (eds.), *Interventional Neuroradiology,*
Techniques in Interventional Radiology,
DOI 10.1007/978-1-4471-4582-0_8, © Springer-Verlag London 2014

Femoral Artery Puncture

Vessel Dissection

- This can occur in patients with atherosclerosis.
- Using "J"-shaped wires rather than straight-tip wires while introducing the femoral sheath reduces this complication.
- Introduce the wire under fluoroscopy in high-risk patients.

Postoperative Hematoma

- This complication occurs due to inadequate compression of femoral artery post-procedure.
- Regular observation in the recovery area of the puncture site.
- Extra care given to patients who have had anticoagulants and aspirin is necessary.

Retroperitoneal Hematoma

- The risk of retroperitoneal hematoma is very high if the puncture site is above the inguinal ligament.
- Computed tomography (CT) scan or ultrasound of the abdomen should be performed to confirm the diagnosis, and a vascular surgeon should be consulted.

Pseudoaneurysm

- Can be treated with compression but sometimes will need surgical intervention (Fig. 1)

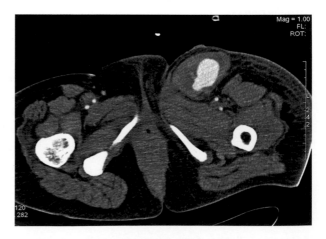

Fig. 1 Left femoral pseudoaneurysm

Catheterization of Cerebral Vessels

Dissection

- Arterial dissection can occur during catheterization of the cerebral vessels with the guiding catheter.
- Patients with atherosclerotic plaques are prone to this.
- Patients with tortuous vessels where distal access is needed are also at a higher risk.
- To reduce the risk, a soft-tip guiding catheter should be used.
- For distal access (e.g., to position the tip of the guiding catheter in the petrous segment of the internal carotid artery (ICA)):
  - The guide catheter can be pushed over the microcatheter/guidewire combination rather than over a Terumo wire.
  - Another technique is to push the guide catheter over a softer (125 cm) vertebral or SIM catheter or catheters such as the Chaperon.

Management

- Small dissection does not usually require any further management.
- If dissection is large enough to cause distal flow compromise, the dissected segment can be crossed with a microcatheter/guidewire combination.
- Stenting the affected segment should then be considered.
- Precaution with anticoagulants has to be considered if the patient subsequently needs treatment of ruptured aneurysm (Fig. 2a–d).

Thromboembolic Complications

- These types of complications can occur while positioning the guide catheter or performing precoiling cerebral angiogram.
- Thrombus can build up within the guide catheter if adequate heparinized saline flush is not maintained. Always check the pressure and flow in the heparinized saline infusion bags to maintain a steady flow.
- Embolic thrombus can be a problem when passing guide catheters past atherosclerotic lesions at the ICA origin. In this scenario:
  (a) Place a self-expanding or balloon expandable stent at the stenosis.
  (b) Position the guide catheter in the common carotid artery (CCA), preferably with additional support with a long sheath (i.e., Destination or Arrow long sheath).
- Treat the thrombus with IV aspirin and full-dose heparin once the aneurysm is secure. Occasionally, mechanical thrombectomy may be required in large clots.
- Small embolic thrombus can cause distal vessel occlusion during angiogram. This is extremely rare if proper technique and care is used during catheter angiogram (Fig. 3a, b).

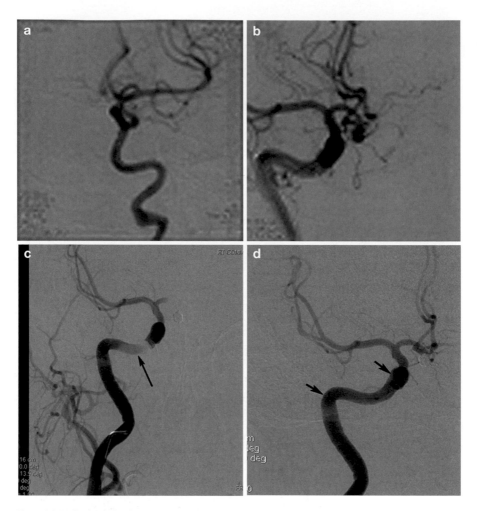

Fig. 2 (**a**) Left ICA injection demonstrates small dissections which occurred during microcatheterization in patient with Ehlers-Danlos connective tissue disorder. (**b**) Guide catheter placed in the petrous segment of ICA in order to get stability for balloon-assisted coiling of ACOM aneurysm. (**c**) Angiogram post-coiling shows dissection caused by guide catheter. (**d**) Angiogram in same patient shows post-stenting

Iatrogenic Vasospasm

- Induced mainly while catheterizing the intracranial vessels using guide catheter. To reduce the risk:
  - Use soft-tip guide catheters like the Neuron with Terumo wire if vasospasm is expected.
  - If distal access with the guide catheter is required, advance the catheter over microcatheter/guidewire combination rather than Terumo wire (Fig. 4a–c).

Fig. 3 (**a**) Demonstrates parietal hypoperfusion during precoiling angiogram. (**b**) Small embolus in M2 branch during placement of guide catheter and angiogram

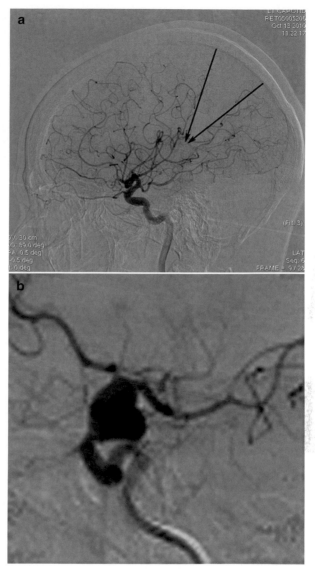

Aneurysm Coiling

- Most feared complications are intraprocedural iatrogenic aneurysm rupture and thromboembolic complications.
- Studies report 2–5 % intraprocedural rupture rate while coiling aneurysms post subarachnoid hemorrhage.

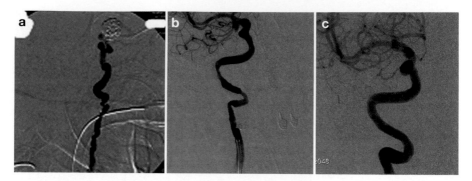

Fig. 4 (**a**) Demonstrates extreme vasospasm caused while trying to achieve distal guide catheter access in tortuous vessel. (**b**) Severe vasospasm of ICA post-catheterization with a guide catheter (different case). (**c**) Increasing the dose of nimodipine and 30 min wait restored normal vessel architecture, and the aneurysm was coiled

- Large series have reported procedural thromboembolic complications leading to mortality or morbidity of around 6 % in ruptured aneurysm and 1–3 % in treatment of unruptured aneurysm.
- Incidence of silent thromboembolic events is higher and is in the region of 15–30 %.
- Can be detected while performing diffusion-weighted magnetic resonance imaging (MRI).

Aneurysm Rupture

Due to Guidewire

- Can occur while catheterizing the aneurysm and usually occurs due to increased forward tension in the microcatheter resulting in "jump" of the guidewire.
- There is increased risk when small distal aneurysms are catheterized in tortuous vessels (vessel tortuosity increases tension in the microcatheter).
- Risk can be reduced by using soft-tip wires and avoiding touching the vessel wall with the wire.
- Controlling the tension and "slack" in the microcatheter is another important technique (Fig. 5a–c).

Due to Microcatheter

- Perforation can occur while catheterizing the aneurysm (see above).
- Catheter can cause perforation during coiling and is most likely due to forward "jump" of catheter, which is often seen immediately after coil detachment.
- Occurs when there is sudden release of forward force that has built up in the catheter.

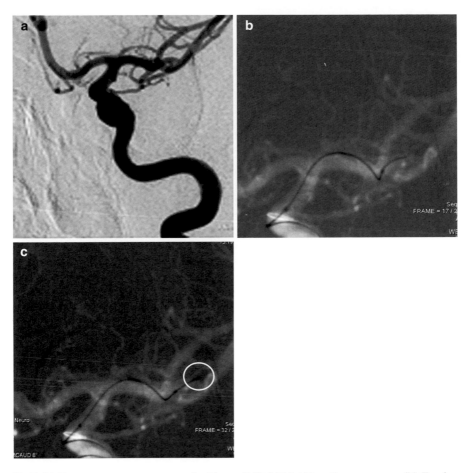

Fig. 5 (**a**) Demonstrates tortuous vessel with small Rt MCA bifurcation aneurysm. (**b**) Tension buildup in the microcatheter is demonstrated by the position of the catheter against the wall. At this stage there is increased risk of guidewire and catheter "jumping" forward. (**c**) Demonstrates guidewire perforation (*circled*)

- Extreme diligence should be given in monitoring the forward movement of the microcatheter, and any slack or tension in the system should be removed before coil detachment.

Due to Coil Loops

- Coil loops can cause perforation going into small daughter sacs or blebs which are potential points of rupture of aneurysm.
- Other potential cause of rupture: while pushing coils out of microcatheters, which are opposed to the walls of the aneurysm. This is because the distal marker of the microcatheter is obscured by previously inserted coils.

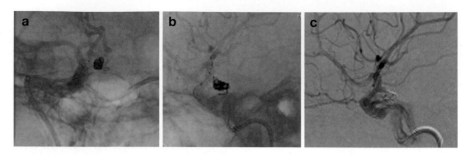

Fig. 6 (**a**) Demonstrated coil loop outside the aneurysm. However, the patient did not have contrast extravasation and no morbidity. (**b**) Endovascular coiling of PCOM aneurysm post-SAH shows coil loops protruding outside the aneurysm inferiorly. (**c**) Same patient showed contrast extravasation on angiography. The aneurysm was then completely occluded with further coils under balloon inflation. Patient developed new 3rd nerve palsy post-coiling

- The position of the distal marker can be judged by assessing the position of the proximal marker and noting its movements during the procedure.
- Another technique is to introduce further coils under negative road map once the first coil is deployed (Fig. 6a–c).

Iatrogenic Rupture

Follow the four *C*s.

Stay *C*alm (easier said than done!).

*C*onfirm rupture angiographically.

*C*ancel heparin.

*C*ontinue packing the aneurysm.

- Risk factors for intraprocedural rupture: small aneurysm, previous aneurysm rupture, vessel tortuosity.
- Intraprocedural rupture associated with 33 % increased risk of death and 5 % disability.
- These risks are much lower if one immediately proceeds to densely pack the aneurysm and this will stop the bleeding.
- Priority is to reverse the heparin and obtain dense packing.
- If catheter tip has gone through the wall of the aneurysm, there are few options:
  − In our center we tend to deploy few loops of coil in the subarachnoid space and then very carefully withdraw the catheter into the aneurysm and continue coiling.
  − Another technique is to insert a second catheter and complete the aneurysm coiling.
  − The final option is to treat the rupture using liquid embolic agents like Onyx 500. We do not use this in our center.
  − Try and avoid repeat angiographic runs as this causes contrast extravasation.

Thromboembolic Complications

- Morbidity and mortality due to thromboembolic complication is 5 % in ruptured aneurysms and in 2 % in unruptured aneurysms.
- Risk factors include previous rupture, age of patient, difficult access, and background atherosclerotic disease.
- In our experience, use of adjuvant devices like balloons slightly increases the complications, but this is controversial.

Coil Protrusion into Parent Vessel

- Occasionally while packing aneurysms coil loops or coil tail from previous coils can prolapse into parent vessel.
- Inflating a balloon to push the protruding coil back into the aneurysm and then inserting further coils under continued balloon inflation can anchor the coil in the aneurysm.
- If there is continued loop prolapse, there is potential for thrombus formation.
- In our center, we give intravenous aspirin 500 mg and slightly increase the mean arterial blood pressure for these patients once the aneurysm is secured.
- Single loop prolapse usually does not cause problems, and using stents to push the loop back is not always necessary.
- Stenting might be needed if several loops of coil protrude into the parent vessel (Fig. 7).

Coil Migration

- Coil migration from aneurysm is a rare complication of coiling but can occur due to various reasons.
- Risk factors include wide-necked aneurysm with a small dome: neck ratio I.
- If the coil is small (i.e., 2 by 2 mm), it usually will not cause any flow compromise and giving IV aspirin will usually suffice.
- Larger coils will eventually cause flow compromise, and hence coil retrieval has to be considered.
- Devices like the EV3 snare or alligator device can be used to retrieve such coils.

Use of Adjuvant Like Balloons and Stents

There is increased incidence of thromboembolic complications while using these adjuvant techniques. To reduce these complications, patients can be preloaded with antiplatelet regime when unruptured aneurysms are treated. However this is not possible in acutely ruptured aneurysm treatment where use of balloons and stents should be carried out with caution.

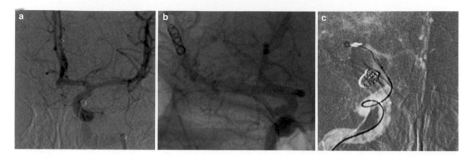

Fig. 7 (**a**) While detaching the last 2 by 2 mm coil in a PCOM aneurysm, the coil migrated from the aneurysm into the left A2. After giving 500 mg IV aspirin and waiting for 30 min, no thrombus formation noted and hence no further intervention required. (**b**) Large first coil deployed with remodelling balloon. Initially stable displaced distally after some minutes causing impeded flow. The coil was then retrieved using a snare. (**c**) Anothe displaced coil being retrieved using an alligator device

Technical Complications

Case Study 1

A 42-year-old female presents with a sudden onset of headache, photophobia, and right diplopia. CT scan demonstrated grade 1 SAH, and CTA (CT angiography) demonstrated a right PCOM (posterior communicating) aneurysm. It was decided to treat the patient by endovascular coiling.

Equipment

- Standard 6-French (F) sheath
- 6-F Neuron guide catheter
- 9 mm Eclipse Balloon across the neck of the aneurysm
- Headway 17 Advanced catheter into the aneurysm using Traxcess wire

The aneurysm was then densely packed with several coils. However towards the end of the procedure while trying to pack the neck of the aneurysm, the last coil did not detach even after multiple attempts. It was decided to retrieve the coil, but, while gently pulling the coil into the microcatheter, the coil detached.

Management Options

(a) To pull the coil out using a snare
(b) To grab the coil using a snare and stretch it into the ECA
(c) Placing a stent to jail the portion of the coil lying outside the aneurysm (Fig. 8a–c)

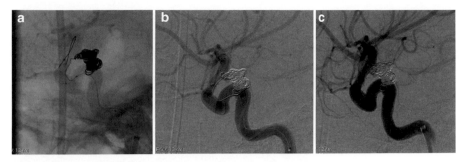

Fig. 8 (**a**) Detachment of the coil while being pulled back into the microcatheter. (**b**) Decision was made to use a stent to oppose the portion of the coil outside the aneurysm against the wall of the parent vessel. Figure shows a Prowler Select Plus catheter placed across the aneurysm neck. (**c**) Angiogram post-stent deployment

Case Study 2

A 52-year-old female presents with sudden headache and vomiting. Patient had previous SAH and coiling of basilar tip aneurysm. CT scan demonstrated grade 1 SAH, and CTA demonstrated recurrence of previously treated aneurysm. It was decided to re-treat the patient by endovascular coiling and stenting.

Equipment

- Bilateral Standard 6-F sheath in CFA
- 6-F Neuron guide catheter in left vertebral and 5 F in fight vertebral artery
- 9 mm Eclipse Balloon across the neck of the aneurysm into the left P2 segment
- Headway 17 Advanced catheter into the aneurysm using Traxcess wire

The aneurysm was then densely repacked with several coils. After achieving dense packing, it was decided to "Y" stent the neck to prevent recurrence. Post-coiling CT however demonstrated further SAH and contrast extravasation even though there was no demonstrable contrast extravasation during the procedural angiograms. One of the complications of using the stents and balloons is wire perforation of small perforating vessels. Great care must be taken with the position and placement of the distal wire while stenting and using balloons. Also one needs to observe the late phase of the angiogram carefully to look for contrast leak (Fig. 9a, b).

Fig. 9 (**a**) The angiogram
shows the stent guidewire
possibly within a perforator.
(**b**) Post-"Y" stenting did not
demonstrate contrast
extravasation

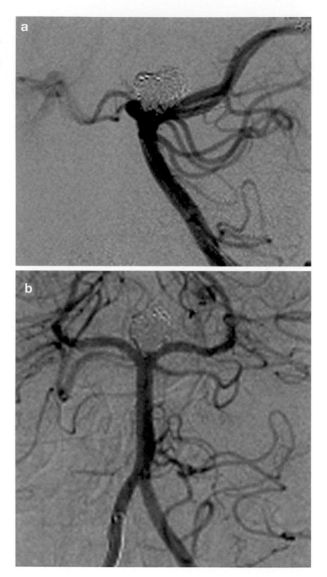

Conclusion

Endovascular technique for coiling of aneurysm is a safe method for treatment of intra-cranial aneurysms. However a good understanding of the possible complications is mandatory.

Key Points

› Formal training in neuroendovascular procedures is mandatory before undertaking cerebral aneurysm coiling.
› Understanding normal and variant cerebral vascular anatomy including dangerous ECA-ICA anastomosis and collateral cerebral perfusion.
› Good technical skill and knowledge of the uses and limitations of various catheters and wires and adjuncts like balloons and stents.
› Keeping up to date with new developments and treatment options in the field of neurointervention.

Avoidance and Treatment of Vasospasm

Martin G. Radvany and James Chen

Abstract

Cerebral vasospasm is caused by subarachnoid hemorrhage (SAH) most often secondary to aneurysm rupture. Other less common causes of SAH include hemorrhage from an arteriovenous malformation, vasculitis, reversible cerebral vasoconstriction syndrome as well as cerebral trauma.

Keywords

Vasospasm • Avoidance • Treatment • Cerebral vasospasm • Subarachnoid hemorrhage • Aneurysm rupture • Arteriovenous malformation • Vasculitis • Reversible cerebral vasoconstriction syndrome • Cerebral trauma

Introduction

Cerebral vasospasm is caused by subarachnoid hemorrhage (SAH) most often secondary to aneurysm rupture. Other less common causes of SAH include hemorrhage from an arteriovenous malformation, vasculitis, reversible cerebral vasoconstriction syndrome (RCVS) as well as cerebral trauma.

M.G. Radvany, MD (✉) • J. Chen, BS
Division of Interventional Neuroradiology, The Johns Hopkins Hospital,
Baltimore, MD, 21287, USA
e-mail: mradvan2@jhmi.edu

K. Murphy, F. Robertson (eds.), *Interventional Neuroradiology,*
Techniques in Interventional Radiology,
DOI 10.1007/978-1-4471-4582-0_9, © Springer-Verlag London 2014

Clinical Features

Delayed cerebral ischemia (DCI) from cerebral vasospasm is most common cause of secondary morbidity and mortality following aneurysmal subarachnoid hemorrhage (SAH).

Pathophysiology

- Blood products in subarachnoid space trigger contraction of smooth muscle cells leading to ischemia and eventual infarction.
- The precise signaling cascades responsible for this phenomenon remain to be fully elucidated.

Risk of Vasospasm

- Studies have shown higher risk of vasospasm with increasing Hunt and Hess grade and CT characteristics including the initial presence, volume, density, and duration of hemorrhage.
- 70 % SAH patients will demonstrate angiographic vasospasm.
- 20–30 % of these patients develop symptomatic vasospasm.
- Up to half of these patients suffer neurologic deficits or death.
- Early diagnosis and treatment is essential to preserve neurologic function in this group.

Time Course

Most commonly occurs 3–14 days following hemorrhage, peaking around day 7.

Diagnostic Evaluation

Clinical Assessment

- No definitive prediction algorithm exists so vigilant clinical monitoring is essential, particularly for patients in the high-risk time window.
- Any of the following signs and symptoms should raise concern:
  New focal motor deficits
  Sudden changes in mental status

Nonfocal neurologic changes: confusion, increasing somnolence, and combativeness
- Consider and rule out other potential causes of symptoms:
Hydrocephalus
Seizures
Delirium

Patients who are neurologically impaired or comatose from initial SAH may not have a meaningful clinical exam and be more dependent on radiographic monitoring.

Laboratory

There are no laboratory studies to diagnose cerebral vasospasm. Vigilant clinical assessment with radiographic imaging is required.

Imaging

The goals of imaging patients during the high-risk vasospasm window:

- Rule out other pathologies.
- Detect vasospasm.
- Assess severity of vasospasm.

Transcranial Doppler (TCD) Ultrasonography

- First-line modality for monitoring for vasospasm and excellent triaging tool

Advantages: Noninvasive, inexpensive, easily performed at bedside, and high specificity for proximal vessel spasm.
Disadvantages: Sensitivity decreases in more distal vascular territories and can vary with adequacy of vessel insonation and operator experience.

Non-contrast Head Computed Tomography (NCCT)

- Initial evaluation in patients with altered clinical exam and/or TCD findings
- Provides rapid survey for established infarctions and rules out other etiologies of neurological deterioration before subsequent interventions are considered

Computed Tomography Angiography (CTA)

- Highly sensitive for severe vasospasm (>50 % luminal reduction) and excellent negative predictive value

Computed Tomography Perfusion (CTP)

- Provides rapid perfusion evaluation to compliment demonstration of vasospasm by CTA and TCD
- Measured parameters include mean transit time (MTT), cerebral blood volume (CBV), and cerebral blood flow (CBF).
- The following patterns of abnormal perfusion are observed in the setting of vasospasm:
  Benign oligemia: Increased MTT, normal CBF, and normal or increased CBV
  Penumbra: Increased MTT, decreased CBF, and normal or increased CBV
  Irreversible ischemia: Increased MTT, decreased CBF, and decreased CBV

The balance between the amount of salvageable penumbra and established infarct in a territory determines whether aggressive intervention should be pursued.

Magnetic Resonance Angiography (MRA) and Perfusion-Weighted

Magnetic Resonance (MR) Imaging

- Generally not as widely adopted as CT-based modalities given the logistical challenges of MR imaging in acutely ill patients

Digital Subtraction Angiography (DSA)

- DSA remains the gold standard for evaluating cerebral vasospasm and is the foundation for endovascular treatments.
- Highly sensitive and specific for vasospasm, provides real-time hemodynamic assessment.
- Minimal risk of iatrogenic complications.
- Its cost and resource requirements, however, make it impractical as a screening tool; patients should usually only be triaged to catheter angiography based on suggestive noninvasive imaging findings.

Indications for Intervention

Once you have identified a patient with symptomatic vasospasm whose imaging findings suggest the presence of a salvageable territory, they should be promptly triaged toward medical or endovascular therapy.

Medical Therapy

- First-line therapy for the majority of patients with symptomatic vasospasm.
- HHH (hypervolemia, hypertension, and hemodilution) therapy has been shown to be effective for improving perfusion and clinical outcomes.

- It will not prevent vasospasm in all cases, and up to 19 % of patients may still develop major neurologic deficits or death due to vasospasm despite medical treatment.

Endovascular Therapy

Modalities:

- Intra-arterial (IA) vasodilator infusion
- Transluminal balloon angioplasty
- Combination of both

   Candidates for endovascular therapy include:

- Patients who are unable to tolerate prolonged courses of hemodynamic therapy due to underlying medical comorbidities (e.g., cardiac or renal insufficiency)
- Patients who have a poor response to medical therapy

Contraindications

The presence of a sizeable infarct core in the vasospasm territory precludes any aggressive therapies as the risk of reperfusion hemorrhage outweighs the potential benefits of recovering the penumbra region.

   Relative contraindication to angioplasty of recently clipped or coiled vessels as fatal rupture can occur.

Anatomy

- Prior to performing any interventions, the patient's baseline anatomy on DSA should be reviewed carefully, with attention to the vessel morphology and diameter.

   Note: the presence of normal variants; hypoplastic segments should not be confused for vasospasm (common locations: A1 segment, intradural vertebral artery, P1 segment, posterior communicating artery).
   Note: the location of coils and clips as angioplasty in these regions is associated with a higher risk of iatrogenic rupture:

- Location and degree of vasospasm have important implications for treatment planning.
- Proximal vasospasm can be addressed with balloon angioplasty, which is generally thought to provide a more durable effect.
- Distal vasospasm can be treated with IA vasodilator infusion.

Equipment

Intra-arterial Vasodilators

Calcium channel blockers (CCBs) are the most commonly used agents due to excellent safety profiles and efficacy. They act primarily by inhibition of voltage-gated calcium channels on smooth muscle cells, but there is also evidence of indirect neuroprotective effects. The use of these agents currently remains off-label.

Commonly used CCBs:

- Nicardipine – T½ ~ 16 h
- Verapamil – T½ ~ 7 h
- Nimodipine – T½ 8–9 h

Catheters/Balloons

The use of balloon angioplasty for treatment of vasospasm has been studied for over half a decade. Mechanical flattening of smooth muscle and endothelial cells produces a durable patency of the spastic vessel segment. Coronary balloons were used historically, but more compliant, trackable, dedicated intracranial systems have since been developed.

Intracranial balloon catheter systems:

- Hyperglide (ev3 Neurovascular, Irvine, California)
- Hyperform (ev3 Neurovascular, Irvine, California)

Balloon inflation syringe:

- 1-ml Cadence syringe (ev3 Neurovascular, Irvine, California)

Procedure

Perform baseline cerebral angiography of anterior and posterior circulation to assess for vasospasm. Compare with prior angiogram if available and determine if treatment will involve proximal vessels (Distal ICA, M1, and A1) or distal vessel (M2, A2, etc.).

Treatment Plan and Technique

- Proximal vessel treatment – angioplasty and/or vasodilator infusion (Fig. 1)
- Distal vessel treatment – vasodilator infusion (Fig. 2)

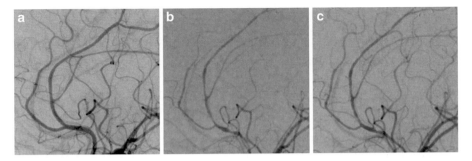

Fig. 1 Fifty-three-year-old female who presented with "thunderclap" headache and a negative CT scan. Lumbar puncture demonstrated RBCs that did not clear, and patient was transferred for presumed SAH. (**a**) Baseline angiography demonstrated a few scattered areas of stenosis. The differential diagnosis included vasculitis and RCVS. The patient subsequently developed an intracerebral hemorrhage, and her neurological exam deteriorated while being treated for vasculitis. Brain biopsy was negative for vasculitis. (**b**) Repeat angiography demonstrated progressive segmental narrowing in the pericallosal and callosomarginal arteries. (**c**) Angiography post-infusion of 2 mg of nicardipine demonstrated improvement in the appearance of the blood vessels helping to confirming the diagnosis of RCVS. Despite a slow nicardipine infusion, the patient required pressor support during and after the infusion

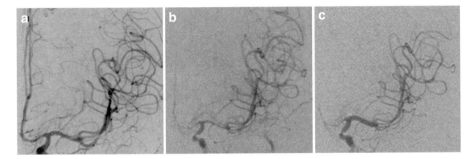

Fig. 2 Forty-three-year-old female with history of SAH secondary to ruptured ACOM aneurysm. Eight days post-aneurysm clipping the patient began to have deterioration in her neurological status. Cerebral angiogram demonstrated bilateral MCA and ACA vasospasm. Both MCAs were treated with angioplasty and infusion of nicardipine (2 mg). ACAs were not treated with angioplasty due to small size and recent aneurysm clipping. (**a**) Baseline left ICA diagnostic angiogram prior to clipping. (**b**) Angiogram from left common carotid demonstrating severe vasospasm of left A1 and M1 segments. (**c**) Control angiogram status post-angioplasty of left M1 segment with underinflated 4 mm × 7 mm HyperForm balloon

Vasodilator Infusion

Infusion Site

- Proximal infusion site from the internal carotid artery or vertebral artery is used for mild to moderate vasospasm in the anterior or posterior circulations, respectively.

- Superselective injections have been performed for severe vasospasm, but there is no evidence in the literature to support the efficacy of this strategy versus proximal infusion.
- Consider systemic heparinization when performing prolonged infusion (ACT > 250).

Infusion Rate

Nicardipine

- Dilute to concentration of 0.1 mg/ml
- 0.5–1 mg nicardipine per minute
- Total dose 0.5–6.0 mg per arterial tree

Verapamil

- Dilute to concentration of 0.1 mg/ml
- 0.5–1 mg verapamil per minute
- Total dose 1–3 mg per arterial tree

Nimodipine

- Dilute to concentration of 0.1 mg/ml
- 1–4 mg nimodipine per hour
- Total dose 0.5–3 mg per arterial tree

Arterial pressures should be titrated carefully:

- Infusion should be stopped when a drop in the mean arterial pressure (MAP) of >15 mmHg or systolic blood pressure of >25 mmHg occurs.
- Infusion can be resumed after pressures return to baseline.

After infusion, control angiography should be performed to evaluate response to treatment (Fig. 1).

Potential Side Effects

- It is important to monitor patient vitals carefully during the infusion to avoid complications from hypotension or elevated intracranial pressure.
- Vasopressor support may occasionally be needed if there is a severe reduction in mean arterial pressure.

Balloon Angioplasty

Balloon diameter should be purposefully undersized from the projected normal caliber of the target vessel segment to reduce the risk of acute vessel rupture.

Administer heparin to achieve ACT > 250 s prior to advancing guidewire and balloon.

The balloon should be advanced to the distal portion of the segment to be treated and angioplasty performed from distal to proximal. Though it may require more dilations, a shorter balloon may be easier to advance through a tight carotid siphon.

Balloons should be inflated with a 50/50 mixture of 300 mg/ml iodinated contrast and saline. A calibrated syringe can be used to inflate the balloon catheter. When using balloon catheter systems in which the guidewire occludes the distal catheter opening, one must be careful not to retract the guidewire into the catheter once the system is in place. Backflow of blood into the balloon lumen dilutes the contrast thereby reducing balloon opacification, which can lead to unintentional overinflation.

Perform control angiography to assess response to treatment and evaluate for complications (Fig. 2).

A vasodilator may be administered prior to angioplasty to help prevent catheter-induced vasospasm prior to angioplasty.

Results

The rate of clinical improvement following balloon angioplasty has been reported in case series at a mean of 62 %, with a range of 11–93 %. There remains no efficacy data from randomized controlled trials to further clarify these results.

Studies have suggested that the rate of clinical improvement when angioplasty is performed within two hours of vasospasm may be higher than outside that window, but further evidence is necessary to fully clarify the ideal window to initiate therapy.

The efficacy of IA vasodilator infusions has also only been described in clinical series, which have reported rates of clinical improvement of up to 76 %. Infusion doses and rates have varied between studies, and a definitive protocol remains to be established.

Complications

Acute vessel rupture occurs in approximately 1 % of cases. This risk has been reduced from the past with the adoption of more compliant, dedicated neurovascular balloon systems and increased technical experience. Severe vessel spasm can still present a challenge due to limited distal visualization – particular care should be taken in these cases to avoid iatrogenic perforation.

Reperfusion injury is a relatively uncommon complication and should be avoided with appropriate analysis of noninvasive studies and avoidance of large infarcts.

Follow-Up

The effect of IA vasodilators is generally not as durable as angioplasty so the critical care team should be aware of the potential for recurrent vasospasm.

Alternative Therapies

Medical therapy should be instituted first in patients with symptomatic vasospasm.

Key Points

> Do not pursue aggressive treatment in patients with significant infarct cores.
> Review baseline angiographic appearance with attention to normal variants during treatment planning.
> Balloon diameter should be undersized with respect to normal vessel caliber.
> Patients may require retreatment, especially if treated only with vasodilators.

Suggested Reading

1. Avitsian R, Fiorella D, Soliman MM, et al. Anesthetic considerations of selective intra-arterial nicardipine injection for intracranial vasospasm: a case series. J Neurosurg Anesthesiol. 2007;19:125–9.
2. Feng L, Fitzsimmons BF, Young WL, et al. Intraarterially administered verapamil as adjunct therapy for cerebral vasospasm: safety and 2-year experience. AJNR Am J Neuroradiol. 2002;23:1284–90.
3. Janardhan V, Biondi A, Riina HA, et al. Vasospasm in aneurysmal subarachnoid hemorrhage: diagnosis, prevention, and management. Neuroimaging Clin N Am. 2006;16:483–96.
4. Jestaedt L, Pham M, Bartsch AJ, et al. The impact of balloon angioplasty on the evolution of vasospasm-related infarction after aneurysmal subarachnoid hemorrhage. Neurosurgery. 2008;62:610–7, discussion 610–7.
5. Lysakowski C, Walder B, Costanza MC, et al. Transcranial Doppler versus angiography in patients with vasospasm due to a ruptured cerebral aneurysm: a systematic review. Stroke. 2001;32:2292–8.

6. Tejada JG, Taylor RA, Ugurel MS, et al. Safety and feasibility of intra-arterial nicardipine for the treatment of subarachnoid hemorrhage-associated vasospasm: initial clinical experience with high-dose infusions. AJNR Am J Neuroradiol. 2007;28:844–8.
7. Wintermark M, Ko NU, Smith WS, et al. Vasospasm after subarachnoid hemorrhage: utility of perfusion CT and CT angiography on diagnosis and management. AJNR Am J Neuroradiol. 2006;27:26–34.
8. Wolf S, Martin H, Landscheidt JF, et al. Continuous selective intraarterial infusion of nimodipine for therapy of refractory cerebral vasospasm. Neurocrit Care. 2010;12:346–51.

Part III

Intracranial Embolization

Endovascular Treatment of Cerebral Arteriovenous Malformations

Shelley Renowden and Fergus Robertson

Abstract

Brain arteriovenous malformations (AVMs) are rare and heterogeneous vascular abnormalities. AVMs are formed of a tangled anastomosis of arteries and veins without intervening capillaries located within the brain parenchyma (90 % supratentorial) with pathologic shunting of blood from the arterial to the venous side. Prevalence is approximately 18 per 100,000 adults with an incidence of approximately 1.3 per 100,000 adults per year. Most cases are sporadic – cause unknown and probably multifactorial with genetic and environmental factors.

Keywords

Cerebral aneurysm • Permanent occlusion • Preservation • Parent artery sacrifice • Occlusion • Constructive technique • High risk • Giant aneurysm • Blister aneurysm • Trapping aneurysmal segment • Deconstructive technique • Arteriovenous malformation • Bleeding

S. Renowden, BSc, MRCP, FRCR (✉)
Department of Neuroradiology, Frenchay Hospital, Bristol, UK
e-mail: shelley.renowden@nbt.nhs.uk

F. Robertson, MA, MBBS, MRCP, FRCR
Department of Neuroradiology, National Hospital for Neuroradiology and Neurosurgery, Queen Square, London, UK

K. Murphy, F. Robertson (eds.), *Interventional Neuroradiology,*
Techniques in Interventional Radiology,
DOI 10.1007/978-1-4471-4582-0_10, © Springer-Verlag London 2014

Clinical Features

- Brain arteriovenous malformations (AVMs) are rare and heterogeneous vascular abnormalities.
- Formed of a tangled anastomosis of arteries and veins without intervening capillaries located within the brain parenchyma (90 % supratentorial) with pathologic shunting of blood from the arterial to the venous side.
- Prevalence approx. 18 per 100,000 adults and incidence approx 1.3 per 100,000 adults per year.
- Most cases are sporadic – cause unknown and probably multifactorial with genetic (>900 genes are involved in the pathogenesis) and environmental factors. Minority associated with congenital and hereditary syndromes: Rendu-Osler-Weber, Wyburn-Mason, and Sturge-Weber. Rare familial cases not associated with syndromes are also described.
- Biologically active lesions can grow or regress. Following obliteration they can rarely recur – most recurrences in children.

Clinical Presentation

- Intracranial hemorrhage (ICH) parenchymal subarachnoid or intraventricular bleed (incidence of AVM-related ICH is approx. 0.50 per 100,000 person-years).
- Seizures (focal or generalized – most respond well to antiepileptic drugs – intractable seizures rare).
- Headaches (no distinctive features – the yield of AVMs in patients investigated for headache is very low).
- Progressive neurological deficit, arterial steal, or venous hypertension.
- Pulsatile tinnitus.
- Typical presentation is ICH in young adult, but many now detected incidentally and majority of cerebral AVMs now present unruptured.

Natural History

Ruptured AVM

- The Columbia database suggests for patients with recent AVM-related ICH that 47 % of those have no deficit, an additional 37 % remain independent, 13 % are moderately disabled, and 3 % are severely disabled. The long-term crude fatality rate is around 1–1.5 % per annum and the annual rates of severe morbidity around 1.4 %.

Unruptured AVM

- Unclear – some data suggests that interventions may lead to worse outcomes than natural history – ARUBA trial is underway.

Diagnostic Evaluation

Clinical

- Comprehensive medical, neurological, cognitive, and radiological assessment is essential. Where relevant, consider other specific assessments, i.e., ophthalmological and psychiatric.

Laboratory

- Basic blood screening includes full blood count, urea and electrolytes, coagulation profiles, and blood group and save; electrocardiography (ECG), chest radiograph etc., as required.

Imaging

Magnetic Resonance Imaging (MRI)

MRI is vital to establish AVM location, relationship to eloquent cortex, evidence of old ICH, and parenchymal changes of gliosis or edema (latter often reflects venous hypertension).

Cerebral Angiography

Cerebral angiography is the gold standard to evaluate arterial and venous anatomy and is crucial for planning treatment: 6-vessel angiography should always be considered, particularly when there has been a previous cerebral intervention, as unexpected (i.e., dural) collaterals are more likely.

Table 1 Major risk factors
for hemorrhage and annual
bleeding risk (Stapf 2006
from columbia database)

Major risk factors for hemorrhage	Annual bleeding risk (%)
1. Previous ICH	4.5
2. Deep location	3.1
3. Exclusively deep venous drainage	2.5

Indications

Management is often challenging and controversial, particularly in unruptured AVMs. Treatment decisions should be made on case-by-case basis with multidisciplinary input with all treatment modalities represented. Risks of invasive treatment must be balanced against natural history, but unbiased natural history data is currently limited.

Suggested Indications for Treatment

- Intracranial hemorrhage (ICH)
- Progressive neurological deficit attributable to the AVM
- Intractable seizures (surgical excision renders 80 % seizure-free)
- Other disabling symptoms likely to be improved by treatment (i.e., dural headache)

Risk Stratification for Future Hemorrhage

Annual bleeding risks: 0/3 risk factors are 0.9 %; 3/3 factors may be as high as 34.4 % (Table 1).

Other risk factors often considered to predict future hemorrhage:

- Stenotic/occlusive changes in the draining vein
  - Single draining vein
  - Intranidal aneurysms
  - Small nidal size
- Some estimate risk the lifetime of bleeding by subtracting age from 105.

Contraindications

- Difficult access – including tortuous/occluded proximal arterial anatomy
- Iodinated contrast allergy
- Severe renal impairment

Anatomy

Thorough angiographic assessment should consider each of the following:

Arteries

- Type and number of feeding arteries
- Aneurysms (remote, feeding vessel, or intranidal)
- Induced collaterals from adjacent vascular territories (may be misinterpreted as part of the nidus)

Shunt

- Nidus compact or diffuse
- Presence of fistula – fast/slow?

Veins

- Numbers – deep/superficial
- Stenosis/ectasia
- Degree of congestion

Spetzler-Martin Grading (Grades I–V) (Table 2 and 3)

- Widely used – primarily reflects surgical risk but broadly reflects embolization; risk large complex AVMs require multiple procedures
- Higher risk with those related to eloquent cortex, deep feeders, and deep venous drainage
- BUT does NOT consider perforator arterial supply, compact on diffuse nidus, associated aneurysms, and, importantly, the experience of the neurosurgeon/interventionalist

Equipment

- Biplane angiography is considered essential.
- 6-F guide catheter with heparinized saline flush.
- Microcatheter: DMSO compatible for Onyx usage.
- Microwire.

Table 2 Spetzler-Martin grade

A point is allocated for size, location, deep venous drainage	
Eloquent cortex is sensorimotor, language, visual cortex, hypothalamus, internal capsule, brainstem, cerebellar peduncles, and deep cerebellar nuclei	
A separate SM grade VI is considered inoperable	
Size	**Point**
Small (<3 cm)	1
Medium 3–6 cm	2
Large >6 cm	3
(Usually at the time of diagnosis, 30% is <3 cm, 60% 3–6 cm, and 10% >6 cm).	
Location	
Non-eloquent	0
Eloquent	1
Venous drainage	
Only superficial	0
Deep (any)	1

Table 3 Incidence of postoperative deficit by AVM SM grade

	Minor	Major
I	0	0
II	5	0
III	12	4
IV	20	7
V	10	12

Cerebral AVM treatment recommendations: North American Guidelines
Surgical excision is the single treatment of choice for Spetzler-Martin grades I and II
STRS is preferred single treatment for those <3 cm diameter if the vascular anatomy is unsuitable for surgery and in anatomically difficult locations
A combined approach with embolization (which may be staged) prior to surgery/STRS may be considered in II–V
Surgery alone is unsuitable for grades IV and V (require multidisciplinary discussion – intervention may carry greater risk than natural history)
Palliative embolization is beneficial when a reduced arterial inflow is required in view of venous outflow obstruction or true steal (controversial)

Embolic Agents

- Liquid embolic agents – penetrate deeply into the AVM achieving permanent embolization – n-butyl cyanoacrylate (NBCA) and Onyx
- Detachable coils – may be helpful adjunct to slow flow in fistulous components
- Particles generally ineffective – high rate of recanalization

NBCA/Histoacryl/"Glue"

- NBCA is a liquid monomer that undergoes a rapid exothermic polymerization catalyzed by nucleophiles found in blood and on the vascular endothelium, to form a solid adhesive.
- NBCA provokes an inflammatory response in the vessel wall and surrounding tissue, leading to vessel necrosis and fibrous ingrowth.
- Recanalization is very uncommon after an adequate embolization.
- The rate of polymerization is adjusted by diluting NBCA with lipiodol, which is also radiopaque, and allows visualization during injection.
- Higher concentrations of lipiodol will reduce the rate of polymerization and increase the viscosity of the embolic material. Dilute NBCA penetrates deeper into the nidus but with greater risk of escape into the venous system.
- Tantalum powder may be added to provide greater radiopacity and is essential where very high concentrations of glue (>90 %) are required.

Positive: NBCA may be preferred to Onyx in some fistulous AV shunts, perforating arteries, leptomeningeal collaterals, en passant feeders, and when the catheter position is away from the nidus.

Negative: NBCA is generally considered less predictable than Onyx, even in experienced hands.

Onyx

- Onyx is ethylene vinyl copolymer (EVOH) dissolved in dimethyl sulfoxide (DMSO) and made radiopaque with tantalum powder.
- A nonadhesive, cohesive liquid – on contact with blood, the DMSO solvent rapidly diffuses away causing precipitation and solidification of the polymer, a permanent spongy material (complete within 5 min).
- Solidification is slower than with NBCA, allowing prolonged controlled injections.
- Precipitation progresses from the outer surface inward, forming a skin with a liquid center that continues to flow (like lava) as the solidification continues.
- Rate of precipitation of copolymer is proportional to concentration of EVOH.

- Onyx 18 (6 % EVOH) is less viscous (viscosity 18 cP), will generally flow further from the catheter tip, and is often used for embolization of the plexiform nidus.
- Onyx 34 (8 % EVOH) is more viscous (viscosity 30 cP) and is generally used for higher flow fistulas.

Positive

- Better nidal penetration from a single pedicle.
- Multidirectional nidus penetration with retrograde filling of other feeders.
- Control angiography possible mid-injection to assess nidus and draining veins.
- More pliable/less inflammatory than NBCA – easier surgical manipulation.

Negative

- DMSO toxic effects include vasospasm, angionecrosis, arterial thrombosis, and vascular rupture. Toxicity directly related to the volume infused and endothelial contact time. To avoid angiotoxicity: *Use SLOW DMSO infusion rate not exceeding 0.25 ml/90 s.*
- Limited to DMSO-compatible microcatheters/syringes, etc.
- Tantalum may cause sparking with bipolar cautery during surgery.
- Artifact on CT but not MRI (hypointense on T1- and T2-weighted sequences).

Pre-procedure Medications

The author uses dexamethasone 12 mg intravenously at the beginning of each procedure to limit any inflammatory response that might be induced by the embolic agent.

The Procedure

Access

- Transfemoral catheterization of the parent vessel (internal carotid, vertebral, or occasionally external carotid artery) with a 6 F guide catheter with continuous heparinized saline flush.
- If the AVM is supplied by >2 vascular territories, e.g., posterior and middle cerebral, the author places guide catheters in both parent vessels (vertebral and ICA) to control the whole arterial territory during embolization.

Angiography and Assessing the Lesion

A minimum of four-vessel angiography should be repeated at the start of each session of embolization. External carotid artery injections should be considered wherever dural supply is possible – superficial lesion/previous intervention.

Provocative Testing

- Involves the selective injection of a short-acting anesthetic into the territory in question in the awake patient followed by neurological testing of that region – amobarbital and methohexital are injected into brain arteries and lignocaine to test cranial nerves in external carotid branches.
- Why? Absence of visible normal vessels on superselective angiography does not guarantee embolization without deficit.
- A negative result is not 100 % predictive – technique not in widespread usage.

Treatment Plan and Technique

- Ultimate goal is usually cure/obliteration – often requiring multimodality approach.
- Any residual early venous filling risks subsequent ICH.
- Partial treatment may increase hemorrhagic risk.
- Invasive treatment in unruptured AVMs may be more risky than natural history (a Randomized Trial of Treatment of Unruptured Brain AVMs (ARUBA) attempts to address this).
- Management requires a careful, experienced multidisciplinary approach.
- Treatment options include conservative management, surgery, stereotactic radiosurgery (STRS), and embolization in any combination.
- No randomized trials have compared treatment types with one another or with natural history.

Consider

Patient factors: presentation, age, comorbidity, occupation, and lifestyle
AVM factors: location, size, and angioarchitecture
Technical factors: local experience/expertise

Embolization Strategies

There must be a clear and realistic embolization strategy from the outset.

Cure

Series report embolization cure rates 15–73 % (mostly around 15–20 %). Cure rates probably better in nidal size <3 cm, supply by 3 or less arterial pedicles, fistulous rather than plexiform, no en passant feeders, superficial venous drainage, cortical location.

Partial Targeted to Suspected Bleeding Source

Aneurysm, venous ectasia, etc.

Pre-STRS Adjunct

- *Volume reduction*: (>70 % often achievable) aim < 4 cm (Table 4)
- *Target aneurysm(s)*: remain a risk for ICH until AVM obliterated
- *Target arteriovenous fistulae*: refractory to STRS

Presurgical Adjunct

Many small AVMs do not require preoperative embolization – exceptions are those grade I and II AVMs with deep arterial feeders that are difficult to access surgically and some grade III AVMs located either deep or involving eloquent cortex. For grade IV and V lesions, staged embolizations often performed at intervals of 3–4 weeks can improve surgical outcome. Advantages of presurgical embolization include targeting of difficult feeders, reducing operative blood loss and operative time, and decreasing nidal volume and blood flow. Staged embolization may reduce risk of normal pressure breakthrough bleeding (NPBB).

Palliation

To relieve symptoms secondary to shunting – arterial steal/venous hypertension, for example, headache, may be transiently improved by targeted treatment of dural feeders;

Table 4 Nodal diameter and treatment

Nidal diameter (cm)	Treatment
<4	No evidence embolization + STRS better than STRS alone
4–6	90 % can be reduced for STRS
>6	50 % can be reduced for STRS

Adapted from Gobin YP, Laurent A, Merienne L, et al. Treatment of brain arteriovenous malformations by embolization and radiosurgery. J Neurosurg. 1996;85:19–28
STRS stereotactic radiosurgery

neurological deficits and (medically intractable) seizure activity may improved by partial embolization.

Caution: Palliative embolization does not seem to improve the eventual outcome in incurable AVMs and may even worsen the subsequent clinical course. Partial treatment of AVMs may increase the risk of subsequent ICH.

Embolization Technique: Onyx

- Should only be undertaken by experienced practitioners – proctor supervision is strongly recommended in initial cases for inexperienced users.
- Biplane angiography is essential with patient under general anesthesia.
- Some operators advocate systemic heparinization – but no consensus.

Preparing to Inject

- Onyx must be shaken vigorously on the mixer for at least 20 min to fully suspend tantalum. Mixing must continue until just before injection to ensure optimal opacification.
- Select DMSO-compatible microcatheter, including UltraFlow, Marathon, Apollo, Echelon (all ev3-Covidien), and Sonic (Codman).
- Detachable tip microcatheters should be considered. The amount of reflux permitted with the detachable tip catheters (Apollo, ev3; Sonic, Balt) will vary according to the length of detachable tip chosen and relates to the microangiographic anatomy.
- All DMSO-compatible microcatheters usually require microguidewire navigation – e.g., SilverSpeed 10 (0.010 in.) and Mirage (0.008 in.) (both ev3-Covidien) and Traxcess (0.014 in. – good with Marathon) (MicroVention).
- The microcatheter is navigated distally in a supplying arterial pedicle (care to avoid perforation) under road map guidance.
- Microcatheter angiography is vital to assess:
  - Arterial anatomy *proximal* to catheter tip – identifying any branches that might be compromised by reflux of embolic agent.
  - Arterial anatomy *distal* to catheter tip – en passant feeders, distal territory supply, flow dynamics within the pedicle, aneurysms, etc.
  - Segment of *nidus* filling from this pedicle includes aneurysms/venous drainage.
  - *Transit* time from arterial to venous phase.
- Select angiographic projections that elongate the microcatheter and do not overlap with the nidus or draining vein. This allows better visualization of reflux/less risk of occluding proximal branches or catheter retention.
- Flush the microcatheter with saline to clear contrast.
- Check the dead space of the microcatheter from the manufacturer's literature and fill the dead space of the microcatheter and hub with that volume of DMSO drawn up in a compatible syringe (volumes – UltraFlow 0.22 ml; Marathon and Apollo 0.23 ml; Echelon 10 0.034 ml).

Onyx Injection

- Onyx drawn up in a DMSO-compatible syringe.
- An interface device can be used to reduce initial mixing of the DMSO/Onyx in the hub making emerging Onyx easier to see fluoroscopically.
- Inject Onyx under road map guidance slowly – 0.25 ml over 90 s to replace the DMSO in microcatheter and then at a similar rate.
- Initial aim is to form a dense plug at the catheter tip, promoting subsequent antegrade flow into the nidus.
- If reflux occurs, stop and wait 20–45 s before resuming injection (waits of longer than 2 min may result in Onyx solidification in the microcatheter).
- After each pause, reset the road map to visualize the "fresh" Onyx.
- The stop-start cycle often needs to be repeated several times (occasionally up to 35–40 min).
- Onyx will eventually go forward to penetrate the nidus.
- The amount of reflux permitted with the detachable tip catheters will vary according to the catheter. The length of detachable tip chosen depends upon angiographic anatomy.
- Precipitation of Onyx in one part of the nidus often redirects newly injected Onyx into other arterial territories; therefore, it can reach many arterial territories from one feeder.
- Long injections involving several milliliters of Onyx may take 40–60 min.
- Author recommends occluding no more than approximately 30 % of the volume of nidus per session – excessive embolization risks ICH.
- Perform control angiography at intervals through the guide catheter to assess nidus occlusion, status of draining veins, etc.
- Control blood pressure during the procedure, maintaining a systolic pressure around 100–110 mmHg. (Some premedicate with a beta blocker.)
- Indeed, if the passage of contrast through the nidus is high flow, it might help to reduce arterial blood pressure during the initial injection until flow is slowed.

Avoid

1. Stasis in the AVM – occluding the draining vein until the very end of entire embolization program when arterial inflow is minimal.
2. Excess reflux >2 cm marathon – risks catheter retention (see later). The amount of tolerated reflux will depend upon location of proximal branches, caliber and tortuosity feeders, and density of refluxed Onyx.
3. Forceful injection of Onyx – excess resistance may herald catheter rupture.

Removing the Microcatheter

- At the end of the injection, gently aspirate the microcatheter to disengage the tip from the Onyx cast and apply gentle traction on the microcatheter – aim for 2–3 cm of catheter stretch, hold for a few seconds, release, and repeat until the catheter is retrieved. Occasionally, this may take some minutes and in some cases may be impossible.

- Do not retrieve at all costs; leaving the catheter is simple and almost always the safest option – symptomatic complications are very rare – catheter endothelialized within a few weeks.

Managing a Retained Microcatheter

1. Cut retained microcatheter hub from its shaft (sterile scissors better than blade especially in braided microcatheters).
2. Open guide catheter hemostatic valve widely (accept back bleeding) so that the microcatheter moves freely within it.
3. Gently withdraw guide catheter over retained catheter while screening the microcatheter tip (to ensure the guide is not transmitting traction to the microcatheter tip).
4. Once guide catheter is fully removed, pull gently on microcatheter to straighten its course in the cerebral arteries and apply gentle traction.
5. Cut microcatheter shaft as close to hub of groin sheath as possible.
6. Push back end of microcatheter though sheathed into femoral artery using sheath introducer/vascular dilator (screen to confirm it is in artery and not retained in sheath).
7. Mention the retained microcatheter in procedural report (appearances on subsequent imaging can be alarming!).
8. Aspirin 75–250 mg/day for 3 months where possible.

Modification of Technique for NBCA/Histoacryl/"Glue"

- Mix NBCA with lipiodol to the appropriate concentration on a separate table to avoid contact with blood or other ionic agent that will cause premature polymerization.
- Use of color-coded syringes is recommended.
- At NBCA concentrations >90 %, it is recommended that tantalum powder is used to improve opacification of the NBCA/lipiodol mixture.
- Dilution should be chosen according to flow dynamics and angioarchitecture.
- NBCA can be injected through any microcatheter.
- Purge the microcatheter with 5 % dextrose before injecting NBCA.
- Inject under long angiographic digital subtraction angiography run.
- Injections usually take between 1 and 3 s, but occasionally longer injections are appropriate.
- When NBCA cast is achieved, gently aspirate microcatheter and briskly remove from the patient.
- Perform immediate guide catheter angiography to evaluate the nidus, draining veins, and complications.

Management of Associated Aneurysms

- If aneurysms are present on a feeding vessel, consider aneurysm occlusion first because embolization of the feeding pedicle will increase the perfusion pressure and may risk aneurysm rupture. Removal of the microcatheter after embolization also risks traction on the aneurysm.

Post-procedural Care

- *Hydration*: Keep the patient well hydrated – 2L N saline in 24 h.
- *Close monitoring*: Patient may be extubated immediately post-procedure; they optimally should be monitored in Neuro ITU or HDU for 24 h.
- *Blood pressure control*: Keep mildly hypotensive. General rule is to decrease post-procedural mean arterial pressure by 20 % to minimize NPBB (see later). Nicardipine and labetalol are the recommended antihypertensive agents.
- *Steroids*: Consider dexamethasone 4 mg qds for 3 days in larger AVMs, reducing over 1 week to reduce risk of perilesional edema/inflammatory response.
- *Antithrombotics*: Heparin may be considered for sluggish venous outflow which could otherwise lead to venous thrombosis. Some use aspirin and some anticoagulate for 3–6 months post-procedure. (The author does not anticoagulate but keeps the patients well hydrated for 24 h post-procedural with intravenous fluids.)
- After Onyx, the patient may notice a garlic-like taste, which may last for hours, and a characteristic odor, which may last for 1–2 days.

Complications

- The reported incidence of procedure-related complications (similar using either Onyx or NBCA) varies between 3 and 25 % and almost certainly reflects the complexity/grading of the AVM. Many deficits improve with time.
- Permanent deficit is around 8–10 % (*per patient*) (*probably higher with grade IV and V*).
- Procedure-related mortality is around 2–4 % (*per patient*) (*largely due to ICH*).

Hemorrhage (ICH)

Reported in 2–18 % using Onyx (similar using NBCA) and usually happens within hours to days post-procedure:

- Clinical picture ranges from asymptomatic to headaches to severe/life-threatening. Emergency craniotomy may be required – prompt surgical backup is essential.
- Many potential causes of post-procedural hemorrhage (Table 5).

Ischemia

Ischemia usually results from reflux of embolic material into normal arteries (despite heparinized flushes). Rarely due to microcatheter rupture – can result in proximal deposition of embolic material/closure of nontarget arteries.

Table 5 Potential causes of post-procedural hemorrhage

Cause	Prevention
Intranidal aneurysm rupture	Target intranidal aneurysm
Subtotal nidal occlusion with venous outflow obstruction/thrombosis	Avoid venous escape of embolic material
	Consider continuing to complete obliteration if venous outflow blocked
	Hemodilution/consider IV heparin
Substantial eradication of the AVM leading to venous stasis/thrombosis	Do not embolize more than 1/3 AVM volume at a time
	Hemodilution/consider IV heparin
Vessel perforation during navigation	Do not put microguidewire out through the catheter tip near to the nidus
Forceful microcatheter angiogram	Gentle microcatheter angiography/avoid injecting at bends
Tearing vessel on catheter retrieval	Use detachable tip microcatheter/be prepared to leave microcatheter in situ
Normal perfusion pressure breakthrough[a]	Suppress cerebral perfusion pressure by reducing arterial pressure
Vascular inflammation/necrosis secondary to embolic material	Steroids may help?

[a]NPPB tends to occur following excessive embolization in patients with high-flow, large AVMs with multiple large feeders and is considered due to a sudden increase in perfusion pressure in the surrounding normal brain parenchyma which has impaired autoregulation due to chronic hypoperfusion. Avoid by limiting embolization to 30 % of the nidus per session and actively managing periprocedural blood pressure

Microcatheter Retention

Reported in <3 % of embolizations with either Onyx or NBCA – attempts to retrieve catheter result in unacceptable deformity of cerebral arteries/hemodynamic changes/vasospasm:

- More common with:
  - Long injections
    - 2 cm reflux
  - Tortuous distal arterial loops
- Microcatheter retention may be less likely to occur with the newer detachable tip catheters (Apollo, Sonic).

Radiation Injury

Prolonged intranidal injections and multiple staged procedures especially those with Onyx are associated with high radiation doses which may cause transient hair loss or erythema. Try to alter the embolization projection for subsequent procedures/modify imaging parameters where possible.

Follow-Up

Angiographically "cured" lesions require catheter angiography at 3–6 months after final embolization. Where Onyx is the primary embolic agent, the author considers 1-year/ 5-year catheter angiography as late recurrences have been described.

Imaging follow-up after STRS/surgically treated lesions varies between centers.

At the author's center, early postoperative angiography is only performed if there are surgical concerns. Otherwise, a single angiogram is obtained at 3 months.

Following STRS, MRI/A is performed 2 years post-STRS. If the AVM appears obliterated, cerebral angiography is performed. If obliterated, stop. If not, the process is repeated at 3 and if necessary, 4 years. If not obliterated beyond 3 years, other treatment options are considered, according to the Sheffield protocol. In our experience, if the AVM has not substantially changed by 2 years, it is unlikely to obliterate by 4 years. Angiographic cure is considered obliteration of early venous drainage (some abnormal vessels usually persist).

Alternative Treatments

Stereotactic Radio Surgery (STRS) (Gamma Knife)

STRS generates vascular injury and induces subsequent thrombosis.

- Useful for small AVMs (<10 ml volume, <3 cm diameter) especially in critical areas of the brain where the surgical risk is high.
- May improve seizure control – 2/3 may be seizure-free.
- Major disadvantage of STRS is the persistent risk of ICH until the lesion obliterates (up to 4 years).
- Adverse effects – radiation necrosis, intracranial arterial stenoses, and cranial nerve injury – more likely with increasing dose/deep AVMs.
- Permanent treatment-related deficits reported in around 6–12 %.
- Transient deficits occur in an additional 6 %.
- Mortality rates are 4–9 %.
- The estimated cure at 2 years 80–88 % for AVMs <10 ml.
- Cure rate for larger AVMs considerably lower.
- Post-STRS, absence of residual angiographic AVM nidus or AV shunting may not equate with definite permanent AVM obliteration – suspect tiny residuum if enhancement is demonstrated on gadolinium-enhanced MRI.

Surgical Resection

This is usually an elective procedure, even following ICH. The surgical risks in expert hands are outlined in the Spetzler-Martin grading system (Tables 1 and 2) and reported in a review on AVMs (Baskaya et al. 2006). Angiographic cure rate is quoted as 94–100 %.

Key Points

> Management of cerebral AVMs requires a strategy agreed upon by an experienced neurovascular MDT.

> Treatment of unruptured AVMs is controversial and risk of treatment may outweigh natural history particularly for Spetzler-Martin grades IV and V.

> Indications for treatment include primarily ICH, but also progressive neurological deficit, intractable seizures, and other disabling symptoms.

> Annual bleeding risks vary from 0.9 to 34.4 % and depend upon presentation, location, and venous drainage.

> Embolization alone cures a small number of AVMs (usually <3 cm, small number of feeding pedicles, etc.) and is more often performed as a preoperative adjunct or to reduce the size to facilitate STRS. Palliative embolization is controversial.

> Liquid embolics are preferred. Onyx is more predictable and controllable than NBCA.

> In general, embolize less than 1/3 of the volume at each session to avoid NPPB and venous stasis/thrombosis.

> Complications as a result of embolization occur in up to 25 % of procedures resulting in on average 8–10 % permanent deficit per patient (probably higher in SM IV and V) and 2–4 % mortality (Fig. 1).

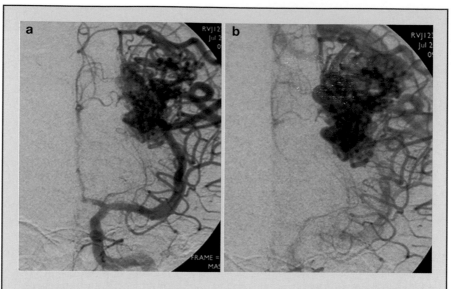

Fig. 1 These images demonstrate serial embolization of an unruptured left occipital AVM in a 17-year-old boy with seizures who wanted treatment. He had been discussed at a neurovascular MDT, and all risks had been thoroughly explained prior to starting the first embolization. The aim here was to reduce the size of the AVM to facilitate STRS and so achieve complete obliteration. The AVM is supplied by distal branches of the left MCA (**a–d**) and temporal branches of the left PCA (**e, f**). Enlarged collaterals from the distal PCA to MCA also supplied the AVM (**e, n**). Venous drainage is superficial. There were no venous stenoses. Intranidal aneurysms were seen in a medial component supplied by the left temporal branch of the PCA (**e**, *arrow*). A Marathon microcatheter (ev3-Covidien) was navigated down a distal left MCA feeder and a satisfactory position obtained very close to the nidus, without any normal branches arising in the vicinity (**g, h**). The position allowed 2 cm Onyx reflux without compromise of any arterial branches supplying normal brain. The best projection for Onyx injection was frontal (**g**). The path of the microcatheter distally is well demonstrated and is clear of the nidus allowing reflux to be readily visualized. During the first embolization, approximately 4 ml Onyx 18 was injected without complication obliterating a little under one-third of the AVM (**i**). Note the Onyx cast filling the nidus (**j**). It was intended to occlude the intranidal aneurysm component during the second session (*arrow*, **k**), but a satisfactory position from the temporal PCA feeder could not be achieved; there were too many normal vessels supplying normal brain in the vicinity (**l, m**). Superselective injections into the distal PCA-MCA collaterals also suggested that this route also was not amenable to safe, adequate embolization (**n**). A satisfactory position for the second embolization was therefore achieved by selective catheterization of another MCA feeder (**o, p**). Five milliliter Onyx 18 was injected again using the frontal projection as the optimal projection for assessing nidal embolization, Onyx reflux, etc. It is interesting to note that during this embolization, Onyx passed from the MCA component of the AVM into the temporal PCA component obliterating this component and the intranidal aneurysms (**q**). At the end of the second embolization, there was residual supply from PCA-MCA collaterals (**q**) and distal MCA feeders (**r**). Progressive AVM thrombosis was demonstrated in the interval between the second and third embolizations. Compare (**r**) with (**s**) and (**q**) with (**t**). After the third embolization, the patient was referred for STRS as the AVM had now been significantly reduced in size and the demonstrated intranidal aneurysms had been obliterated

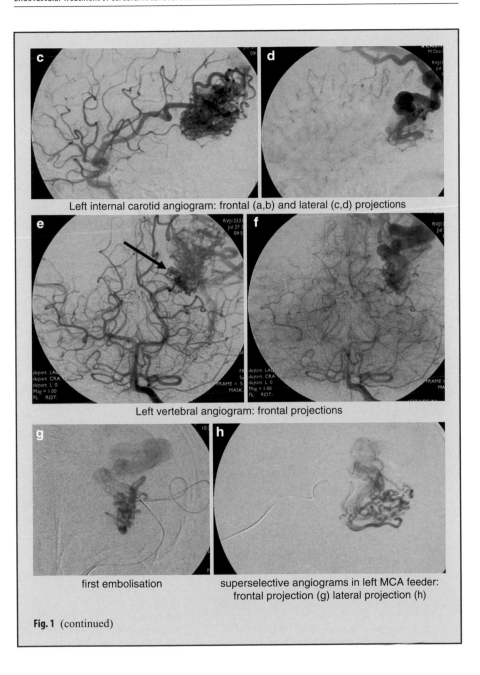

Left internal carotid angiogram: frontal (a,b) and lateral (c,d) projections

Left vertebral angiogram: frontal projections

first embolisation   superselective angiograms in left MCA feeder:
                              frontal projection (g) lateral projection (h)

Fig. 1 (continued)

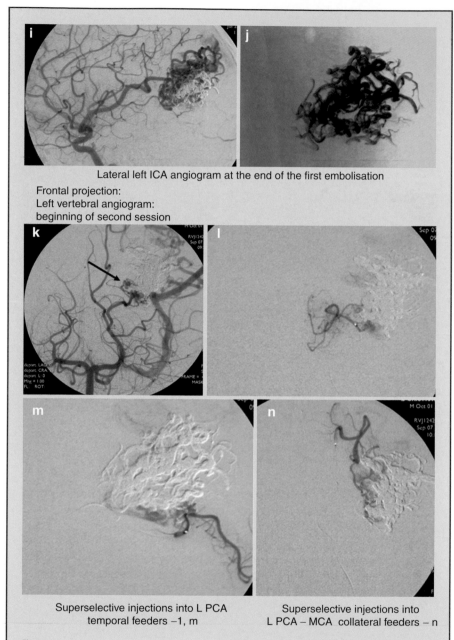

Lateral left ICA angiogram at the end of the first embolisation

Frontal projection:
Left vertebral angiogram:
beginning of second session

Superselective injections into L PCA
temporal feeders –1, m

Superselective injections into
L PCA – MCA collateral feeders – n

Fig. 1 (continued)

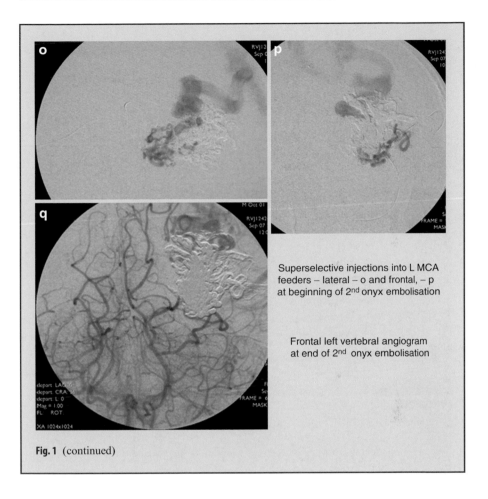

Superselective injections into L MCA
feeders – lateral – o and frontal, – p
at beginning of 2nd onyx embolisation

Frontal left vertebral angiogram
at end of 2nd onyx embolisation

Fig. 1 (continued)

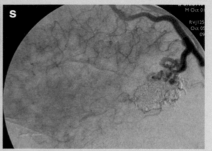

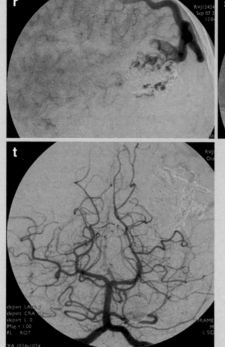

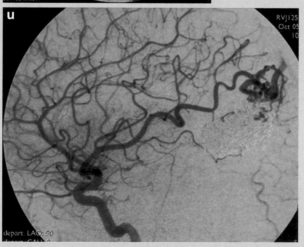

Lateral projection left ICA
angiogram - (r:)
at end of 2nd onyx embolisation

Lateral projection left ICA
angiogram - (s,) and frontal
projection left vertebral
angiogram - (t,)
before 3rd onvx embolisation

Lateral projection left ICA angiogram at end of
final (3rd) onyx embolisation. Suitability for
STRS has been achieved (u)

Fig. 1 (continued)

Suggested Reading

1. Baskaya MK, Jea A, Heros RC, Javahary R, Sultan A. Cerebral arteriovenous malformations. Clin Neurosurg. 2006;53:114–44.
2. Gobin YP, Laurent A, Merienne L, et al. Treatment of brain arteriovenous malformations by embolization and radiosurgery. J Neurosurg. 1996;85:19–28.
3. Kim LJ, Albuquerque FC, Spetzler RF, McDougall CG. Postembolization neurological deficits in cerebral arteriovenous malformations: stratification by arteriovenous malformation grade. Neurosurgery. 2006;59:53–9.
4. Liebman KM, Severson MA. Techniques and devices in neuroendovascular procedures. Neurosurg Clin N Am. 2009;20:315–40.
5. Liu L, Jiang C, He H, Li Y, Wu Z. Periprocedural bleeding complications of brain AVM embolization with onyx. Interv Neuroradiol. 2010;16:47–57.
6. Ross J, Al-Shahi Salman R. Interventions for treating brain arteriovenous malformations in adults (review). Cochrane Database Syst Rev. 2010;7:Art No:CD003436.
7. Stapf C, Mast H, Sciacca RR, et al. Predictors of haemorrhage in patients with untreated brain arteriovenous malformation. Neurology. 2006;66:1350–5.
8. Strake RM, Komotar RJ, Otten M, et al. Adjuvant embolization with N-butyl-cyanoacrylate in the treatment of cerebral arteriovenous malformations: outcomes, complications and predictors of neurological deficit. Stroke. 2009;40:2783–90.
9. Strozyk D, Nogueira RG, Lavine SD. Endovascular treatment of intracranial arteriovenous malformations. Neurosurg Clin N Am. 2009;20:399–418.

Intracranial Dural Arteriovenous Fistulas

Robert Lenthall

Abstract

The term dural arteriovenous fistula (DAVF) incorporates a wide variety of durally based vascular lesions occurring in different locations, at different ages with characteristics that vary between demographic groups. This chapter will review intracranial DAVF occurring in the adult population with key information summarized and highlighted.

Keywords

Intracranial dural arteriovenous fistulas • Vascular lesion • Demographics • Adults • Acquired lesion • Isolated • Trans-arterial venous embolization • Surgical resection • Disconnection of pial venous drainage • Radiosurgery • Multidisciplinary management • Pathogenesis • Cortical vein • Thrombophilia • Venous hypertension • Angiogenesis • Genetics • Vascular biology • Location

Introduction

The term dural arteriovenous fistula (DAVF) incorporates a wide variety of durally based vascular lesions occurring in different locations, at different ages with characteristics that vary between demographic groups. This chapter will review intracranial DAVF occurring in the adult population with key information summarized and highlighted.

R. Lenthall, MBBS, FRCR
Department of Diagnostic Imaging, Nottingham University Hospital NHS Trust, Nottingham, UK
e-mail: robert.lenthall@nuh.nhs.uk

K. Murphy, F. Robertson (eds.), *Interventional Neuroradiology,*
Techniques in Interventional Radiology,
DOI 10.1007/978-1-4471-4582-0_11, © Springer-Verlag London 2014

DAVFs Are Rare

- Incidence is unknown.
- Acquired lesions presenting later in life.
- Usually isolated.

Treatment Options

- Trans-arterial (TA) or transvenous (tv) embolization
- Surgical resection or disconnection of pial venous drainage
- Radiosurgery

Due to anatomical location and access, some DAVFs represent the most technically challenging vascular lesions in interventional practice. Management decisions should be multidisciplinary, tailored to individual patients, and based on optimal balance of risk/benefit.

Pathogenesis

- Thrombus within the dural sinus or cortical vein
- Higher incidence of thrombophilia in patients with DAVF than in the general population
- Venous hypertension
- Angiogenesis
- Possible influence of genetics and vascular biology

Location

- Transverse/sigmoid sinus in 50–63 %
- Cavernous sinus in 12–16 %
- Tentorium in 8–12 %
- Superior sagittal in 7–8 %
- Anterior cranial fossa in 4–6 %
- Others in <5 %

Diagnostic Evaluation

Clinical

History, particularly past medical history of prothrombotic tendency:

- History of venous or arterial thrombotic events (DVT, pulmonary embolus (PE), etc.) both for pathogenesis of the DAVF and for prophylaxis against possible admission-related extracranial thrombotic events
- History of trauma, temporal bone infection, or surgery

Neurological Features

- Ocular symptoms: chemosis, diplopia, and visual loss
- Vestibular symptoms: tinnitus and vertigo
- Focal neurology: focal deficit (related to venous congestion or hemorrhage)
- Global symptoms: headache, seizures, dementia, and myelopathy
- Asymptomatic incidental imaging finding

Laboratory

Clotting screen if there is a relevant history

Imaging

Dependent on clinical presentation
CT/CTA
MRI/DWI/MRA
Catheter angiography

Imaging Signs

Hemorrhage
Parenchymal edema
Venous infarction
Calcification
Dilated vessels
Leptomeningeal enhancement

Anatomy

See Lasjaunias.

Key Questions

Is there evidence of current or previous intracranial hemorrhage?
What is the dural supply to the DAVF?
Is the origin of the ophthalmic (retinal) artery conventional?
Are there any dangerous external carotid artery (ECA)/internal carotid artery (ICA) or ECA/vertebral artery (VA) anastomoses?
What is the venous drainage pathway of the DAVF?
What is the venous drainage pathway of the normal brain?

Classification of DAVF by Venous Drainage Pathway

Djindjian and Merland (1977)

I	Dural sinus (or meningeal vein)
II	Sinus drainage with reflux into cerebral veins
III	Cortical veins only
IV	Supra- or infratentorial venous lake

Cognard (1995)

I	Antegrade drainage via a dural sinus
IIa	Retrograde drainage into sinus only
IIb	Retrograde venous drainage into cortical veins only
IIa+b	Retrograde drainage into sinus and cortical veins
III	Direct drainage into cortical vein, no ectasia
IV	Direct drainage into cortical vein, plus ectasia
V	Direct drainage into spinal perimedullary veins

Borden (1995)

I	Antegrade dural sinus/meningeal vein flow (benign)
II	Antegrade dural sinus flow but retrograde cortical vein drainage (aggressive)
III	Direct retrograde cortical vein drainage (aggressive)

Lasjaunias (2008)

Ventral, dorsal and lateral epidural venous shunts

Natural History

- Spontaneous resolution.
- Transformation to a different grade 2 %.
- Increased inflow.
- Venous outflow restriction by stenosis or thrombosis.
- Estimated annualized risks of aggressive lesions.
- Annual mortality in 10 %.
- Hemorrhage in 8 %.
- Nonhemorrhagic neurological deficit in 7 %.
- Difference in annualized bleeding rate depending on hemorrhagic or nonhemorrhagic presentation.
- Presence of "high-risk" angiographic features may be less significant in asymptomatic patients.
- Annualized hemorrhage rate for CVR in patients without hemorrhage or nonhemorrhagic neurological deficit in 1.5 %.

Factors Associated with an Aggressive Clinical Course

- Cortical venous drainage
- Venous varicosities
- Venous stenosis
- Galenic drainage
- Location
- Previous intracerebral hemorrhage (ICH)

Factors Associated with DAVF Regression

- Reducing inflow (manual compression)
- Thrombosis of venous outflow
- Recanalization of venous outflow
- Hemorrhage
- Trauma (Natural history of lesions may differ)
- Angiography

Factors Associated with DAVF Progression

- Stenosis or thrombosis of venous outflow
- Increased arterial inflow
- Recruitment of new AV shunts
- Ineffective treatment

Treatment Options

- Conservative
- Curative
- Partial treatment

Conservative Management

- Natural history risk<treatment risk.
- Patients with "low risk" transverse/sigmoid sinus DAVF have a low annual hemorrhage risk and are encouraged to live with their symptoms if tolerable. Patients with indirect CCF, orbital drainage, and normal ocular pressures may also be managed conservatively, particularly if other comorbidities (diabetes or ischemic heart disease) alter their operative risks.
- Spontaneous resolution of DAVF is uncommon but well recognized.
- Measures that may improve prospect of spontaneous resolution:
    - Intermittent manual compression of supplying artery
    - Avoiding aspirin and other antiplatelet/anticoagulant agents

Interventional Neuroradiology

- Biplane angiographic facilities.
- Trans-arterial or transvenous approach or both, either as a single modality treatment or in combination with other treatments.
- Trans-arterial approach:
    - Proximal arterial occlusion is unlikely to be effective due to the rich collateral dural arterial blood supply.
- Use of liquid embolic agents in arterial territories that supply the dura is associated with the risk of cranial nerve injury and stroke (ECA/ICA and ECA/VA collaterals).

Onyx

- This liquid agent spreads through compartments of the DAVF and precipitates as the solvent diffuses out of the liquid.
- Distal access close to the fistula point.
- Microcatheter tip positioned in straight arterial segment (visualize reflux).
- Slow injection to establish Onyx plug.
- Intermittent injection to control direction of flow.
- Gradually fill supplying arteries, diseased sinus compartment, and proximal draining vein.
- Possible to reflux Onyx into other supplying arterial pedicles from a single injection.
- Check imaging to confirm progressive cast and exclude dangerous reflux.
- Possible to achieve cure in a single session.

Specific Risks

- Cranial nerve injury or stroke
- Catheter retention due to excessive proximal reflux (detachable tip catheter)
- Radiation injury from prolonged screening times
- DMSO toxicity

NBCA

- Requires significant user experience, meticulous preparation, and precise technique (microcatheter wedged or not)
- Potential uses dependent on user experience
- High flow AV shunts (+/− coils to slow the flow)
- Adjunctive treatment option
- Challenging material to use
- Relatively short time to polymerization
- Fragmentation of glue bolus by parallel arterial inflows
- Distal glue migration (outflow occlusion)
- Uncontrolled proximal reflux (particularly when wedged in small access vessels)
- Catheter adhesion/retention
- May require multiple procedures
- Declining clinical experience since the introduction of Onyx

PVA Particles

- Unlikely to be curative when used in isolation
- Adjunctive option to transiently reduce arterial inflow in combination with surgery or radiosurgery
- Palliative option for symptom control

Transvenous Approach

A transvenous approach may be used to:

- Sacrifice the involved section of dural sinus
- Occlude the involved venous compartment adjacent to or within a dural sinus
- Disconnect a "high-risk" venous drainage pathway and downgrade the shunt (possibly without occluding it)

Transvenous access to the venous circulation may be indirect from femoral, cubital, or jugular puncture or direct via surgical bur hole access, orbitotomy, or direct cavernous sinus puncture. Trans-arterial access to the venous compartment is also possible in the presence of larger AV shunts.

The diseased venous segment may be closed with coils (bare platinum, fibred, or hydrogel) or Onyx.

Transvenous treatment may be very effective. It is essential to identify the venous drainage of the adjacent brain before occluding major veins or dural sinuses.

Advantages

- Where arterial supply is challenging, via multiple small distal vessels.
- Access may be relatively simple.
- Single session treatment possible.
- Relatively low risk of ischemic stroke or cranial nerve injury.

Scenarios where a transvenous approach may not be possible:

- Isolated segment of dural sinus
- Distal access via tortuous small, stenosed, or ectatic veins

Scenarios where venous occlusion may be associated with an increased hemorrhage risk:

- Functioning draining pial vein occluded
- Venous outflow occlusion with persistent supply to ectatic shunt-related vessels

Technique-specific risks:

- Inadvertent occlusion of normal pial veins
- Isolation of sinus segments, potentially inducing cortical reflux and upgrading the lesion

Transvenous Treatments with a Sinus Preserving Strategy

Stenting

- Radial force
- Close shunts in dural sinus wall
- Restore antegrade venous drainage
- Can be technically challenging
- Relatively small case experience

Balloon and Onyx

- E.g. 8 mm RC copernic balloon (Balt) inflated in sings to preserve lumen during trans-arterial onyx injection

Transvenous Treatments with Sinus Recanalization

Crossing previously occluded segments of dural sinus/recanalizing a thrombosed sinus segment to gain access to treat the DAVF or simply to restore antegrade venous drainage and downgrade the shunt classification (Malek, Murphy)

Surgery

Surgical options include:

- Skeletonization of the diseased sinus
- Disconnection of the draining vein
- Combined treatments with other modalities

Sites where a surgical option should be considered:

- Anterior cranial fossa
- Tentorial DAVF
- Superior sagittal sinus

Stereotactic Radiosurgery

- May be effective as a primary option or as part of a staged approach.
- Series have reported higher occlusion rates in patients with indirect CCF and in patients treated with both embolization and radiosurgery.

Advantages

- Less invasive and low complication rates

Disadvantages

- Ongoing natural history risk during time to treatment effect, e.g., DAVF occlusion (may be several years).
- Presence of cortical venous reflux is a relative contraindication to primary treatment with radiosurgery.

Treatment Options Based on DAVF Location

- Lesion location
- Symptom pattern
- Risks
- Treatment options

Transverse/Sigmoid Sinus

- Antegrade venous drainage (benign pattern): manage conservatively unless intractable symptoms impair quality of life.
- Retrograde dural sinus drainage without CVR: manage conservatively with clinical follow-up (possibility of raised ICP in longer term).
- Retrograde dural sinus drainage with CVR: treat.

Cavernous Sinus

- Indirect CCF only.
- Conservative management may be an option.
- Prospect for spontaneous thrombosis.
- Indications to treat – progressive orbital/cerebral symptoms.
- TV approaches 1st line.

Tentorium

- Drain via cortical veins (Cognard III or IV).
- High risk of hemorrhage (Cognard 1995).
- Deep location.
- Difficult access.
- Require complete occlusion.
- Venous disconnection remote from the shunt caries significant hemorrhage risk.
- ?Surgery if no TA or TV access.
- ?SRS if elderly/major comorbidities.

Superior Sagittal

- Frequently associated with restricted or occluded antegrade dural sinus drainage.
- Frequently associated with CVR.
- Both TV and TA access may be challenging.
- Surgery:
    – SRS

Anterior Cranial Fossa

- Drains directly into cortical veins.
- Bleeding.
- Dementia.
- Conventional wisdom = surgical disconnection.
- Access to the dural supply from the anterior/posterior ethmoidal circulation via the ophthalmic artery is challenging but possible.

Cases

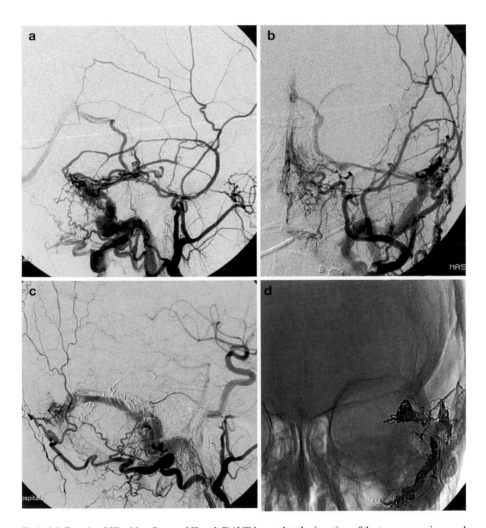

Fig.1 (**a**) Case 1a: 55F with a Cognard II a + b DAVF located at the junction of the transverse sinus and superior petrosal sinus (SPS). Middle meningeal artery (MMA) supply. Retrograde filling of the petrosal vein and basal vein of Rosenthal. (**b**) Case 1b: AP view of left ECA run. (**c**) Case 1c: lateral image following left MMA access and delivery of Onyx. The deep venous drainage via the left SPS and petrosal vein has been disconnected. (**d**) Case 1d: AP image after combined trans-arterial and transvenous sacrifice of the left transverse and sigmoid sinus resulting in complete occlusion of the DAVF

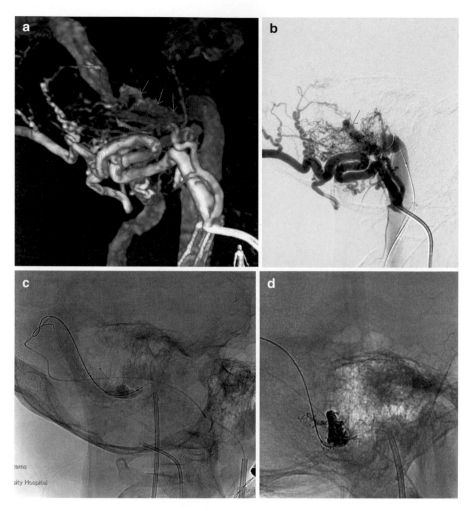

Fig. 2 (**a**) Case 2a: 74F with multiple DAVF. Sigmoid sinus compartment (*arrows*) with antegrade drainage causing severe pulsating bruit. (**b**) Case 2b: unable to access arterialized pouch (*arrow*) trans-arterially or via the right IJV. (**c**) Case 2c: Retrograde microcatheter access from the left IJV, via the torcula. Onyx compatible balloon delivered from the right IJV. Test inflation before Onyx injection. (**d**) Case 2d: Onyx cast occluding the arterialized pouch. Runs confirmed occlusion and the bruit resolved completely. The remaining asymptomatic DAVFs were not treated

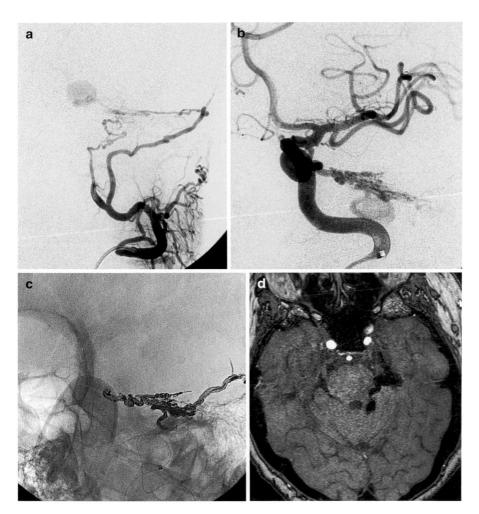

Fig. 3 (**a**) Case 3a: 65F with SAH. Left SPS DAVF supplied by the MMA and accessory meningeal artery, draining via the petrosal vein and deep venous system. (**b**) Case 3b: left ICA run showing filling of the DAVF from the meningo-hypophyseal trunk via the basal tentorial circulation. (**c**) Case 3c: Onyx cast following trans-arterial injections from both the MMA and the basal tentorial arteries. (**d**) Case 3d: Follow-up MRA showing the Onyx cast in the basal meningeal vessels and the draining petrosal and perimesencephalic vein

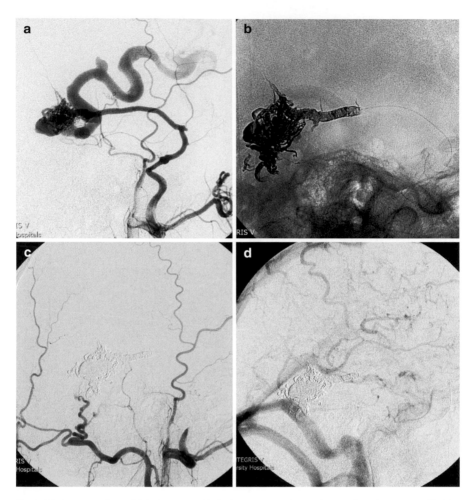

Fig. 4 (**a**) Case 4a: 48M with left temporal lobe hemorrhage from a Cognard IV DAVF supplied by the MMA draining into the vein of Labbe. (**b**) Case 4b: Onyx cast following trans-arterial treatment via the left MMA. (**c**) Case 4c: Left ECA run confirming occlusion of the DAVF. (**d**) Case 4d: Late venous phase of left ICA run showing pseudo-phlebitic appearance due to prolonged hemispheric venous hypertension associated with the DAVF

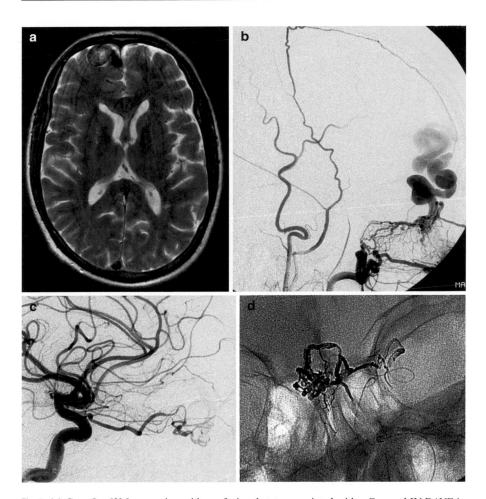

Fig. 5 (**a**) Case 5a: 63M presenting with confusional state associated with a Cognard IV DAVF in the anterior cranial fossa. Axial T2 image shows dilated/aneurysmal medial frontal veins. (**b**) Case 5b: Right ECA run showing filling of the DAVF via nasal septal vessels and the MMA. (**c**) Case 5c: Left ICA run showing filling of the DAVF from the anterior ethmoidal circulation arising from the left ophthalmic artery. (**d**) Case 5d: Midline PA view. A microcatheter was advanced into the distal left ophthalmic artery (beyond the retinal supply) and an Onyx cast was delivered to occlude the shunt. The patient recovered from his confusional state completely

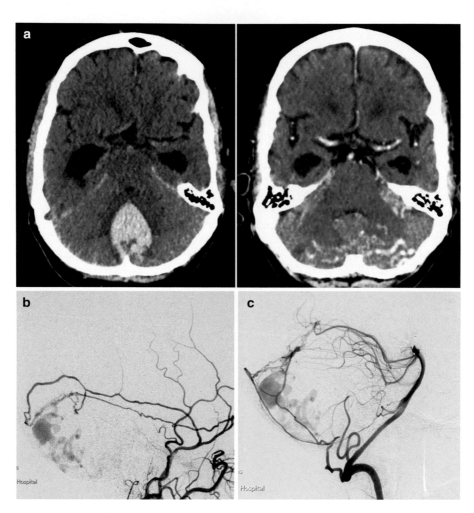

Fig. 6 (**a**) Case 6a: 75M presenting with vermian hemorrhage and hydrocephalus (*left*). Delayed CT (*right*) shows dilated cerebellar veins raising the possibility of DAVF. (**b**) Case 6b: MMA supply to a tentorial DAVF draining into aneurysmal vermian veins. (**c**) Case 6c: VA run showing posterior fossa dural supply to the tentorial DAVF draining into aneurysmal vermian veins. (**d**) Case 6d: Trans-arterial treatment with Onyx via the MMA. ECA run confirming complete occlusion of the DAVF. Note the artery of the free margin of the tentorium is no longer visualized

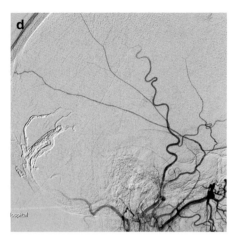

Fig. 6 (continued)

Key Points

> Intracranial DAVFs are relatively rare.
> Patients with intracranial DAVF should be referred to neuroscience centers and treated by experienced multidisciplinary teams.
> The spectrum of intracranial DAVFs ranges from simple shunts with benign clinical features to complex lesions that carry significant clinical risks.
> The presence of reflux into cerebral/pial veins is associated with increased clinical risk, particularly if patients present with intracranial hemorrhage.
> Many intracranial DAVF can be managed conservatively with clinical follow-up.
> Intracranial DAVF can be treated by neurointerventional techniques, surgery, radiosurgery, or combinations of these approaches.
> Neurointerventional techniques may involve trans-arterial, transvenous, percutaneous, or combined techniques using a variety of embolic materials.

Suggested Reading

1. Cognard C, Gobin YP, Pierot L, Bailly AL, Houdart E, Casasco A, Chiras J, Merland JJ. Cerebral dural arteriovenous fistulas: clinical and angiographic correlation with a revised classification of venous drainage. Radiology. 1995;194(3):671–80.
2. Cognard C, Houdart E, Casasco A, Gabrillargues J, Chiras J, Merland JJ. Long-term changes in intracranial dural arteriovenous fistulae leading to worsening in the type of venous drainage. Neuroradiology. 1997;39(1):59–66.

3. Cognard C, Januel AC, Silva Jr NA, Tall P. Endovascular treatment of intracranial dural arteriovenous fistulas with cortical venous drainage: new management using Onyx. AJNR Am J Neuroradiol. 2008;29(2):235–41.

4. Davies MA, Saleh J, Ter Brugge K, Willinsky R, Wallace MC. The natural history and management of intracranial dural arteriovenous fistulae. Part 1: benign lesions. Interv Neuroradiol. 1997a;3(4):295–302.

5. Davies MA, Ter Brugge K, Willinsky R, Wallace MC. The natural history and management of intracranial dural arteriovenous fistulae. Part 2: aggressive lesions. Interv Neuroradiol. 1997b;3(4):303–11.

6. Guedin P, Gaillard S, Boulin A, Condette-Auliac S, Bourdain F, Guieu S, Dupuy M, Rodesch G. Therapeutic management of intracranial dural arteriovenous shunts with leptomeningeal venous drainage: report of 53 consecutive patients with emphasis on transarterial embolization with acrylic glue. J Neurosurg. 2010;112(3):603–10.

7. Kim DJ, terBrugge K, Krings T, Willinsky R, Wallace C. Spontaneous angiographic conversion of intracranial dural arteriovenous shunt: long-term follow-up in nontreated patients. Stroke. 2010;41(7):1489–94.

8. Luciani A, Houdart E, Mounayer C, Saint Maurice JP, Merland JJ. Spontaneous closure of dural arteriovenous fistulas: report of three cases and review of the literature. AJNR Am J Neuroradiol. 2001;22(5):992–6.

9. Piske RL, Campos CM, Chaves JB, Abicalaf R, Dabus G, Batista LL, Baccin C, Lima SS. Dural sinus compartment in dural arteriovenous shunts: a new angioarchitectural feature allowing superselective transvenous dural sinus occlusion treatment. AJNR Am J Neuroradiol. 2005;26(7):1715–22.

10. Roy D, Raymond J. The role of transvenous embolization in the treatment of intracranial dural arteriovenous fistulas. Neurosurgery. 1997;40(6):1133–41, discussion 1141–4.

11. Söderman M, Pavic L, Edner G, Holmin S, Andersson T. Natural history of dural arteriovenous shunts. Stroke. 2008;39(6):1735–9.

12. Zipfel GJ, Shah MN, Refai D, Dacey Jr RG, Derdeyn CP. Cranial dural arteriovenous fistulas: modification of angiographic classification scales based on new natural history data. Neurosurg Focus. 2009;26(5):E14 (Review).

Endovascular Management of Direct Carotid-Cavernous Fistula

Marcus Bradley

Abstract

Direct carotid-cavernous fistula (CCF) is a direct connection between the internal carotid artery (ICA) and the cavernous sinus (CS) caused by a rent in wall of cavernous carotid artery. It is usually a rapid fistula with arterial pressure of the ICA transmitted to the CS and its venous drainage pathways. CCF is uncommon in the developed world.

Keywords

Direct carotid-cavernous fistula • Internal carotid artery • Cavernous sinus • Connection • Arterial pressure • Developed world • Prevalence • Traumatic • Spontaneous • Clinical presentation • Malignancy

Clinical Features

- Direct carotid-cavernous fistula (CCF) is a direct connection between the internal carotid artery (ICA) and the cavernous sinus (CS) caused by a rent in wall of cavernous carotid artery (Table 1).
- Usually rapid fistula with arterial pressure of ICA transmitted to the CS and its venous drainage pathways.
- Uncommon in developed world.

M. Bradley, BSc, MBBS, MRCP, FRCR
Department of Neuroradiology, Frencham Hospital, Bristol, UK
e-mail: marcus.bradley@nbt.nhs.uk

K. Murphy, F. Robertson (eds.), *Interventional Neuroradiology,*
Techniques in Interventional Radiology,
DOI 10.1007/978-1-4471-4582-0_12, © Springer-Verlag London 2014

Table 1 Venous connections of the cavernous sinus

Intercavernous sinuses
Inferior petrosal sinus
Superior petrosal sinus
Pterygoid plexus
Superior ophthalmic vein
Sphenoparietal sinus
Basilar venous plexus
Middle cerebral vein

Cause

Traumatic

- Majority follow severe head injury – e.g., skull base fracture or deep penetrating wound to the orbit (Fig. 1).
- Signs of direct CCF may be masked and diagnosis delayed due to patient being obtunded with facial injuries and swelling or sometimes delay in fistula opening (Fig. 1).

Spontaneous

- Usually acute presentation due to rupture of asymptomatic cavernous ICA aneurysm (Figs. 2 and 3)
- May be underlying vascular disorder (e.g., Ehlers-Danlos syndrome, fibromuscular dysplasia, ICA dissection)
- Rarely direct CCFs are slow flow with milder presenting features similar to a slow-flow indirect fistula (B, C, D) (Table 2)

Clinical Presentation

- Eye signs (most): proptosis, ophthalmoplegia, extraocular muscle congestion or cranial nerve palsy, chemosis, red eye, and visual loss (signs may be unilateral or bilateral)
- Headache and bruit

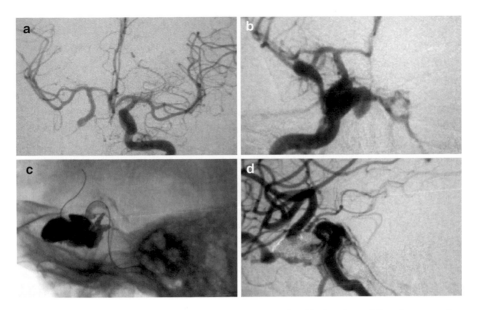

Fig. 1 Forty-three-year-old male with stabbing injury into left orbit showing a delayed presentation of a CCF and use of high-density Onyx® with balloon protection to partially treat the CCF which subsequently closed spontaneously. (**a**) Initial left ICA angiography shows retrograde flow in right ICA as the penetrating injury crossed the midline and occluded the right ICA; (**b**) Two weeks later a right CCF occurred as right ICA recanalized; (**c**) Microcatheter placed into CS via arterial route with ICA balloon protection; (**d**) Incomplete occlusion of CCF sufficient for later spontaneous occlusion

- Neurological deficit – cerebral hypoperfusion (arterial steal), intracranial hemorrhage, or edema (significant retrograde cortical veins causing venous hypertension)
- Variable venous anatomy – CS often compartmentalized, e.g., ophthalmic veins may be isolated from fistulous point within CS – may be no eye signs despite high-flow fistula with cortical venous reflux, intracranial hemorrhage, or cerebral edema possible with no prior overt signs of fistula

Natural History

- Usually progress to malignant lesion – often rapidly
- Spontaneous resolution very unusual

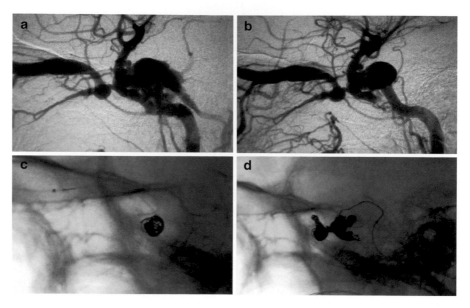

Fig. 2 Seventy-eight-year-old female with a CCF due to a ruptured cavernous ICA aneurysm demonstrating how angiography can change without treatment and how several routes of access to CS can be used to occlude a CCF. (**a**) Initial angiogram shows drainage of CS via SOV and IPS; (**b**) IPS drainage closed a few days later before treatment; (**c**) Initial transvenous coil embolization via SOV; (**d**) Further coil embolization of CS via arterial route through rent in ICA

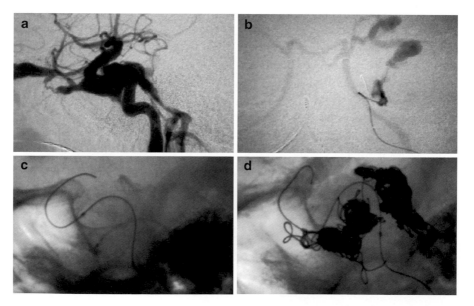

Fig. 3 Seventy-four-year-old female with a ruptured cavernous ICA aneurysm showing several venous routes into the CS, how balloon protection may be needed to retain coils, and that multiple treatments may be needed. (**a**) CS drainage via IPS and SOV; (**b**) Transvenous access to CS via IPS also showing SOV and facial veins; (**c**) Balloon protection of ICA during IPS coil embolization; (**d**) CCF reopened 3 days later and needed further coiling via IPS

Table 2 Barrow spontaneous carotid-cavernous fistula classification

Spontaneous carotid-cavernous fistulas are classified into the following groups
A. Direct high-flow shunt between ICA and cavernous sinus, often from ruptured cavernous ICA aneurysm
B. Indirect low-flow dural shunts between meningeal branches of the ICA and the cavernous sinus
C. Indirect low-flow dural shunts between meningeal branches of the ECA and the cavernous sinus
D. Indirect low-flow dural shunts between meningeal branches of both the ICA and ECA and the cavernous sinus
Another way to consider carotid-cavernous fistulas is by whether they are direct or indirect
Direct
Traumatic
Barrow Type A
Torn wall of cavernous carotid artery (collagen vascular disease)
Indirect
Barrow Types B–D

Barrow DL, Spector RH, Braun IF, et al. Classification and treatment of spontaneous carotid-cavernous fistulas. J Neurosurg. 1985;62:248–56

Diagnostic Evaluation

Clinical

- Clinical features of pulsatile proptosis, orbital congestion, ophthalmoplegia, visual loss, headache, raised intraocular pressures, and bruit strongly point to the diagnosis of a CCF (Table 3)
- Full ophthalmological assessment – baseline eye movements, visual acuity, fundi, and intraocular pressures
- Need high index of suspicion in head trauma patients

Laboratory

- Routine blood tests including renal function, electrolyte profile, blood count, and coagulation profile

Imaging

Cross-Sectional Imaging (Computed Tomography (CT)/Magnetic Resonance Imaging (MRI))

- Proptosis/orbital edema/engorged extraocular muscles
- Enlarged superior ophthalmic vein (SOV) (Fig. 4)

Table 3 Signs, symptoms, and radiological features of a direct carotid-cavernous fistula

Symptoms
Bulging eye
Double vision
Red eye
Headache
Visual loss
Facial numbness
Signs
Proptosis
Ophthalmoplegia
Chemosis
Reduced visual acuity
Dilated episcleral veins
Raised intraocular pressure
Cranial nerve palsy (CN 3–6)
Papilloedema
Radiological features on cross-sectional imaging
Proptosis
Orbital edema
Enlarged extraocular muscles
Dilated superior ophthalmic vein
Enlarged cavernous sinus

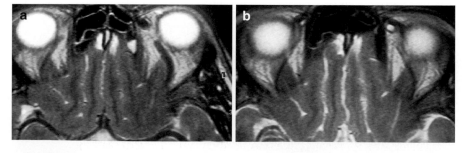

Fig. 4 MRI of 33-year-old female diabetic patient with an indirect CCF showing evidence of a CCF on cross-sectional imaging. (**a**) Dilatation of left SOV prior to treatment with a normal right SOV; (**b**) Left SOV appears normal after closure of CCF

Table 4 Angiographic assessment

Direct or indirect (dural)
High flow or slow flow
Cerebral perfusion
Retrograde filling of distal ICA to the fistula
Fistula point
Venous drainage
Routes of access to the cavernous sinus
Danger signs (varicosities, retrograde cortical venous filling)
Risk of carotid artery sacrifice

- Enlarged CS with engorgement of other venous connections to CS
- Decreased caliber of the supraclinoid ICA
- Rarely intracranial hemorrhage due to cortical venous reflux

CT or MR Angiography Shows Venous Anatomy

- May show cavernous sinus/draining veins filling early to indicate presence of a fistula

Catheter Angiography (Gold Standard)

- 6 vessel injections: bilateral internal and external carotid and vertebral arteries (Table 4)

Indications for Treatment

Direct CCFs often require urgent treatment and most will ultimately to progress to more aggressive lesions, often suddenly – urgent or semi-urgent treatment is usually recommended for all. Urgent indications and indications for treatment are listed in Tables 5 and 6, respectively.

Contraindications

All are *relative* in the absence of a viable non-endovascular treatment alternative

- Difficult access – including tortuous/occluded proximal arterial anatomy
- Severe vasculopathy – Ehlers-Danlos Type IV
- Iodinated contrast allergy
- Severe renal impairment

Table 5 Urgent indications

Malignant proptosis (cornea exposed)	Orbital venous congestion
Visual loss or impending visual loss	Raised intraocular pressure and/or papilloedema
Ophthalmoplegia	Extraocular muscle congestion/cranial nerve palsy
ICH/risk of ICH	Evidence of cortical venous hypertension/venous ectasia
Intractable severe headaches	Venous hypertension/orbital congestion
Distressing bruit[a]	Rapid shunt

[a]The resolution of bruit in untreated CCF is often an ominous sign indicating occlusion of the normal inferior petrosal drainage pathways of the sinus and redirection of arterialized venous drainage into ophthalmic/cortical veins

Table 6 Indications for treatment

Risk of intracranial hemorrhage
Visual loss or risk of visual loss
Raised intraocular pressure
Malignant proptosis
Intractable pain
Intractable tinnitus

Anatomy

Systematic angiographic assessment should consider each of the following:

Arteries

- Confirm direct versus indirect CCF – single ICA supply/no dural supply
- Distal arterial territory supply – may be no antegrade flow in the ICA distal to fistula – cerebral hypoperfusion
- Collateral arterial circulation – feasibility of ipsilateral carotid sacrifice
- Underlying cause – vasculopathy/ruptured aneurysm, etc.

Shunt

- Identify fistulous point – often difficult due to rapid flow, helped by:
- High acquisition frame-rate (6–7.5 frames per second)
- Manual compression of ipsilateral ICA during vertebral artery or contralateral ICA injection shows fistula point by retrograde flow
- Temporary balloon occlusion (Fig. 5)

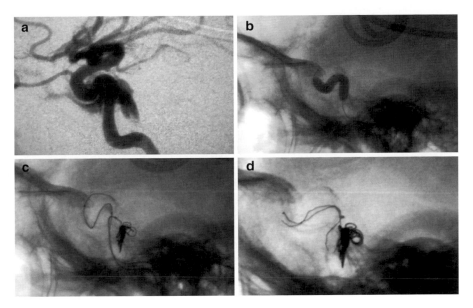

Fig. 5 Fifty-five-year-old female with a head injury and fixed dilated pupils which was due to a CCF (not brain death) showing how to identify the fistula point and also demonstrating that an ICA stent may be needed to retain coils. (**a**) Precise site of fistula difficult to identify; (**b**) Balloon inflated to identify fistula point in poster ascending cavernous ICA; (**c**) Coils placed in CS via arterial route proximal to balloon; (**d**) Stent subsequently placed in ICA to prevent coil prolapse

Veins

- Venous drainage pathways – cortical venous drainage and ectasia are risk factors for intracranial hemorrhage (ICH)
- Potential venous access routes to CS for endovascular treatment
- Compartmentalization of cavernous sinus

Treatment Strategies and Technique

Conservative Treatment

Rarely an option for direct CCFs – if suitable, regular ophthalmological follow-up for visual acuity and intraocular pressures is essential to ensure lesion is not progressing.

Noninvasive Treatments

Anecdotal treatments with simultaneous manual compression of the ipsilateral ICA and jugular vein

Invasive Treatments

Endovascular occlusion is now the first-line treatment (historically surgical techniques have been employed, some quite elaborate).

Endovascular Strategies

- The goal is to occlude fistula while preserving the ICA.
- Most effectively achieved by occluding the CS adjacent to the fistula.
- Preferred access to the CS is via arterial route.
- Access via the various venous routes, by direct puncture, or even surgically assisted access required in some cases – precise method determined by indication, venous anatomy, size of the fistula, and local expertise.
- Many described techniques including carotid sacrifice, detachable balloon occlusion, coil embolization, Onyx embolization, and stent repair.

Patient Preparation

- Patient consent should include standard information about risk of stroke, hemorrhage, and death similar to any neurointerventional procedure.
- Eventualities include failed/incomplete treatment – carotid artery sacrifice.
- Outcome – high success rate in resolving many of the eye signs, particularly proptosis and pain – lower levels of success in reversing cranial nerve palsy or visual loss.
- Best performed under general anesthetic, with full IV heparinization.
- Full cerebral angiography as described above – to assess arteries, fistula, and venous drainage patterns.
- Occlusion of the fistula can be achieved via a single common femoral artery using a 6-French guide catheter using a transarterial approach – a second femoral artery puncture may be required to evaluate other vessels, particularly if ICA sacrifice considered – for venous approaches, common femoral vein used alongside arterial access.

Detachable Balloon Occlusion (see Chap. 6)

- Historically commonly used endovascular device for occluding direct CCFs – directed via arterial route, through rent in the ICA and into the CS (Fig. 6) transfemoral guide catheter (7 F)/6 F Cook shuttle placed into ICA.
- Deflated Goldbal (Balt) balloon is mounted onto the balloon delivery microcatheter (see manufacturer's instructions).
- Balloon navigated into the fistulous segment and flow carries to venous side.
- Often minimal inflation facilitates flow-directed passage of balloon across fistula into CS.

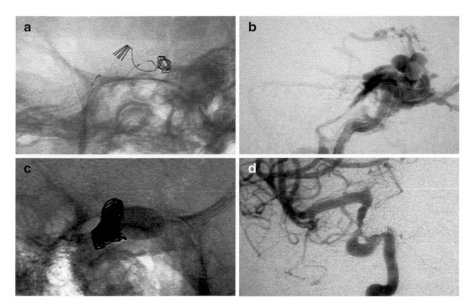

Fig. 6 Forty-five-year-old male with a head injury following a road traffic accident demonstrating the combined use of coils and detachable balloons and how ICA appears irregular after occlusion of the fistula. (**a**) Initial attempts at coiling CS via arterial route resulted in coil prolapse; (**b**) 6.2 A detachable balloon was retained successfully with CS to close CCF; (**c**) 6.3 CCF recurred after a few days as balloon migrated and coils used as adjunct to occlude the residual fistula sitting around the edge of the balloon; (**d**) 6.4 CCF closed with irregularity and stenosis in ICA at end of treatment

- Some place a shaped wire inside the balloon (care not to damage balloon).
- Once inside the CS, balloon inflated until the fistula is occluded.
- Balloon detached by gentle progressive traction on balloon delivery microcatheter.
- Additional balloons may be needed to achieve complete closure.

Advantages

- Rapid closure of fistula
- High success rates
- Inexpensive

Disadvantages

- Premature detachment and distal arterial embolization
- Imprecise inflation may increase size of the rent in ICA
- Balloon pressure effects – (worsening) cranial nerve palsies

- May deflate over subsequent weeks with fistula recurrence if CS has not fully thrombosed (inflation with polymers/silicone described to avoid this, but increases incidence of cranial nerve palsies and authors have no experience)
- Limited availability of detachable balloons

Detachable Coil Embolization with Arterial Remodeling Balloon Protection

- Preferred method at our institution is delivering detachable coils to the cavernous sinus via the arterial route (or combined arterial and venous approach) with protective remodeling balloon in ICA to prevent coil prolapse.
- Guide catheter (6-French or above) with a triple-port rotating haemostatic valve navigated into ICA.
- Microcatheter passed into CS via the arterial route.
- Second remodeling balloon microcatheter positioned in ICA across the rent to be inflated during coil placement (Fig. 2).
- Direct CCFs frequently have a large defect in the wall of the ICA and a protective remodeling balloon (i.e., Hyperform, Covidien/EV3) is often necessary to prevent coil prolapse.
- Coils placed into the CS until there is occlusion – often requires dense coil packing to achieve this.
- For ruptured cavernous aneurysms, coiling of the aneurysm alone may suffice.
- Fibred coils (i.e., Vortex, Stryker) or hydrogel-coated coils (HydroCoil, MicroVention) may facilitate thrombosis of the CS, although bare platinum is usually adequate.
- Advantages – coils widely available in all centers performing neurointerventional procedures, widespread expertise, effective and versatile, wide range of sizes, can also be inserted via the venous route (Figs. 2 and 3), and useful adjunct to balloons for residual fistula (Fig. 6).
- Disadvantages – more costly than detachable balloons; coil compaction may result in recurrence of fistula.

Venous Approaches

- CS is heavily loculated – access via a preferred venous route may not be sufficient to access the entire CS and occlude the fistula – most straightforward route into CS is via inferior petrosal sinus (IPS) (Fig. 3).
- Guide catheter placed in jugular bulb and microcatheter navigated beyond this point – even without drainage of the CS via the IPS (Fig. 2) it may be possible to access CS using knowledge of venous anatomy.
- May not be able to occlude entire CS and completely occlude the fistula, may be necessary to enter the CS via the SOV or via other route (Figs. 2 and 3), and may require direct puncture or surgical exploration.

Other Treatment Considerations

- If rent in ICA is large, a stent may be needed to prevent coil prolapse into the ICA (Fig. 5) – microcatheter jailed or placed through the interstices of the stent – dual anti-platelet therapy required in these circumstances.
- Covered stents have been used, but in practice they are usually very stiff and navigation through the carotid siphon is frequently not possible.
- Various other techniques have been used to occlude the CS including high-density Onyx (Fig. 1).
- Sacrifice of the ICA may be the only option – most patients tolerate occlusion of an ICA; some require surgical bypass procedure beforehand – ensure segment where fistula originates is also occluded; majority of fistulae occur in horizontal segment of the cavernous ICA or just proximal to this at the junction of the posterior ascending and horizontal segments; some occur just proximal to the ophthalmic artery origin; occluding just the petrous segment will not suffice as fistula will remain patent due to retrograde flow via circle of Willis.
- Ideal end point of treatment is complete closure of the fistula in single setting – further explorations of CS may be required often using alternative routes to the fistula (Figs. 2, 3, and 6).
- Marked reduction in flow of the fistula may be sufficient to remove high-risk features and allow final remnant to close spontaneously (Fig. 1; Fig. 3 in chapter "Type 1: Dural Arteriovenous Fistula").
- When complete occlusion of fistula is achieved, ICA often appears irregular and sometimes stenosed (Fig. 6).
- Follow-up guided by clinical progress – serial assessments of visual acuity and intra-ocular pressures are important – early angiography if any deterioration or lack of improvement; all cases require follow-up angiography to ensure fistula remains occluded; there may be complete resolution of the symptoms with clinically occult, but dangerous, cortical venous drainage or venous ectasia prompting further treatment due to the risk of intracranial hemorrhage.
- May be immediate improvement in clinical features following occlusion of fistula – severe cases can take several days to see progress – any deterioration of cranial nerve palsies may respond to steroids.

Key Points

> Direct CCFs infrequent and are often associated with severe head injury.
> Need urgent treatment to preserve vision and prevent cerebral complications.
> Various treatment approaches including transarterial, transvenous balloon, and/or coil occlusion or parent artery sacrifice.
> Symptomatic recovery can be delayed and/or incomplete.

Suggested Reading

1. Arat A, Cekirge S, Saatci I, Ozgen B. Transvenous injection of Onyx for casting of the cavernous sinus for the treatment of a carotid-cavernous fistula. Neuroradiology. 2004;46: 1012–5.

2. Archondakis E, Pero G, Valvassori L, Boccardi E, Scialfa G. Angiographic follow-up of traumatic carotid cavernous fistulas treated with endovascular stent graft placement. Am J Neuroradiol. 2007;28:342–7.

3. Barrow DL, Spector RH, Braun IF, Landman JA, Tindall SC, Tindall GT. Classification and treatment of spontaneous carotid-cavernous sinus fistulas. J Neurosurg. 1985;62:248–56.

4. Berlis A, Klisch J, Spetzger U, Faist M, Schumacher M. Carotid cavernous fistula: embolization via a bilateral superior ophthalmic vein approach. Am J Neuroradiol. 2002;23:1736–8.

5. Chun GFH, Tomsick TA. Transvenous embolization of a direct carotid cavernous fistula through the pterygoid plexus. Am J Neuroradiol. 2002;23:1156–9.

6. Debrun G, Lacour P, Vinuela F, Fox A, Drake CG, Caron JP. Treatment of 54 traumatic carotid-cavernous fistulas. J Neurosurg. 1981;55:678–92.

7. Goto K, Hieshima GB, Higashida RT, Halbach VV, Bentson JR, Mehringer CM, Pribram HF. Treatment of direct carotid-cavernous sinus fistulae. Various therapeutic approaches and results in 148 cases. Acta Radiol Suppl. 1986;369:576–9.

8. Gutpa AK, Purkayastha S, Krishnamoorthy T, Bodhey NK, Kapilamoorthy TR, Kesavadas C, Thomas B. Endovascular treatment of direct carotid cavernous fistulae: a pictorial review. Neuroradiology. 2006;48:831–9.

9. Higashida RT, Hieshima GB, Halbach VV, Bentson JR, Goto K. Closure of carotid-cavernous fistulae by external compression of the carotid artery and jugular vein. Acta Radiol Suppl. 1986;369:580–3.

10. Kobayashi N, Miyachi S, Negoro M, Suzuki O, Hattori K, Kojima T, Yoshida J. Endovascular treatment strategy for direct carotid-cavernous fistulas resulting from rupture of intracavernous carotid aneurysms. Am J Neuroradiol. 2003;24:1789–96.

11. Morón FE, Klucznik RP, Mawad ME, Strother CM. Endovascular treatment of high-flow carotid cavernous fistulas by stent-assisted coil placement. Am J Neuroradiol. 2005;26:1399–404.

12. Van Rooij WJ, Sluzewski M, Beute GN. Ruptured cavernous sinus aneurysms causing carotid cavernous fistula: incidence, clinical presentation, treatment, and outcome. Am J Neuroradiol. 2006;27:185–9.

13. Wang C, Xie X, You C, Zhang C, Cheng M, He M, Sun H, Mao B. Placement of covered stents for the treatment of direct carotid cavernous fistulas. Am J Neuroradiol. 2009;30:1342–6.

Part IV

Spinal Embolization

Type 1: Dural Arteriovenous Fistula

John S. Millar

Abstract

Spinal dural arteriovenous fistula with perimedullary venous drainage (SDAVF) is a treatable, potentially reversible form of myelopathy that continues to be overlooked by clinicians and radiologists. It is still unfortunately the case that the diagnosis may only come to light when the spinal images of a patient with failed back surgery are reviewed by a neuroradiologist. An understanding of spinal cord vascular anatomy and pathology of SDAVF is essential to the safe and effective treatment of the condition.

Keywords

Spinal dural arteriovenous fistula • Perimedullary venous drainage • Myelopathy • Back surgery • Spinal cord vascular anatomy • Pathology • Treatment • Anatomy • Embryology • Pathoanatomy • Classification

Introduction

Spinal dural arteriovenous fistula with perimedullary venous drainage (SDAVF) is a treatable, potentially reversible form of myelopathy that continues to be overlooked by clinicians and radiologists. It is still unfortunately the case that the diagnosis may only come to light when the spinal images of a patient with failed back surgery are reviewed by a neuroradiologist. An understanding of spinal cord vascular anatomy and pathology of SDAVF is essential to the safe and effective treatment of the condition.

J.S. Millar, MRCP, FRCR
Department of Neuroradiology, Wessex Neurological Center,
University Hospital Southamptom, Southampton, UK
e-mail: john.millar@suht.swest.nhs.uk

K. Murphy, F. Robertson (eds.), *Interventional Neuroradiology,*
Techniques in Interventional Radiology,
DOI 10.1007/978-1-4471-4582-0_13, © Springer-Verlag London 2014

Clinical Features

- SDAVF is a rare disease, but it is the commonest spinal vascular malformation (60–80 %) encountered in routine clinical practice.
- Patients are usually middle-aged men (5M:1F), presenting with a progressive myelopathy. Autonomic disturbance is common, particularly urinary symptoms and erectile dysfunction but are often dismissed as age related.
- Symptoms of pain in the back or legs and gait disturbance induced by exercise lead to the common misdiagnosis of lumbar canal stenosis in these patients. The clinical picture may mimic a polyneuropathy or polyradiculopathy. Upper motor neuron signs exclusively or in addition to lower motor signs should alert the clinician to the possibility of SDAVF.
- Untreated, symptoms usually progress over months or years, leading to wheelchair confinement and urinary incontinence. Progression may however be rapid, occurring over days, hours, or even minutes, and presumably the result of venous infarction in the cord.
- The clinical features and MRI appearances of venous hypertensive myelopathy are usually found in the lower thoracic region and lumbar expansion of the spinal cord. There are particular aspects of spinal cord venous anatomy that predispose to this.

Anatomy

Embryology and Normal Anatomy

- Radicular arteries arise bilaterally at each segmental level of the spine and give rise to a dural branch that accompanies the respective nerve root sheath.
- The radicular arterial contributions to the longitudinal arterial network of the spinal cord are arranged in a myelomeric fashion, i.e., the radiculomedullary (anterior spinal axis) and the radiculo-pial (posterior spinal axis) follow the course of their respective nerve root, through the same dural opening, to reach the spinal cord. This arrangement gives rise to the characteristic hairpin appearance of radicular arterial branches.
- The spinal cord drains in a centripetal fashion to the pial venous network, which in turn drains to anterior and posterior longitudinal collecting veins – the anterior and posterior spinal cord veins. The pial venous network and the longitudinal collecting veins together comprise the so-called perimedullary veins. The longitudinal spinal cord veins are usually single in the cervical and lumbar regions but are duplicated or triplicated in the thoracic region. They drain to the epidural venous plexus via emissary bridging veins (Fig. 1).
- Drainage in the thoracic region is bidirectional – cranial superiorly, caudal inferiorly. This, in combination with the convergent venous network described above, predisposes to venous stagnation in the thoracic region.
- The longitudinal veins of the spinal cord drain to the epidural venous plexus and paravertebral veins via emissary bridging veins that are not linked to a myelomere. Consequently, they follow a different course to the nerve root and radiculomedullary/pial artery, which may be horizontal, cranial, or caudal in direction (Fig. 2). It may drain through the same dural opening as an adjacent nerve root or it may be completely separate.

Fig. 1 Triplicated, thoracic longitudinal venous collecting system, also known as the perimedullary venous plexus. Convergence to the single longitudinal collectors of the cervical and lumbar regions and the possibility of bidirectional flow predisposes to stagnation in this region. Subsequent drainage through multiple emissary bridging veins to the epidural venous plexus and paravertebral veins (Image courtesy of Dr Norman McConachie, QMC Nottingham)

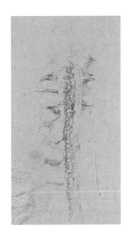

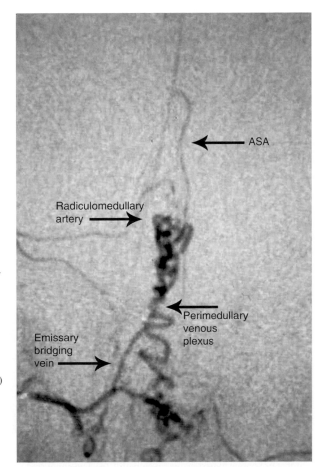

Fig. 2 Common radicular origin of a radiculomedullary artery and SDAVF illustrates that in contrast to segmental spinal arterial contribution, the direction and orientation of the intradural vein (draining the fistula retrogradely to the perimedullary venous plexus) do not follow the course of the spinal nerve root, i.e., segmental spinal arteries are linked to a myelomere, the emissary bridging veins are not

Pathoanatomy

- A SDAVF with perimedullary venous drainage drains retrogradely to an emissary bridging vein to reach the perimedullary veins surrounding the spinal cord, which results in congestion of normal spinal cord venous drainage and venous hypertensive myelopathy. The perimedullary venous congestion is usually posterior but may be anterior to the cord (Fig. 3a, b).
- Postmortem studies have suggested that radicular arteriovenous fistulas (AVFs) may actually be quite common. Even if these were to cause radicular symptoms, they would however be difficult to detect on MRI. Consequently, SDAVF are only likely to come to attention when they lead to venous hypertensive myelopathy.

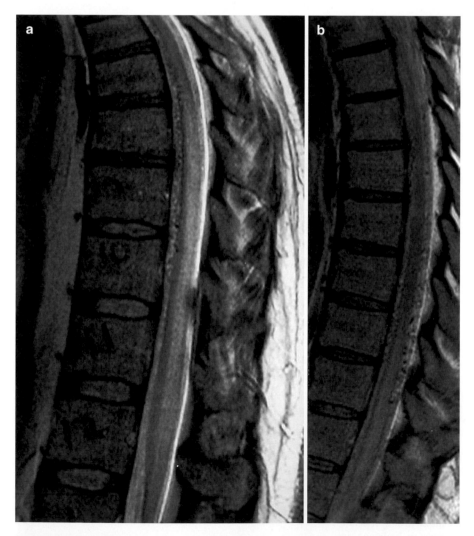

Fig. 3 T2W MRI of SDAVF exhibiting cord swelling and edema, which correlate with the clinical features of venous hypertensive myelopathy. (**a**) The congested veins of the perimedullary venous plexus are usually dorsal, (**b**) but may be predominantly or exclusively ventral

- SDAVF are low volume arteriovenous (AV) shunts. The postmortem observation of thrombosis or fibrosis resulting in narrowing of emissary bridging veins, presumed to occur with aging, has led to the proposition that SDAVFs become symptomatic as a result of outflow restriction of the normal spinal cord venous drainage.
- Multiple SDAVF may occur in up to 5 % of cases.

Classification

- There are a number of different classification systems of spinal vascular malformations (SVM), some of which group is spinal dural arteriovenous fistula with perimedullary venous drainage (SDAVF) together with AVMs and AVFs of the spinal cord (SCAVM), and emphasize differences from their cranial counterparts. SCAVM and SDAVF drain to the veins of the spinal cord, which results in an overlap in clinical presentation and features on noninvasive imaging, but there are important differences between the two conditions.
- SCAVM, by definition, arise from the pial arterial network of the spinal cord. They drain to the veins of the spinal cord.
- SDAVF arise from the dural branch of a radicular artery. Although the radicular artery supplying the SDAVF may also give rise to a radiculomedullary or radiculo-pial branch of the spinal cord, this is a random association and the two are not linked.
- AVF of the spinal meninges may be extradural or intradural. A variety of patterns of venous drainage incorporating extradural and/or intradural venous drainage are possible. In this respect, they are not so different from cranial dural AVF.
- A spinal AVF may be exclusively extradural in location and venous drainage, analogous to a type 1 (Borden/Cognard) cranial dural AVF (CDAVF). It may be extradural with extradural drainage and intradural reflux (cf. CDAVF type 2) (Fig. 4). The commonest clinical scenario, an SDAVF with exclusively intradural venous drainage, would therefore be analogous to a type 3 CDAVF (Fig. 5).
- It has been suggested that the pattern of venous drainage of dural arteriovenous shunts, both cranial and spinal, is related to the embryological derivation of the adjacent bone anatomy. Understanding the existence of three embryologically distinct epidural venous spaces, linked to the development of the overlying bone (membranous vs. cartilaginous) within the spinal and cranial cavities may explain certain commonly observed patterns of venous drainage of dural arteriovenous shunts at various cranial and spinal locations.

Diagnostic Evaluation

Magnetic Resonance Imaging (MRI) and Magnetic Resonance Angiography (MRA)

- Sagittal T2W MRI demonstrates swelling and edema, usually affecting the lower thoracic and lumbar expansion of the cord (Fig. 3) regardless of the site of the fistula. The reasons for this are explained above. It is usually accompanied by T2W signal void in prominent vessels over the cord, representing congestion in the perimedullary veins.

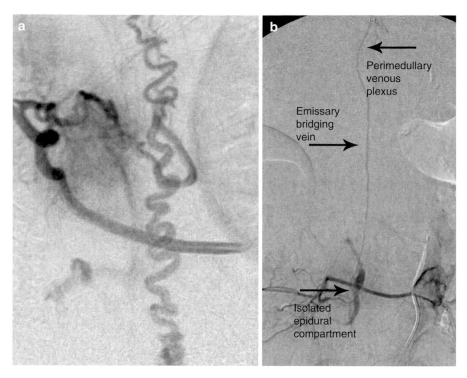

Fig. 4 Spinal AVF involving the epidural venous plexus associated with intradural reflux to the perimedullary venous plexus. These might therefore be considered analogous to type 2 cranial DAVF. (**a**) Illustrates a case with simultaneous epidural and intradural venous drainage. (**b**) Illustrates a fistula to an isolated compartment of the epidural venous plexus with secondary intradural reflux

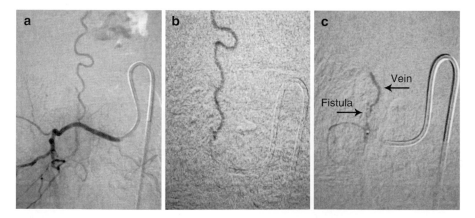

Fig. 5 (**a**) Selective and (**b**) superselective angiography of a SDAVF. (**c**) Curative embolization (25 % NBCA/lipiodol) achieved by occlusion of the fistula and the proximal 2 cm of the intradural (emissary bridging) vein

Fig. 6 Fat suppressed, contrast-enhanced T1W MRI illustrating characteristic features of SDAVF with venous congestion of the perimedullary venous plexus and intramedullary enhancement

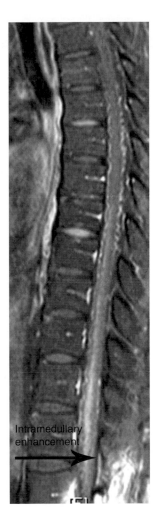

- The cervical cord may be affected, usually as a result of fistula of the skull base or craniovertebral junction.
- The imaging features of swelling and edema in the cord correlate with the clinical features of venous hypertensive myelopathy (Fig. 3). Contrast enhancement in the affected portion of the cord is commonly seen (Fig. 6).
- Prominent vessels may only be apparent on contrast-enhanced T1W MRI. Applying a fat saturation sequence will greatly enhance their conspicuity and increase the likelihood of detection (Fig. 6).
- Normal spinal cord vessels may be detected, usually over the lumbar expansion, spanning approximately 1–2 vertebral segments. In the appropriate clinical setting, vessels extending over 3 or more vertebral levels should raise the suspicion of SDAVF.

- Contrast-enhanced MRA is a useful means of localization of the site of the fistula, considerably reducing the dose of radiation, contrast, and time spent performing diagnostic spinal angiography.
- SDAVF may be present without prominent vessels detectable on MRI. Conversely, an SDAVF with prominent perimedullary veins but without clinical features of myelopathy or imaging findings of cord edema may also occur.

Cerebrospinal Angiography

- Full anticoagulation with heparin monitored by ACT after placement of a femoral sheath.
- Bilateral selective injection of all segmental arteries supplying the vertebral column, including cervicocerebral angiography, may be necessary to diagnose and localize the site of a spinal dural arteriovenous fistula. Contrast-enhanced MRA may help direct spinal angiography exactly or close to the level supplying the fistula.
- The commonest reason for failure to localize a SDAVF with typical MRI features is usually due to poor or incomplete angiographic technique. Meticulous record of the levels injected must be kept to avoid omission or repetition. The aim is to perform an unwedged ostial injection avoiding arterial dissection or high-pressure injection in a radiculomedullary feeder.
- Choice of catheter shape will depend on the size and tortuosity of the aorta. Cobra and coronary Judkins configurations are well suited to the selective catheterization of most intercostals and lumbar segmental arteries. Simmonds configurations are useful in the ectatic, tortuous aorta in addition to the pelvic vessels including the median sacral and internal iliac arteries. Flush aortography covering the abdomen and pelvis may be helpful.
- Stable ostial injections may be difficult to achieve and the catheter will usually have to be stabilized at the groin during the run to prevent the tip flipping into the aorta. A frame rate of 1 or 2/s is usually sufficient, and this may be spaced out to 1 every 2 s in the venous phase.
- Angiography under general anesthetic is preferred, particularly if embolization is contemplated. This allows for respiratory arrest and permits detailed, high-quality magnified runs to look for small radiculomedullary or radiculo-pial contributors at the same level as the fistula.
- It is insufficient to record a level as adequately assessed with only arterial phase imaging. Similarly, the temptation to tick off adjacent levels, opacified by aortic reflux from a single pedicle injection, must be avoided. Selective injection of these incompletely opacified levels may subsequently reveal the site of a fistula.
- The most reliable indicator of an adequately assessed level is demonstration of the respective hemivertebral blush. Multiple levels opacified from a single injection, e.g., supreme intercostal artery and adjacent arteries connected by intersegmental or retrocorporeal anastomoses, should be recorded as adequately assessed only if a hemivertebral blush is demonstrated at these levels.

- The angiographic run should continue well into the venous phase in order to detect very slow flow and, in particular, epidural AVF.
- In practice, SDAVF are most commonly encountered in the thoracolumbar region and consequently, spinal angiography will usually commence and concentrate in this region. If the fistula is not found in this region, then the search is extended to the pelvic vessels and subsequently the vessels supplying the craniocervical dura. This requires six-vessel cerebral angiography together with selective subclavian, costocervical, and thyrocervical injections centered on the cervical spine including the craniocervical junction and upper thoracic spine.
- Once the fistula is located, fast-frame rate angiography (2 fps or greater) is acquired at maximum magnification and with respiratory arrest and carefully scrutinized for a radiculomedullary or radiculo-pial contribution.
- A minimum of bilateral segmental injections at two levels above and below is performed to look for adjacent spinal cord contribution.
- A lateral run and large field of view AP imaging at the level of the fistula, encompassing the full cranial and caudal extent of the intradural veins, is acquired. If these do not correlate with the vessels depicted on MRI, then suspicion of a second fistula is raised.
- The main radiculomedullary contribution of the affected region should be identified, which is usually the artery of Adamkiewicz. If this is found before the level harboring the fistula, the venous phase should be included, which, if visible, is typically delayed >20 s in the presence of SDAVF due to venous congestion.
- Fast-frame rate angiography (2 fps or greater) at the level of the fistula, acquired at maximum magnification and with respiratory arrest, will help define the angioarchitecture of the fistula and the radiculodural branch supplying it. Oblique views may help, but it is often the case that overlapping muscular and osseous branches make it difficult to identify, and it is not until superselective angiography is performed that the branch to the fistula is finally revealed.
- Occasionally, a fistula may only be revealed by a superselective microcatheter injection, which may be indicated and directed by strongly positive MRI/MRA in spite of negative, selective spinal angiography.

Mimics

- Slightly prominent vessels over the cord associated with signal change may be seen with an arterial infarct. Inflammatory myelopathies may mimic SDAVF and prominent vessels supplying a vascular tumor, e.g., hemangioblastoma or ependymoma, may persist even after successful tumor resection.
- In all such cases, perimedullary veins, corresponding to the vessels depicted on MRI, will opacify after the capillary phase of the spinal cord angiogram (injection of the artery of Adamkiewicz). Depending on the pathology, the venous opacification may be early or normal and the capillary phase may be prominent, but there is no evidence of an arteriovenous shunt.

- In SDAVF, the spinal cord venogram is delayed (>20 s) or is undetectable. Veins demonstrated in the venous phase of the spinal cord angiogram (Adamkiewicz) will differ from the perimedullary veins that drain the fistula, as revealed by MRI or angiographic depiction by injection of the fistula.
- A type 1 (no dilatation of the spinal arterial axis) perimedullary AV fistula, an AVF of the conus medullaris or a micro SCAVM may mimic SDAVF clinically and radiologically. In this case, the AV shunt is supplied by the spinal arterial axis and demonstrated on the spinal cord (Adamkiewicz) angiogram (Fig. 7). Presenting in a similar age group to SDAVF, it may be the case that venous outflow restriction results in decompensation and presentation of these previously asymptomatic, congenital lesions.

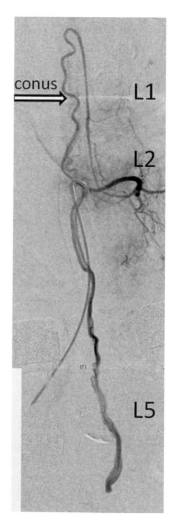

Fig. 7 An AV fistula of the filum terminale may mimic SDAVF clinically and on MRI. In this situation a slightly hypertrophied radiculomedullary artery (RMA-Adamkiewicz) arises from the L2 segmental artery and contributes to the ASA. Its continuation as the artery of the filum terminal supplies the fistula on the filum at the L5 level. It is imperative to recognize the difference between the typical hairpin of the RMA/ASA and not confuse this with the more tortuous course of an emissary bridging vein and perimedullary venous plexus of an SDAVF. The small cranial continuation of the ASA is just visible and helps distinguish these two entities

Indications for Embolization

- Embolization is successful in approximately 50 % of cases. Provided the correct level is identified, surgery is more likely to cure a SDAVF (98 %). Consequently, the indications for embolization are:
  − It may be performed under the same anesthetic, following diagnostic spinal angiography.
  − Embolization permits immediate post-procedural anticoagulation, whereas it is conventional to wait a period of time (24 h) following surgery to reduce the risk of postoperative hemorrhagic complications.
  − In a frail or elderly patient, from an anesthetic point of view, embolization may be preferable.
  − Local expertise and patient preference.

Contraindications for Embolization

Absolute

- Spinal cord supply (radiculomedullary or radiculo-pial) arising on the same segmental branch as the fistula.

Relative

- Spinal cord supply (radiculomedullary or radiculo-pial) arising on an adjacent or contralateral segmental branch as the fistula. Embolization from a proximal position could risk penetration through intersegmental/retrocorporeal collaterals. Achieving distal microcatheterization with the tip close to point of the fistula diminishes this risk.

Procedure

- Particulate embolization is likely to be only palliative and is not recommended. Embolization with liquid embolic agents is preferred.
- The procedure is performed under general anesthesia. A 6 F femoral arterial sheath is placed and full heparinization is commenced with ACT monitoring.
- A stable guide catheter position is essential for distal microcatheter placement, which is necessary for safe and effective embolization. A 4F diagnostic catheter (min 0.38″ lumen) is usually adequate, and in any case, the segmental or intercostal artery is often too small or may be stenotic at the origin to permit anything larger. A 6F guide catheter (e.g., renal curve) may be employed in some instances.

- On continuous heparinized saline flush and using a hydrophilic guidewire (0.35″), the tip of the 4F catheter is advanced along the segmental branch. It is easy to dissect the vessel at this stage, so great care must be taken to avoid this. Aortic tortuosity and the shape and orientation of the segmental branch, however, will ultimately determine the position that can be achieved with the guide catheter.
- The guide catheter will usually be in a wedged position at this stage and consequently runs for angiography, or road mapping must be performed very slowly and gently to avoid vessel rupture.
- The size and tortuosity of the dural branch will influence the choice of microcatheter. Both braided and flow-directed microcatheters may succeed in reaching the site of the fistula. The flow in SDAVF is never rapid enough to utilize the flow directing properties of the latter, but the greater suppleness is useful in negotiating tight loops. In both cases navigation with an appropriate microguidewire will be necessary. Once again, great care must be taken not to dissect the vessel during distal navigation.
- Magnified, superselective angiography with respiratory arrest should be performed prior to distal placement in the dural branch as a final check against a small spinal cord branch not identified on selective angiography. Identification at this stage would require termination of the procedure.
- The tip of the microcatheter is placed as close as possible to the point of the fistula and superselective angiography is performed. The closer the tip is to the vein, the higher the chance of success. Flow control or a wedged microcatheter tip position is preferable at this stage. Competitive in flow from intersegmental or retrocorporeal anastomoses resulting in marked dilution of contrast and poor opacification of the intradural vein may predict poor venous penetration of the liquid embolic and failure of the procedure.
- The aim is to occlude the fistula and the proximal 2 cm of the intradural vein using a liquid embolic agent, which may be NBCA/lipiodol or Onyx™. If venous penetration is not achieved, or is insufficient, the fistula is likely to persist. Fragmentation or pushing too much embolic material into the perimedullary veins risks venous infarction.
- The concentration and type of liquid embolic material employed will be a matter of experience and personal preference. Dilute glue (e.g., 20–25 % NBCA/lipiodol) or Onyx 18™ are typically used. Preparation of the microcatheter with 5 % dextrose (approx 3–5 ml) in the case of NBCA or DMSO (according to dead space of the microcatheter) in the case of Onyx™ is performed prior to injection of the embolic agent.
- Having identified the target for embolization, and with a blank road map to aid visibility, slow injection of the liquid embolic is performed until the required cast is achieved (Fig. 7). Great care should be taken to avoid excessive arterial reflux of the embolic material as this carries the risk of occluding a proximal spinal cord branch that might have been overlooked. Reflux may be more likely with Onyx than cyanoacrylate glue.
- If liquid embolization does not proceed for any of the reasons outlined above, it is useful to place a coil in the segmental branch for the purposes of subsequent surgical localization.

Post-procedure and Follow-Up

* Anticoagulation is continued following the procedure to reduce the risk of thrombosis in the dilated perimedullary veins, the patency of which is threatened once they are no longer arterialized.
* The length of time required for anticoagulation is unclear. There are reports of neurological deterioration more than a week following disconnection of SDAVF. Subcutaneous fractionated heparin (enoxaparin) has the advantage that it can be self-administered as an outpatient, and it may be prudent to continue this for up to a fortnight after the procedure.
* If the target 2 cm of intradural venous cast is achieved, T2W and contrast MRI is performed at 3 months. Spinal angiography is not usually required in the follow-up of an adequately embolized SDAVF so long as the MRI features resolve and the patient's symptoms stabilize or improve.
* A partially embolized SDAVF, with glue/Onyx cast within the fistula but little or no venous penetration, may proceed to complete thrombosis, but the probability is low. The decision to proceed to early surgery or wait a period of a few weeks and reassess with MRI will depend on the severity of symptoms and the views of the patient.
* Persistent T2W signal change without cord swelling or persistent enhancing vessels is not uncommon in a successfully treated fistula and probably represents gliosis/myelomalacia secondary to venous infraction.
* Spinal angiography to look for a residual or a second fistula would be indicated if there is persistent edema and swelling of the cord or persistent vessels on contrast-enhanced MRI.

Complications

* Femoral puncture complications: AV fistula, retroperitoneal hematoma, etc.
* Dissection or perforation of segmental artery or branch vessel. The latter may lead to local hematoma – retroperitoneal or retropleural – and, once identified would require reversal of anticoagulation and embolization of the branch.
* Spinal cord infarction leading to paralysis, loss of sensation, dysesthesia, pain, incontinence of bladder and bowel, and loss of sexual function. If immediate, this is most likely arterial and the result of inadvertent embolization of an unrecognized branch supplying the spinal cord. Delayed deterioration is presumed to be the result of a venous infarction due to thrombosis of dilated perimedullary veins.

Key Points

> Magnified, selective, and superselective angiography with respiratory arrest must be performed prior to embolization and carefully scrutinized to look for a small spinal cord branch arising from the same branch.
> The aim of embolization is to occlude the fistula and the proximal 2 cm of the intradural vein using a liquid embolic agent.
> Place the tip of the microcatheter as close as possible to the point of the fistula. The closer the tip is to the vein, the higher the chance of success.
> If the anatomy is unfavorable for stable distal microcatheterization, it is preferable to abandon the procedure in favor of surgery and place a coil in the segmental branch for subsequent localization.
> Anticoagulate following the procedure. Outpatient treatment with low-molecular weight heparin for up to 2 weeks following the procedure may be prudent.
> Follow-up at 3 months with T2W and contrast-enhanced MRI to ensure resolution of prominent vessels, cord swelling, and edema.

Suggested Reading

1. Geibprasert S, et al. Dural arteriovenous shunts: a new classification of craniospinal epidural venous anatomical bases and clinical correlations. Stroke. 2008;39:2783–94.
2. Jellema K, et al. Spinal dural arteriovenous fistulas: clinical features in 80 patients. J Neurol Neurosurg Psychiatry. 2003;74:1438–40.
3. Jellema K, et al. Spinal dural arteriovenous fistulas: a congestive myelopathy that initially mimics a peripheral nerve disorder. Brain. 2006;129:3150–64.
4. Pierre L, Alejandro B, ter Brugge KG, editors. Surgical neuroangiography, vol. 1. Hamburg: Springer; 2011.
5. Saraf-Lavi E, et al. Detection of spinal dural arteriovenous fistulae with MR imaging and contrast-enhanced MR angiography: sensitivity, specificity, and prediction of vertebral level. AJNR Am J Neuroradiol. 2002;23:858–67.

Part V

Intra-arterial Therapy in Acute Ischaemic Stroke

Acute Stroke: Mechanical Thrombectomy

Tommy Andersson

Abstract

Acute stroke is today the third commonest cause for death in the industrialized world responsible for 10–12 % of overall mortality. It is the single most common cause of permanent disability in adults. Approximately 15 % of acute stroke patients suffer from an intracranial bleed, while the remaining 85 % have an ischemic stroke. Approximately one in four patients die within 1 year of having an initial ischemic stroke and with 15–30 % left permanently disabled.

Keywords

Acute stroke • Mortality • Permanent disability • Intracranial bleeding • Ischemic stroke • Intra-arterial therapy • Recanalization • Reperfusion • Neuroprotection • Supratentorial • Infarction

Introduction

- Acute stroke is today the third leading cause for death in the industrialized world responsible for 10–12 % of the overall mortality. It is also the single most common cause for permanent disability in adults. Only approximately 15 % of acute stroke patients suffer from an intracranial bleed; whereas, the remaining 85 % has an ischemic stroke.

T. Andersson, MD, PhD
Department of Neuroradiology and Clinical Neuroscience,
Karolinska University Hospital and Karolinska Institute, Stockholm, Sweden
e-mail: tommy.andersson@karolinska.se

K. Murphy, F. Robertson (eds.), *Interventional Neuroradiology,*
Techniques in Interventional Radiology,
DOI 10.1007/978-1-4471-4582-0_14, © Springer-Verlag London 2014

- Approximately one out of four patients die within 1 year after having an initial ischemic stroke and 30–50 % of the survivors of stroke do not regain functional independence leaving 15–30 % permanently disabled.
- Neuroprotection has never worked in human clinical trials in spite of promising animal data. Focus therefore shifted towards recanalization strategies enabling reperfusion of the ischemic parts of the brain.
- Fast recanalization is crucial as a large vessel, supratentorial acute ischemic stroke leads to an estimated loss per minute of 1.9 million neurons, 14 billion synapses, and 12 km myelinated nerve fibers.

Evolution of Recanalization Strategies

- Reperfusion of the ischemic brain by recanalization of the occluded artery is the most effective therapy in acute stroke. By restoring blood flow to the threatened tissue before progress to infarction, reperfusion therapies reduce the final infarct size and enable better clinical outcome.
- Recanalization in acute ischemic stroke can be achieved by intravenous thrombolysis, intra-arterial thrombolysis, and mechanical thrombectomy.

Intravenous Thrombolysis with Alteplase

- Intravenous (IV) thrombolysis with alteplase (recombinant tissue plasminogen activator – rt-PA) has proven efficient and safe in several randomized control trials (RCT), initially within 3 h of stroke onset but more recently within 4.5 h.
- Indications for IV alteplase are ischemic stroke within 4.5 h with no bleeding on computed tomography (CT) and <1/3 of the middle cerebral artery (MCA) territory infarcted.
- There are several exclusion criteria beside time and CT appearance, e.g., unclear time of symptom onset, severe stroke, i.e., National Institute of Health Stroke Scale (NIHSS) score >25, history of intracerebral hematoma, recent ischemic stroke, gastrointestinal bleeding, or major head trauma.
- Despite proven clinical efficacy, >50 % of IV-treated stroke patients remain disabled or die. Unfavorable outcome is more likely in patients with severe neurological deficits, higher age, and persistent arterial occlusion.
- Partial or complete recanalization by IV alteplase is especially unlikely in proximal large vessel occlusions, only achieved in 10 % of occluded internal carotid arteries (ICA) and in 25 % of occluded proximal MCAs.
- The numbers needed to treat for death and dependence are high and increases with time: <90 min=4, 90 min–3 h=7 and 3–4.5 h=14.
- Intravenous alteplase in the posterior circulation for basilar artery occlusion (BAO) has bad outcome with high mortality and low percentage of independent patients at 90 days follow-up.

Intra-arterial Thrombolysis

- Intra-arterial (IA) thrombolysis can be performed with alteplase (rt-PA), recombinant prourokinase, urokinase, or streptokinase. The efficacy in MCA occlusions with the infusion starting within 6 h of symptom onset has been studied in three randomized trials (PROACT I, PROACT II and MELT).
- Treated patients in PROACT II had higher recanalization rates and better 90 days outcomes than the control group, but a higher occurrence of symptomatic intracranial hemorrhage (ICH).
- The combination of IV and IA thrombolysis was investigated in the IMS and IMS II studies. In these studies, the patients received IV alteplase followed by the same drug additionally administered IA. Treated patients in both studies had significantly better outcome than placebo-treated patients in a large rt-PA stroke trial (NINDS) and a similar rate of symptomatic ICH compared with actively treated patients from that same trial.
- IA thrombolysis is usually performed so that the tip of a microcatheter (MC) is positioned close to the proximal end of the clot where after the drug is infused. Cautious mechanical manipulation with MC and microguidewire (MGW) as well as repetitive flushing with saline through the MC may augment the lytic effect.
- The main disadvantages are that the procedure takes time, does not always lead to recanalization, and that IA administration of large doses of alteplase may increase the risk for hemorrhagic transformation.
- For BAO, IA thrombolysis has similar bad outcome figures as IV thrombolysis, i.e., high mortality rate and very few independent patients at 90 days follow-up.

Mechanical Thrombectomy

- Potential patients for mechanical thrombectomy are firstly those that are excluded from intravenous treatment, e.g., presenting >4.5 h after ictus or with an unclear time of onset. Secondly, patients in which the intravenous infusion *does not* or *may not* work.
- Patients unlikely to respond to IV treatment are those with NIHSS >12, which is indicative of a large vessel occlusion, especially if the length of the thrombus is >8 mm.
- A thrombus aspiration technique was early on studied in the Penumbra Pivotal Stroke Trial and in the Penumbra Post Trial. Both studies revealed a very high rate of recanalization but the percentage of independent patients at 90 days were relatively low in the Pivotal trial with a high mortality rate comparable to that in Multi-MERCI. The 90 days outcome was markedly improved in the POST trial with also a decreased mortality.
- Mechanical thrombectomy utilizing and old, today obsolete technique ("MERCI retriever"), was initially studied in two prospective, non-randomized trials: the MERCI trial and the Multi-MERCI trial. Both these studies included patients with large vessel occlusion in which mechanical thrombectomy could be started within 8 h after symptom onset. MERCI trial patients were rt-PA ineligible; whereas, the Multi-MERCI trial also included patients that had been unsuccessfully treated with IV rt-PA. These trials showed higher recanalization rates compared with control patients from the PROACT II study, a reasonably good percentage of independent patients at 90 days follow-up, but a higher mortality rate as compared to actively treated patients in PROACT II.

- Modern thrombectomy technique utilizing so-called stent retrievers was proven to be superior to the MERCI retriever in two multicenter, randomized, controlled trials (SWIFT and TREVO 2).
- Old techniques, the MERCI retriever and IA thrombolysis (partly with augmented IA sono-thrombolysis with the EKOS ultrasound/micro-infusion system), were also used in three recently published RCTs in which there was no proven benefit from adding endovascular therapy to IV thrombolysis (IMS 3, SYNTHESIS, MR RESCUE). In addition to using today's obsolete techniques, patients were in the first two studies included without a proven large vessel occlusion. Because of these and several other shortcomings, the three published RCTs do not reflect modern endovascular therapy as it is practiced today. There are also other ongoing national prospective, randomized studies for mechanical thrombectomy with the purpose to study safety and effectiveness, e.g., THRACE in France and MR CLEAN in the Netherlands.
- Up to date endovascular therapy for acute stroke patients, i.e., thrombectomy with stent retrievers, has been studied in recent large multicenter retrospective (Dávalos) as well as prospective (STAR) studies revealing high percentages of recanalization (≥ 84 %) and independent functional outcome (≥ 55 %).
- Extracted data from the MERCI and Multi-MERCI trials as well as several small single center retrospective studies have shown excellent recanalization rates and 90 days outcome after mechanical thrombectomy for BAO. In comparison with the generally bad revascularization rates and 90 days outcome after IV as well as IA thrombolysis, a strategy with mechanical thrombectomy as a first-line treatment for BAO may be considered.

Organization of a Neurointerventional Stroke Center

- As time to treatment is crucial, a good organization is important in order to get the patients *to hospital* fast and to streamline the chain of events *in hospital*. To help with this, it is important to develop a flow chart/protocol that is adapted to local conditions (Fig. 1). It may guide less experienced physicians as well as clarify the structure making it easier to identify weak links in the management of acute stroke patients. All patient transportations should be done with top priority.
- The neurointerventional stroke center should be operational 24/7, the neurointerventionalists and stroke neurologists easily contacted through special phone numbers, preferably having access to telemedicine.
- Referring hospitals should, if possible, be trained to perform CT and CT angiography (CTA) before contacting the stroke center. Patients eligible for IV thrombolysis transferred from referring hospitals may receive the infusion in full concentration (0.9 mg/kg rt-PA with a maximum dose of 90 mg) as bridging therapy and transported acutely with the drip ongoing. It is important that the IV infusion do not delay the transportation to the neurointerventional stroke center, instead it can be administered while the transfer is being organized. It is almost always quite sufficient to have well-trained paramedics looking after the patient during the transportation.

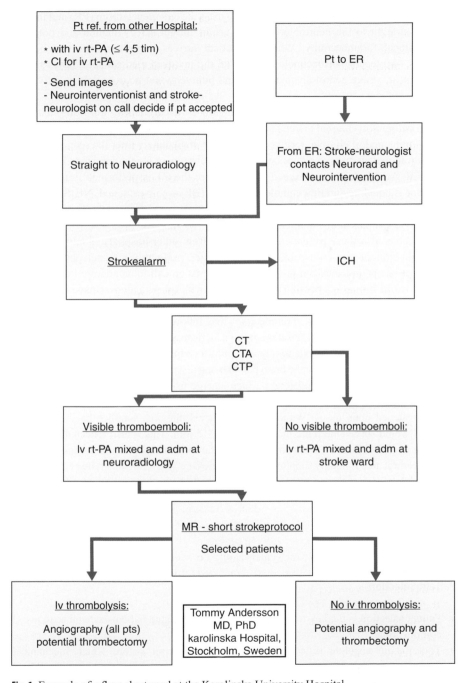

Fig. 1 Example of a flow chart used at the Karolinska University Hospital

- The transferred patients should if possible bypass the emergency room (ER) and instead come straight to the neurointerventional center for further evaluation and potential mechanical thrombectomy. When the patient arrives, representatives (physicians, nurses, and technicians/technologists) for all the involved medical specialities should be present: stroke neurology, diagnostic and interventional neuroradiology as well as anesthesiology.
- Patients that are brought directly to the emergency department of a hospital that perform neurointerventional therapy should have the CT performed at the earliest possible time point, and, if eligible, receive IV treatment immediately after the scan at the neuroradiology department and not be transported elsewhere for the infusion. The time at the ER should ideally not exceed 10 min before the CT is performed; brief medical history is noted, respiration and blood pressure (BP) are investigated, NIHSS is calculated, and potential contraindications for IV treatment are determined. There is no need for blood samples at this moment.
- If possible, also these patients not transferred from other hospitals should instead be brought straight to the neurointerventional center, preferably after telephone contact between the paramedics and the stroke neurologist on call in an attempt to rule out as many stroke mimics as possible. Such patients with other diagnoses have to be transported secondarily to the ER.
- Medical management before thrombectomy may follow standard guidelines as published by the European Stroke Organisation or the American Stroke Association. It is important not to lower a high BP too extensively, accepting a systolic pressure ≤ 200, as this pressure may be necessary to perfuse the brain parenchyma distal to the clot through so-called pial collaterals (Fig. 2). Such collaterals, which emerge from other vascular territories, vary significantly between different individuals and are the structural basis behind the survival of threatened brain tissue. Without pial collaterals, the area supplied by the occluded artery would survive no more than perhaps 10–15 min. This is also reflected in the fact that it is very difficult to avoid basal ganglia infarction in an MCA main stem occlusion. This central area is mainly supplied by end arteries, i.e., the lenticulostriate perforators, in such case obstructed by an MCA (M1) thromboemboli. As there is limited collateral supply to the basal ganglia, an ischemic infarct will consequently develop rapidly.

Patient Selection

- Patient selection is the key to good outcome for the treated patients as well as to avoid complications.
- There is no absolute time limit from symptom onset before which mechanical thrombectomy has to be started. Instead, patient selection should be based on clinical and radiological criteria. In practice, it is however rare that a patient may benefit from thrombectomy if the procedure starts >8 h after onset in the anterior circulation and >24 h after onset in the posterior circulation.

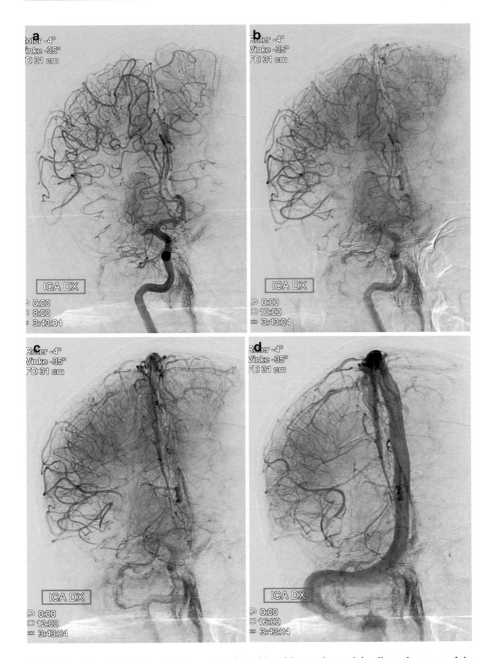

Fig. 2 Thromboembolic M1 occlusion on the right side with prominent pial collaterals retrogradely supplying the MCA territory. (**a**) Late arterial phase (**b**) Early capillary phase (**c**) Late capillary phase, (**d**) Early venous phase. The patient was successfully treated with mechanical thrombectomy resulting in a NIHSS decrease from 19 to 4 in 24 h

Clinical

- Anterior circulation: NIHSS 6–25. If the patient has a score <6, the risk/benefit ratio becomes unfavorable. A lower score may be accepted if the patient has aphasia as this may be viewed as a devastating handicap. If the patient has a score >25, he/she is usually in a too bad condition to be helped by a thrombectomy procedure.
- Posterior circulation: NIHSS is not readily applicable. The selection is especially difficult as even patients in Glasgow Coma Scale (GCS) 3–4 may have a good outcome. Clinical fluctuations are usually a good sign.
- There is no absolute age limit for thrombectomy, but *high biological age* should be a restricting factor as well as *many significant comorbidities*. These may impose anesthesiological problems (e.g., cardiopulmonary restrictions), affect the possibility for recovery and rehabilitation (e.g., contralateral stroke, dementia), and long-time survival (e.g., cancer with bad prognosis).

Radiological

Anterior Circulation

- CT-based radiological protocols for selection of patients with anterior circulation stroke can be recommended to contain a non-contrast enhanced CT, CTA, and CT perfusion (CTP, Fig. 3). The CTA provides invaluable information about the status of the arteries from the aortic arch to the intracerebral circulation. Not only can the exact location of the thromboemboli be determined but obstacles on the way (e.g., carotid stenosis) are discovered making it possible to plan the procedure beforehand. The basal axial images called CTA-SI (source images) can be used not only to estimate the extent of pial collaterals but also to more clearly delineate the infarcted tissue by adjusting the window level and width. As CTP still may be regarded uncertain, for one thing because of difficulties to determine thresholds, the status of the ischemic brain tissue can consequently be supplementary estimated on the basis of CT and CTA, preferably utilizing the so-called ASPECTS score, possible on both non-contrast CT and CTA-SI.
- Alternatively, the protocol may be based on MR and should then, in addition to a CT which is usually always done, consist of at least time-of-flight (TOF), diffusion weighted images (DWI), and T2-weighted images/Flair. MR perfusion is usually not necessary as the focus should be on detecting *brain parenchyma already infarcted*. This means that blood volume in CTP and DWI in MR become especially important. In large vessel occlusions, no extensive infarct present usually means salvageable tissue. Under such circumstances, there are always threatened areas, so-called penumbra, kept alive by pial collaterals. In contrast, large infarcts (>1/3–1/2 of the MCA territory, so-called malignant MCA-pattern) imply bad patient outcome even with successful revascularization and a thrombectomy procedure in that context only adds risk for reperfusion hematomas/hemorrhagic conversion in addition to the risk for complications from the procedure itself.

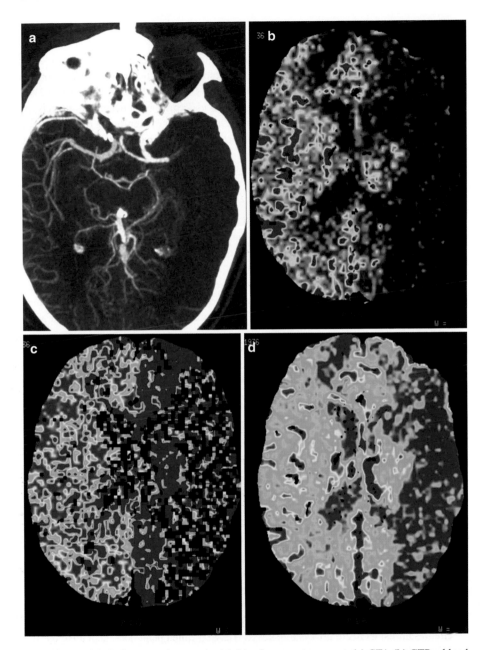

Fig. 3 CTA and CTP from a patient scanned 1.5 h after symptom onset. (**a**) CTA (**b**) CTP – blood flow (**c**) CTP – mean transit time (**d**) CTP – cerebral blood volume. Note the *left-sided* MCA occlusion, lack of pial collaterals, and markedly decreased blood flow and cerebral blood volume in large areas of the MCA-territory. The patient also deteriorated clinically very rapidly and it was decided not to pursue a thrombectomy procedure

Posterior Circulation

- For radiological selection of patients with posterior circulation stroke, usually BAO, it may be recommended to include MR-sequences in the selection process. The protocol can consist of CT, CTA (alternatively MR-TOF), CTA-SI, MR-DWI, and MR-T2WI/Flair. It is crucial to detect brain stem infarcts, especially mesencephalic infarcts, as they are strong predictors for bad outcome. The presence of significant mesencephalic infarcts speaks against thrombectomy as it probably is too late for saving or helping the patient by revascularization.

Treatment Protocol

- If possible, it is preferred to perform the thrombectomy under conscious sedation (CS) instead of general anesthesia (GA) for several reasons. CS is faster and it is possible to have better control of the patient. Most importantly though, the patients always get hypotensive at induction of GA unless the BP drop is counteracted with vasopressors (e.g., noradrenaline/norepinephrine), something that is rarely done for acute stroke patients. As these patients rely on pial collaterals, they need a high-cerebral perfusion pressure and a BP decrease may be deleterious, pushing ischemic/oligemic tissue into manifest infarct. If GA is inevitable, special care should always be taken to meticulously avoid blood pressure drop.
- There is no need for anticoagulation or antiaggregation during a thrombectomy procedure other than a standard dose of heparin in the flushes (e.g., 5 IU/ml) unless the patient is permanently stented. This should, however, be avoided as the necessary medication to keep the stent patent may increase the risk for reperfusion hematomas/hemorrhagic conversion. If it is necessary to leave a stent, Gp IIb/IIIa inhibitors can be used in the acute situation. For example, half bolus of abciximab can be administered IV when the stent is in place followed by a loading dose of clopidogrel (300 mg) and acetylsalicylic acid (ASA) (300–500 mg) after 12–24 h, usually in the next morning. If the patient is resistant to clopidogrel, the dose may be doubled or changed to prasugrel (bolus 60 mg). The patient should be kept on double medication, clopidogrel 75 mg (alternatively prasugrel 10 mg)/ASA 75–325 mg daily for at least 3 months and on ASA alone for another at least 3 months. Alternatively, if the patient is regarded be at a specifically high risk for intracerebral hemorrhage, a loading dose of ASA (300–500 mg) alone may be administered orally, IV, or per rectum (PR) immediately after stent placement. Clopidogrel (or prasugrel) is than added if a 22–36 h post-procedure CT is negative, i.e., with no *symptomatic* intracerebral hemorrhage according to the so-called ECASS definition. This latter pharmacological regime may, however, pose a slightly higher risk of immediate or delayed stent thrombosis.

Basic Procedural Protocol for Thrombectomy with a "Stent Retriever" in the Anterior Circulation

- There are several stent retrievers available today with different advantages and disadvantages. This protocol is applicable to all of them (Fig. 4).

Fig. 4 Thromboemboli removed with various "stent retriever" devices all of which are commercially available today

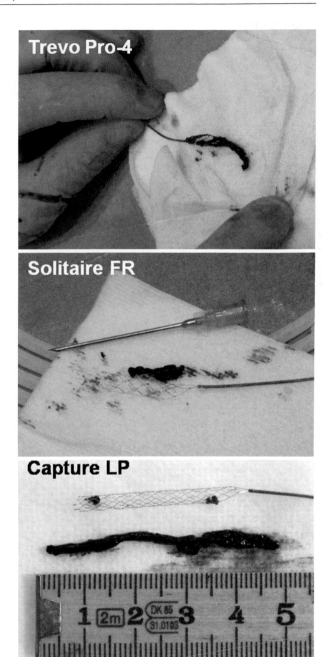

- In the anterior circulation, stent retrievers can, in most patients, be used safely as distal as in the M2-segments. Occasionally, it is possible to use them even further distal but that is generally not recommended and demands utmost care. In the posterior circulation it is rarely needed to perform a thrombectomy more distal than the P1 segment.

- If there are small remaining distal emboli, the first question is whether they should be "chased" or left alone. If the occluded artery supplies an eloquent area and there are no obvious pial collaterals, small doses of IA rt-PA and careful mechanical manipulation can be used as an adjunct to the thrombectomy. If the patient has received IV alteplase, the IA dose can be recommended not to exceed 10 mg. Without preceding IV thrombolysis, as much as 20 mg may be administered IA.
- After groin puncture, preferably a long (80 cm) 8 F introducer sheath is placed with the tip in the common carotid artery (CCA) by the aid of a 5 F diagnostic catheter (DC) and a 0.035″ (0.89 mm) guidewire (GW). As compared to a standard short 8 F introducer, this offers more stability and if the guide catheter for any reason needs to be removed, it is easy to have it regain its position.
- An 8 F balloon guide catheter (BGC) is then positioned with the tip in the internal carotid artery. The possibility for flow reversal with the balloon guide is an advantage compared with standard guide catheters, with less thromboemboli escaping into collateral areas.
- After the position of the clot has been confirmed by contrast injection through the guide catheter, a microcatheter (MC; inner diameter 0.021″ or 0.0165″) is introduced with the aid of a microguidewire (MGW, 0.014″). The thrombus is passed with, if possible, the MC, keeping the MGW retracted. When the tip of the MC is beyond the clot, the position may be confirmed with a gentle infusion of contrast, even though this step can be left out if the stent retriever is positioned based on the proximal end of the thrombus which of course always is defined from the initial angiographic run.
- The stent retriever device is released centered at the clot, preferably slightly more distal than proximal but always covering the proximal clot boundary and left to expand and "incubate" for at least 5 min.
- The MC is then readvanced and the stent retriever partially resheated almost up to the face of the thrombus.
- The balloon is inflated and the stent retriever pulled back as one entity together with the MC with simultaneous aspiration in the BGC. The aspiration is gradually escalated and maximized when the device is entering the orifice of the guide. The retrieval of the device is usually slightly painful for the patient and it is often wise to administer suitable medication for pain relief a few minutes ahead of this maneuver.
- The rotating hemostatic valve (RHV) is then removed and the device taken out on the table and checked for thrombus and potential damage. Further aspiration is then applied directly to the BGC to clear the lumen from any remaining small thrombi before the balloon is deflated.
- The result of the procedure is controlled by contrast injection in the BGC, the device rinsed and cleaned, the RHV reconnected, and the thrombectomy maneuver repeated if necessary. The same stent retriever can usually be used at least three times. If there is a tendency for vasospasm, a calcium antagonist may be administered slowly IA (e.g., 2–3 mg nicardipine or nimodipine).
- The exact same technique may be applied in the posterior circulation with the exception that it may be difficult to advance an 8 F guide catheter into one of the vertebral arteries (VA). In addition, as most patients have two patent VAs, inflating a BGC in one of them does not usually create flow arrest. Instead, the use of a long, *soft* 6–7 F guide catheter (e.g., Navien, Fargo, Neuron), mostly possible to advance even as high as the vertebrobasilar junction, may be recommended for BAO, still though with aspiration applied while pulling back the stent retriever.

Alternative Protocol Using the "Local Aspiration Technique (LAT)"

- This technique takes advantage of a distal access catheter (DAC), either the intermediate catheter named "DAC", or any of the available soft guide catheters, some of which are mentioned above. The "DAC" as well as the soft guides come in different inner diameters and can be introduced directly from a long, 80 cm, introducer sheath. The smaller sizes can also be used together with a BGC or a standard guide catheter in case such has already been positioned in the proximal ICA. Generally, however, it is preferable to use as large a DAC as possible as this increases the possibility to encase the thromboemboli without shaving of small fragments.
- The thrombus is passed with the MC, the stent retriever device is released and then used as an anchor for the DAC that is now advanced over the MC, and the device pusher wire to a position with the tip close to the proximal end of the thrombus.
- The MC is then removed, mainly to improve the aspiration that with this technique is performed through the DAC. After at least 5 min of device "incubation" into the clot, the device is retrieved into the DAC under aspiration, i.e., a more "local" thrombectomy.
- The device is then pulled out of the DAC and checked for thrombus. Further aspiration is applied to the DAC to clear remaining small thrombi that may still be stuck within the lumen. If in doubt, the DAC may be removed, flushed, and reintroduced through the long introducer sheath or guide. With the DAC in place, the MC and stent retriever device can easily be repositioned if needed.
- The disadvantage with this technique as compared to the standard use of a BGC is an increased risk of small fragments escaping and subsequently causing infarcts in the present or collateral vascular territories. As the thromboemboli is equal in size to the occluded artery and the DAC normally is smaller, parts of the clot may be "shaved off" and subsequently transported distal, as there is no reversal of flow. Even though heavy aspiration through the DAC initially may cause flow arrest or even reversal, as soon as the first mm of the thrombus enters the DAC, it will get clogged and that hemodynamic effect is lost.

Post-procedure Protocol

- No anticoagulation or antiaggregation is usually necessary after a successful thrombectomy. If there is an estimated risk for intimal damage, e.g., if several thrombectomy attempts with extensive endovascular maneuvers have been necessary, the patient may receive 250–500 mg ASA, if possible intravenously, otherwise orally or per rectum.
- The patient should preferably be transferred to a specialized stroke ward or a neurointensive care unit. Special attention should be on monitoring the blood pressure where the systolic pressure should ideally be kept ≤140 mmHg. Unless the patient has contraindications (e.g., obstructive pulmonary disease, severe cardiac insufficiency, AV-block II or III), this can usually be achieved by repeated intravenous injections of beta receptor blockers, e.g., 50 mg labetalol administered during 3–5 min.
- A non-contrast CT, or a MR (with minimum sequences DWI, Flair, and T2*WI) should be performed 22–36 h after the procedure, mainly to look for reperfusion hemorrhages/hemorrhagic conversion and infarct size. Small amounts of mixed blood and contrast material can then almost inevitably be seen in infarcted areas on these post-procedure scans. This phenomenon is solely a manifestation of a disturbed and leaking blood brain barrier and

should *not* be interpreted as evidence of a failed procedure and does *not* represent a bad prognostic sign. If the 24 h control is performed with CT, it is advantageous to utilize so-called double energy technique by which blood and contrast agent may be separated.

- If the post-procedure scan is negative, a standard dose of low-molecular heparin can be administered (e.g., 2,000 IU BID or 4,000 IU daily) to avoid venous thrombosis.
- The patient should be evaluated at the outpatient clinic 90 days after the procedure, preferably by an independent neurologist. Patient outcome should then be estimated including assessment of the modified Rankin score. It can be recommended that the patient and his/her relatives also get a chance to meet the neurointerventionalist, either at the same time point or later (suggestively 6 months after the treatment), for one thing because they usually have many questions regarding the procedure itself.

Problems on the Way: Acute Carotid Dissection or Severe Atherosclerotic Carotid Stenosis/Occlusion

Acute Carotid Dissection

- An acute carotid dissection may be the cause for an ICA or MCA thromboemboli. For the majority of the patients, the distal occlusion is then the primary problem as the dissection itself most of the time does not cause hemodynamic impairment.
- Four options can be considered in this situation:
  1. Pass the dissection carefully with a MGW and a 0.014″ MC, follow with a DAC and retrieve into the DAC with the local aspiration technique as described above.
  2. Do a gentle angioplasty of the dissection and advance the guide catheter cautiously across the dissection.
  3. Stent the dissection and position the tip of the guide catheter above the distal end of the stent. The disadvantage with this technique is that the patient needs antiaggregation therapy, which should be avoided in the acute situation because of the risk for hemorrhage.
  4. Perform the thrombectomy through the dissection as it is. If this technique is used, it can be recommended to work under flow reversal, i.e., with an inflated BGC.
- *Never* try to retrieve a stent retriever through an acutely inserted carotid stent as there is a significant risk that the stent retriever gets caught in the mesh.

Severe Carotid Stenosis/Occlusion

- If not too severe, the stenosis may be passed with a BGC or at least with a DAC making the local aspiration technique a good alternative or it may be possible to retrieve through the stenosis. The risk for dislodging thrombus or debris causing distal embolization or for plaque rupture/dissection should, however, be considered and may urge the need for starting the procedure by treating the carotid stenosis. It should, however, always be kept in mind that it is the ICA/MCA thromboemboli that constitute the primary concern and should consequently be prioritized.

- If necessary, the carotid stenosis can be treated with conventional carotid stenting. Distal protection may be utilized but an alternative protection in this setting is to stent through a BGC keeping the balloon inflated with gentle aspiration while passing the stenosis with the stent and possible pre- and postdilatation balloons.
- The disadvantage with primary stenting is that it delays the thrombectomy and, again, that the stent necessitates antiaggregation making it reasonable to consider only performing an angioplasty in this acute phase.
- When a so-called near occlusion becomes complete, there seems to be a risk for distal emboli. There is no other plausible explanation for the rather high percentage of patients that present with so-called tandem occlusions, i.e., obstructions simultaneously in the proximal carotid and the MCA. Even such a completely occluded carotid may, however, be carefully opened (Figs. 5 and 6):
  1. The first attempt is usually to try and pass the carotid occlusion with the MGW/MC.
  2. If that is not successful, the second effort can be to try with a long (110–120 cm) 4–5F DC and a 0.032–38 GW.

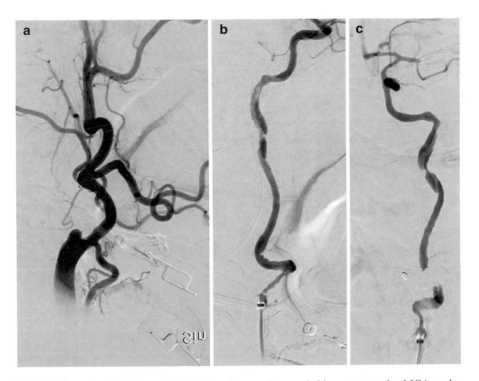

Fig. 5 Stroke patient in whom a CTA disclosed a complete, probably acute, proximal ICA occlusion as well as an MCA (M1) thromboemboli. (**a**) Obstruction of flow in the left ICA (**b**) The ICA occlusion has been reopened by the BGC mandrel and gentle inflation of the balloon (**c**) As the proximal ICA is again open, the M1 occlusion becomes visible

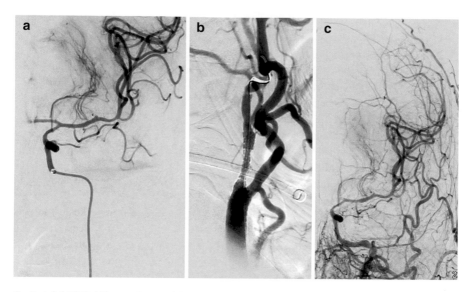

Fig. 6 A 0.057″ DAC was advanced through the reopened ICA, the tip positioned in the distal ICA, and a stent retriever thrombectomy performed. The proximal carotid was subsequently stented. (**a**) Selective injection through the DAC after successful stent retriever thrombectomy (**b**) A carotid stent has been positioned across the previous occlusion (**c**) A final run reveals contrast filling of the ICA and perfusion of the MCA territory. The patient recovered to MRS = 1 at 90 days follow-up

3. Finally, it is also possible to use a shapable BGC mandrel or a stiff GW that is gently advanced, closely followed by the BGC itself. This maneuver may open the carotid occlusion on its own, but if not, careful inflation of the balloon may result in the artery becoming, again, patent.

- If a MC or DC is used, as in 1 and 2 above, this is preferably done in conjunction with a BGC keeping the balloon inflated with gentle aspiration as there may be fresh thrombus distal to the occlusion.

Complications: Reperfusion Hematomas and Directly Procedure-Related Complications

Reperfusion Hematomas

- Significant, symptomatic reperfusion hematomas, in accordance with the ECASS definition, may appear also after a successful thrombectomy. There is a higher risk if the patient is >60 years old, has a high NIHSS, a high blood glucose level, and a low platelet count. To avoid such hematomas, it can be recommended to minimize the use of anticoagulation/antiaggregation and to meticulously monitor and treat elevated BP and glucose levels.

- Significant hematomas are often deleterious and should not, as was previously discussed, be confused with the small amounts of blood mixed with contrast commonly seen in infarcted areas at the post-procedure (22–36 h) CT or MR scans.

Direct Procedure-Related Complications

- Procedure related complications include dissections/ruptures, perforations, and collateral infarcts, i.e., in previously unaffected areas of the brain.
- Such complications are fortunately rare and mostly due to obvious mistakes working in a stressful situation. They can mostly be avoided by diligent patient selection, a good organization and proper protocols, and by not being overaggressive realizing that it is sometimes better for the patient to give up and not pursuing a procedure with unacceptable risks.
- If a stent retriever gets stuck when trying to retract or if it does not behave as expected, it is of utmost importance not to proceed with the attempt by using increased force. Instead, the device should be resheated and removed together with the MC, where after both are checked on the table and possibly exchanged.

Treatment of Acute Ischemic Stroke in the Future

- Ischemic stroke mostly affects older people. With an aging population (at least in the western world) in combination with ongoing campaigns encouraging stroke patients to seek care early, a steady increase of stroke patients can probably be expected. Many of these patients will be potentially treatable with endovascular techniques. This likely, and perhaps dramatic, enlargement of the patient population obviously puts special emphasis on the necessity of proper recruitment and standardized training for an increasing number of neurointerventionalists in the near future.

Key Points

> Acute ischemic stroke is a leading cause for death and disability. Reperfusion by recanalization is the most effective therapy. It can be achieved by pharmacological thrombolysis or mechanical thrombectomy.

> Mechanical thrombectomy is an option for patients not eligible for intravenous therapy and for patients in which such infusion has no effect or is highly unlikely to work, i.e., patients with a large vessel occluded by a long thrombus causing a severe stroke.

> The keys to success for a neurointerventional stroke center are good organization and proper clinical as well as neuroradiological patient selection.

> So-called stent retrievers have been proven safe and effective for mechanical thrombectomy. There are technical variations and preferences but it is important to develop a local treatment protocol aiming for a fast procedure with minimized patient risk.

> Acute carotid dissection or severe atherosclerotic stenosis/occlusion pose an increased treatment difficulty but is a challenge that may be overcome with proper technical maneuvers. However, it is sometimes better for the patient to decline or give up a procedure if it carries unacceptable risks, rather than overaggressively expose him/her for escalating hazards.

> The number of acute ischemic stroke patients is likely to increase and there will consequently be a need for more neurointerventionalists in a not too distant future. This highlights the need for proper recruitment and standardized training already today.

Suggested Reading

1. Andersson T, Kuntze Söderqvist Å, Söderman M, et al. Mechanical thrombectomy as the primary treatment for acute basilar artery occlusion: experience from 5 years of practice. J Neurointerv Surg. 2013;5(3):221–225.
2. Broderick JP, Palesch YY, Demchuk AM, et al. Endovascular therapy after intravenous t-PA versus t-PA alone for stroke. N Engl J Med. 2013;368:893–903.
3. Ciccone A, Valvassori L, Nichelatti M, et al. Endovascular treatment for acute ischemic stroke. N Engl J Med. 2013;368(25):2431.
4. Dávalos A, Pereira VM, Chapot R, Bonafé A, Andersson T, Gralla J, Solitaire group. Retrospective multicenter study of Solitaire FR for revascularization in the treatment of acute ischemic stroke. Stroke. 2012;43:2699–705.
5. Furlan A, Higashida RT, Wechsler L, et al. Intra-arterial prourokinase for acute ischemic stroke. The PROACT II study: a randomized controlled trial. Prolyse in Acute Cerebral Thromboembolism. JAMA. 1999;282:2003–11.

6. Kidwell CS, Jahan R, Gornbein J, et al. A trial of imaging selection and endovascular treatment for ischemic stroke. N Engl J Med. 2013;368(10):914–23.
7. Lees KR, Bluhmki E, von Kummer R, et al. Time to treatment with intravenous alteplase and outcome in stroke: an updated pooled analysis of ECASS, ATLANTIS, NINDS, and EPITHET trials. Lancet. 2010;375:1695–703.
8. Mattle HP, Arnold M, Lindsberg PJ, et al. Basilar artery occlusion. Lancet Neurol. 2011;10:1002–14.
9. Nogueira RG, Lutsep HL, Gupta R, Jovin TG, Albers GW, Walker GA, et al. Trevo versus Merci retrievers for thrombectomy revascularization of large vessel occlusions in acute ischaemic stroke (TREVO 2): a randomized trial. Lancet. 2012;6:1231–40.
10. Pereira VM, Gralla J, Bonafé A, et al; Final results of the Solitaire FR thrombectomy for acute revascularization (STAR) – prospective, multi-centre, controlled trial in EU, Australia and Canada. Abstr. LB7, Int Stroke Conf. 2013.
11. Riedel CH, Zimmermann P, Jensen-Kondering U, et al. The importance of size: successful recanalization by intravenous thrombolysis in acute anterior stroke depends on thrombus length. Stroke. 2011;42:1775–7.
12. Saver JL, Jahan R, Levy EI, Jovin TG, Baxter B, Nogueira RG, et al. Solitaire flow restoration device versus the Merci Retriever in patients with acute ischaemic stroke (SWIFT): a randomized, parallel-group, non-inferiority trial. Lancet. 2012;6:1241–9.

Part VI

Angioplasty and Stenting of Arterial Stenosis

Vertebral Artery Angioplasty/Stenting

Andrew Clifton

Abstract

Posterior circulation stroke accounts for approximately 20–25 % of all strokes. Approximately 25 % of these are due to stenoses in the vertebral and/or the basilar arteries. Atherosclerotic stenosis of the vertebral artery is most common at its origin. Embolization from such lesions is an important cause of posterior circulation stroke. Approximately 1 on 5 posterior circulation strokes occur in the setting of extracranial vertebral artery stenosis. Optimal management of such patients is unclear.

Keywords

Vertebral artery stenosis • Stroke • Restenosis • Vertebral origin stenosis • Balloon-mounted stent • www.vertart.com

Introduction

- Posterior circulation stroke accounts for approximately 20–25 % of all strokes.
- Approximately 25 % of these are due to stenoses in the vertebral and/or the basilar arteries.
- Atherosclerotic stenosis of the vertebral artery is most common at its origin.
- Embolization from such lesions is an important cause of posterior circulation stroke.
- Approximately 1 on 5 posterior circulation strokes occur in the setting of extracranial vertebral artery stenosis.
- Optimal management of such patients is unclear.

A. Clifton, MA, MRCP, FRCR
Department of Neuroradiology, Atkinson Morley Wing, St. George's Hospital, London, UK
e-mail: andrew.clifton@stgeorges.nhs.uk

K. Murphy, F. Robertson (eds.), *Interventional Neuroradiology,*
Techniques in Interventional Radiology,
DOI 10.1007/978-1-4471-4582-0_15, © Springer-Verlag London 2014

Risk of Stroke After Vertebrobasilar Stroke and TIA

- For a long time the prognosis for vertebrobasilar transient ischemic attack (TIA)s was thought to better than that for carotid TIAs.
- Landmark paper by Flossman and Rothwell in *Brain* in 2003.
- Review of 820 abstracts and 304 papers in detail.
- Found no evidence that patients presenting with vertebrobasilar events have a lower risk of subsequent stroke or death compared with patients presenting with carotid TIA or minor stroke.
- The risk of stroke is probably higher in the acute phase, concluded that patients with vertebrobasilar events require active preventative treatment.
- Greater than 50 % vertebrobasilar stenosis is associated with a high early risk of recurrent stroke. Marquardt et al. in *Brain* in 2009.
- Recurrence is highest soon after the initial event, mostly within 20–30 days. Gulli et al. *Stroke* 2009.
- Thus risk profile is similar to that seen in symptomatic carotid stenosis, emphasizing the need for a similarly active treatment strategy.

How Common Is Vertebral Artery Stenosis?

- Two large studies
- Hospital based, Gulli et al., 186 patients without vertebral dissection, 45 % had stenosis, of these 43 % at V1, 35 % intracranially
- Population based, Markquardt et al., 141 patients with vertebrobasilar stoke/TIA, 26 % greater than 50 % vertebral basilar stenosis

Diagnosis and Imaging

- Diagnosis of vertebrobasilar territory stroke and TIA can be unclear – magnetic resonance imaging (MRI) is essential to confirm diagnosis.
- Duplex ultrasound – the vertebral artery origin can often be well delineated, distal stenosis often detected by flow disturbance, but poor sensitivity.
- MR angiography (MRA), contrast enhanced – better views of vessel origin, better signal to noise but caution in renal disease as needs gadolinium, and can overestimate the degree of stenosis.
- Computed tomography angiography (CTA) – quick, open, available, often performed with CT when the patient is admitted with a diagnosis of stroke. *Disadvantages* – radiation, renal impairment, calcium obscuring the lumen.

- Analysis of published data, Khan et al. *JNNP* 2007; contrast-enhanced MRA and CTA were sensitive and specific; duplex was not sensitive but quite specific.
- CTA and MRA good at excluding stenosis, in some cases formal angiography may be needed, e.g., where there is discrepancy in noninvasive imaging.

Treatment

Medical Treatment

- Traditionally considered mainstay of therapy for posterior circulation stoke.
- No randomized trials of the use of different antiplatelet therapies or anticoagulant therapy against antiplatelet therapies in extracranial vertebral arterial disease.
- Intracranial atherosclerosis – few studies, WASID. Stenosis greater than 50 % of a major intracranial artery randomized to receive warfarin or aspirin. Trial halted due to concerns about the safety of patients receiving warfarin. Aspirin-treated patients ischemic stroke 12 % at 1 year, warfarin 11 % but death in 4.3 % of the aspirin group, 9.7 % of the warfarin group.

Invasive Treatment

- Extracranial and intracranial vertebral artery endovascular treatment will be considered separately.

Extracranial Vertebral Artery Stenting

- Evidence only one completed randomized trial, data derived from the Carotid and Vertebral Artery Transluminal Angioplasty Study. 16 patients randomized, 8 to endovascular treatment in association with best medical therapy, and 8 to medical care alone. All symptomatic. Endovascular treatment successful in all 8 patients. 2 TIAs within 30 days, no strokes. Follow-up mean of 4.5 years in the endovascular group and 4.9 years in the medical group. No further vertebrobasilar strokes in either group. No firm conclusions from this report.
- Meta-analysis, Eberhardt O et al. 2006. 60 papers reviewed, 313 with proximal disease, periprocedural stroke risk of 1.3 %, death rate of 0.3 %, recurrent stroke risk of 0.7 % over 14 months, rate of restenosis 25.7 % usually asymptomatic, and no comparison with medical data.
- Results suggest primary stenting of vertebral artery atherosclerosis at the vessel origin has a high success rate, acceptable complication rate, and low rate of restenosis. No comparison with modern antiplatelet, anti-lipid, or antihypertensive therapy.

- Randomized trial currently ongoing, VIST, Vertebral Artery Ischaemia Stenting Trial, St George's Hospital, University of London (*no data reported*).
- To determine whether stenting/angioplasty or best medical treatment is more effective at preventing recurrent events in patients with symptomatic vertebral stenosis.
- 5-year trial period.
  - *Criteria*Vertebrobasilar stroke/TIA in last 6 months
  - Vertebral stenosis greater than 50 % as per MRA/CTA or angiogram
  - Stenosis resulting from presumed atheromatous disease
  - Stenting considered technically feasible
  - Women or men aged 20 years of age or greater
  - Patient able to provide written informed consent
- Study ongoing – contact details VIST@sgul.ac.uk, www.vertart.com

Intracranial Vertebral Artery Stenosis

- Review of evidence Eberhardt O et al. 2006.
- Distal vertebrobasilar lesions with angioplasty and stenting, 107 angioplasties, periprocedural complication rate 7.1 % for stroke and 3.7 % for death. 180 patients undergoing stenting as opposed to angioplasty, similar complication rates, 7.7 and 3.2 % mortality.
- Stenting of symptomatic atherosclerotic lesions in the vertebral or intracranial arteries trial, SSYLVIA, success rate of 95 % in 61 cases; strokes after stent placement occurred in 2 of 22 intracranial cases, 14 % during a 1-year follow-up period. 30-day complication rate and 6.6 % stroke rate.
- Wingspan study. 15 patients, anatomically and clinically adequate results in all patients; initial degree of stenosis 72 % and mean residual stenosis 54 %.
- Randomized trials: The SAMMPRIS trial, angioplasty combined with stenting plus aggressive medical therapy versus aggressive medical therapy alone for intracranial artery stenosis. The trial was stopped on April 11, 2011. 14 % of patients treated with angioplasty combined with stenting experienced a stroke or died within the first 30 days compared to 5.8 % patients treated with medical therapy alone. A highly significant difference. This may limit use of endovascular treatment intracranially until further detail is available or trials are underway.

Technical Aspects

- Patients should be premedicated with antiplatelet agents; regimes vary but the author use recommends aspirin 75 mg a day for at least 7 days prior to the procedure, or a 600 mg loading dose the day before the procedure and 75 mg on the day, plus clopidogrel 75 mg a day for at least 7 days before the procedure, or a 600 mg loading the dose the day before the procedure and 75 mg on the day of the procedure.
- 75 mg of both agents continued for 6 weeks and one agent, usually aspirin, 75 mg/day for life.

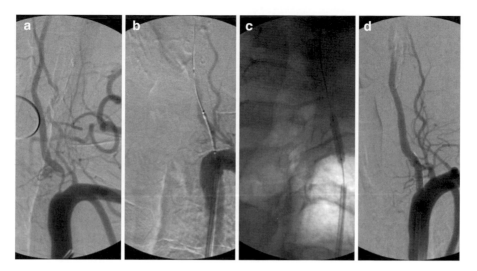

Fig. 1 Left vertebral origin stenosis treated with a balloon-mounted stent. 3.5 mm Pharos balloon expandable stent

- If a platelet functional analyzer such as VerifyNow is available, antiplatelet function should be tested prior to the procedure and dosages adjusted accordingly.

Extracranial Stenting

- Most stenoses at origin. Stenting within the foramina is not generally recommended as neck movement can cause stent fracture and occlusion.
- Stenting at the origin can be performed under local anesthesia +/− sedation. 5 or 6 French groin puncture depending on the size of the guiding sheath needed.
- Full angiography to both subclavian arteries to look at both vertebral origins and collateral flow and views of intracranial circulation.
- 5,000 units of heparin given intravenously before insertion of the guiding catheter.
- Appropriate ACT levels obtained prior to inserting the guiding catheter.
- Usual practice is to use balloon-mounted stents under road mapping; the lesion is crossed with a 014 or 018 wire, depending on the stent selected, and a balloon-mounted stent deployed across the stenosis leaving a few millimeters of stent in the subclavian artery (Figs. 1 and 2).
- Post-dilatation a check angiogram is performed and, if appearance is satisfactory, the delivery system is removed.
- Rarely the lesion needs to be pre-dilated.
- *Technical tip:* Access to the right vertebral can often be difficult, and sometimes using a 7 French sheath with a wire into the subclavian stabilizes the system to gain access.
- Brachial artery puncture using a 5 French sheath is sometimes necessary for access.

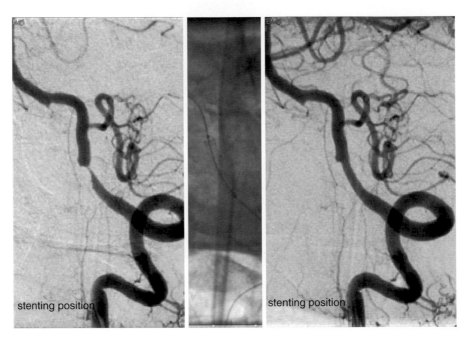

Fig. 2 Left intradural vertebral stenosis treated with a balloon-mounted stent. Intradural vertebral stenosis pre- and post-stenting

Stent Types

- Monorail preferred; various stent types are available including cardiac, renal, and specific intracranial stents such as the Pharos.

Intracranial Stenting

- Premedication as above. Heparinization as above.
- Procedure is ideally performed under general anesthesia.
- Both balloon-mounted Pharos and self-expanding (Wingspan) stents are used. Self-expanding stents usually require pre-dilatation of the lesion using a gateway balloon to approximately 75 % of the diameter of the normal vessel before deployment of the stent. Dilation beyond this risks vessel rupture and catastrophe.

Post-procedure Care

- Extracranial can be managed in a high dependency unit overnight. Heparinization is not necessary for extracranial stents.

- Intracranial stenting – essential the patient has access to an HDU or even an ITU bed overnight for close monitoring of blood pressure and other neurological parameters. Heparinization is usually continued for 24 h after the procedure.
- It goes without saying that all of these patients have atheromatous disease and will be managed by a neurologist or stroke physician with control of risk factors such as hypertension, glucose, and cholesterol.

Imaging Follow-Up

- Unless follow-up is prescribed as part of a trial, noninvasive imaging such as ultrasound, particularly to look at flow through an origin stenosis, or CTA or MRA is recommended.
- Catheter angiography is reserved for those who become symptomatic or as follow-up as part of a trial.

Key Points

> The risk of stroke following vertebrobasilar TIA/minor stroke is as high as for the carotid circulation.
> The risk is highest earliest after TIA.
> CEMRA and CTA provide sensitive screening for vertebral stenosis.
> Stenotic disease occurs in approximately 20–30 %.
> Stenting of vertebral stenosis is technically possible.
> Randomized trials are required to determine efficacy.
> Trials looking at intracranial disease currently favor medical treatment.

Suggested Reading

1. CAVATAS Investigators. Endovascular versus surgical treatment inpatient with carotid stenosis in the Carotid and vertebral Artery Transluminal Angioplasty Study (CAVATAS): a randomized trial. Lancet. 2001;357:1729–37.
2. Chimowitz MI, Kokkinos J, Strong J, et al. The Warfarin – aspirin symptomatic intracranial disease study. Neurology. 1995;45:1488–93.
3. Chimowitz MI, Lynn MJ, Howlett-Smith H, et al. Comparison of Warfarin and aspirin for symptomatic intracranial arterial stenosis. N Engl J Med. 2005;352:1305–16.
4. Clifton A. Vertebral artery occlusive disease (indications for intervention, technical aspects, troubleshooting and current results). In: Thompson MM, Morgan RA, Matsumura JS, Sapoval M, Loftus IM, editors. Endovascular intervention of vascular disease, principles and practice. New York: Informa Healthcare USA Inc.; 2008. p. 193–8.

5. Cloud GC, Crawley F, Clifton AG, McCabe DJH. Vertebral artery origin angioplasty and primary stenting: safety and restenosis rates in a prospective series. J Neurol Neurosurg Psychiatry. 2003;74:586–91.
6. Conners III JJ, Wojak JC. Percutaneous transluminal angioplasty for intracranial atherosclerotic lesions: evolution of technique and short term results. Stroke. 2004;35:1388–92.
7. Coward LJ, Featherstone RL, Brown MM. Percutaneous transluminal angioplasty and stenting for vertebral artery stenosis. Stroke. 2005;36:2047–8.
8. Crawley F, Brown MM, Clifton AG. Angioplasty and stent in the carotid and vertebral arteries. Postgrad Med J. 1998a;74:7–10.
9. Crawley F, Clifton A, Brown MM. Treatable lesions demonstrated on vertebral angiography for posterior circulation ischaemic events. Br J Radiol. 1998b;71:1266–70.
10. Eberhardt O, Naegele T, Raygrotzki S, Weller M, Ernemann U. Stenting of vertebrobasilar arteries in symptomatic atherosclerotic disease and acute occlusion: case series and review of the literature. J Vasc Surg. 2006;43(6):1145–54.
11. Flossman E, Rothwell P. Prognosis of vertebrobasilar transient ischaemic attack and minor stroke. Brain. 2003;126:1940–54.
12. Gulli G-E, Khan S, Markus HS. Vertebrobasilar stenosis predicts high early recurrent stroke risk in posterior circulation stroke and TIA. Stroke. 2009;40:2732–7.
13. Khan S, Cloud GC, Kerry S, Markus HS. Imaging of vertebral artery stenosis; a systematic review. J Neurol Neurosurg Psychiatry. 2007;78:1218–25.
14. Khan S, Rich P, Clifton AG, Markus HS. Non-invasive detection of vertebral artery stenosis: a comparison of contrast enhanced MR angiography, CT angiography and ultrasound. Stroke. 2009;40:3499–503.
15. Marquardt L, Kuker W, Chandratheva A, Geraghty O, Rothwell PM. Incidence and prognosis of greater than 50 % symptomatic vertebral or basilar artery stenosis: prospective population based study. Brain. 2009;132:982–8.
16. SSYLVIA Study Investigators. Stenting of Symptomatic Atherosclerotic Lesions in the Vertebral or Intracranial Arteries (SSYLVIA): study results. Stroke. 2004;35:1388–92.

Part VII

Venous Procedures

Cerebral Venography/Venous Pressure Monitoring/Venous Stenting

Geoffrey D. Parker

Abstract

Cerebral venous sinus stenting (VSS) has been shown to be an effective new form of therapy in some cases of benign intracranial hypertension (BIH), also known as idiopathic intracranial hypertension or pseudotumor cerebri. Cerebral venography with venous pressure measurement (direct retrograde cerebral venography and manometry – DRCVM) is a diagnostic tool used in pre-stenting evaluation of patients with BIH who are unresponsive or intolerant to conventional therapies. DRCVM procedures aim to identify the subset of the BIH patients who have a venous sinus stenosis, elevated venous pressure above the stenosis, and a venous pressure gradient across the stenosis, who might benefit from stenting of the venous sinus to relieve the stenosis.

Keywords

Cerebral venous sinus stenting • Benign intracranial hypertension • Idiopathic intracranial hypertension • Pseudotumor cerebri • Cerebral venography • Direct retrograde cerebral venography and manometry • Diagnosis • Conventional therapy • Venous sinus stenosis • Stenting

Introduction

- Cerebral venous sinus stenting (VSS) has been shown to be an effective new form of therapy in some cases of benign intracranial hypertension (BIH), also known as idiopathic intracranial hypertension or pseudotumor cerebri.

G.D. Parker, BMBS, FRANZCR
Department of Radiology, Royal Prince Alfred Hospital, Camperdown, NSW, Australia
e-mail: geoffp@pnc.com.au

K. Murphy, F. Robertson (eds.), *Interventional Neuroradiology,*
Techniques in Interventional Radiology,
DOI 10.1007/978-1-4471-4582-0_16, © Springer-Verlag London 2014

- Cerebral venography with venous pressure measurement (direct retrograde cerebral venography and manometry – DRCVM) is a diagnostic tool used in pre-stenting evaluation of patients with BIH who are unresponsive or intolerant to conventional therapies.
- DRCVM procedures aim to identify the subset of the BIH patients who have a venous sinus stenosis, elevated venous pressure above the stenosis, and a venous pressure gradient across the stenosis, who might benefit from stenting of the venous sinus to relieve the stenosis.
- VSS is offered to suitable patients with abnormal DRCVM studies, as an alternative to ongoing medical therapies or surgical treatments for BIH.
- Venous sinus stenting is performed to treat venous sinus stenosis and obliterate a venous pressure gradient, thereby relieving cerebral venous hypertension and aiming to allow increased CSF absorption across arachnoid granulations, leading to decreased CSF pressure.

Clinical Features

- Benign intracranial hypertension is also known as idiopathic intracranial hypertension (IIH) or pseudotumor cerebri (PTC).
- Potentially debilitating condition characterized by raised intracranial pressure that most commonly affects young females of childbearing age (female–male incidence ratio 9:1).
- Characterized by:
  - Headache.
  - Visual disturbances (including blurred vision and transient visual obscurations).
  - Papilledema.
  - Can lead to progressive loss of peripheral vision and blindness.
  - The majority of patients are obese.
  - Many describe pulsatile tinnitus.
  - Diplopia can be seen due to 6th-nerve palsies.
  - Other nonspecific symptoms such as numbness of the extremities and generalized weakness, anosmia, and incoordination may also be present.
- The condition was first described in 1895 as "meningitis serosa."
- In the past similar symptoms were frequently seen in patients with chronic mastoiditis and secondary transverse sinus thrombosis.
- The term "otitic hydrocephalus" was used in these patients but it is now known that ventricular dilation is not present and modern diagnostic criteria exclude venous sinus thrombosis as a cause for idiopathic intracranial hypertension.

Diagnostic Evaluation

Clinical and Laboratory

- Diagnosis is based on the Modified Dandy Criteria, amended by Digre and Corbett (Table 1) or the Friedman and Jacobson Criteria (Table 2).

Table 1 Modified Dandy Criteria (amended by Digre and Corbett)

1. Signs and symptoms of raised intracranial pressure (headache, nausea, vomiting, transient visual obscurations, or papilledema)
2. No localizing signs with the exception of abducens (sixth) nerve palsy
3. The patient is awake and alert
4. Normal CT/MRI findings without evidence of venous sinus thrombosis
5. LP opening pressure of >25 cm H_2O and normal biochemical and cytological composition of CSF
6. No other explanation for the raised intracranial pressure

CT computed tomography, *MRI* magnetic resonance imaging, *CSF* cerebrospinal fluid

Table 2 Friedman and Jacobson Criteria for diagnosing idiopathic intracranial hypertension

1. If symptoms are present, they may only reflect those of generalized intracranial hypertension or papilledema
2. If signs are present, they may only reflect those of generalized intracranial hypertension or papilledema
3. Documented elevated intracranial pressure measured in the lateral decubitus position
4. Normal CSF composition
5. No evidence of hydrocephalus, mass, structural, or vascular lesion on MRI or contrast-enhanced CT for typical patients and MRI and MR venography for all others
6. No other cause of intracranial hypertension identified

CT computed tomography, *MRI* magnetic resonance imaging, *CSF* cerebrospinal fluid

Imaging

- Computed tomography (CT) or magnetic resonance imaging (MRI) studies show normal or small ventricles and normal brain parenchyma.
- MRI typically shows flattening of the posterior aspect of the globes, dilatation of the optic nerve sheathes (Fig. 1), with elevation of the optic disc sometimes visible on axial T2-weighted MRI images, and occasionally an acquired Chiari malformation.
- There must be no mass lesion or any obvious cause for elevated intracranial pressure.
- Other features of chronically raised intracranial pressure such as a partially empty sella are frequently present, and cerebrospinal fluid (CSF) leaks are sometimes seen.
- MR venography (MRV) shows that venous sinus stenoses are frequently present in patients with BIH.
- There has been much controversy as to whether these stenoses are primary and causative or secondary to raised intracranial pressure, or possibly both.
- Filling defects due to large arachnoid granulations can also be seen in the transverse sinuses in asymptomatic patients, but it is not correct to assume that such filling defects are *always* incidental.
- Can be done with conventional time-of-flight MRV techniques.

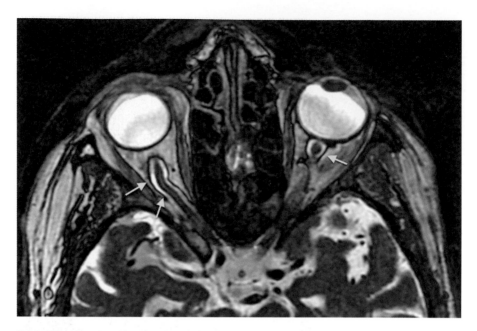

Fig. 1 Dilated optic nerve sheathes seen on thin section T2-weighted FIESTA images in long-standing BIH (*arrows*)

- Artifacts due to saturation frequently impair conventional MRV studies leading to artifactual stenoses or disregarding of real stenoses.
- Much better studies can be obtained using ATECO (auto-triggered elliptic centric-ordered) techniques utilizing gadolinium contrast enhancement to coincide interrogation of the central part of K-space with peak gadolinium concentration and thereby greatly improve the quality of MRV studies.
- Rotating maximum intensity projection images and 3-D modelling allow the cranial venous sinuses to be inspected from almost any angle and the possibility of venous sinus abnormalities can be accurately and noninvasively assessed. Figure 2 shows normal MRV while Fig. 3 shows abnormal MRV.
- Many patients with BIH can be shown to have abnormalities in the venous sinuses. Farb et al. showed that bilateral sinovenous stenoses were seen in 27 of 29 patients with IIH and in only 4 of 59 controls.
- Where these patients can be shown to have increased venous sinus pressure above the stenosis by DRCVM, we hypothesize that relief of venous hypertension could increase CSF absorption and thereby decrease intracranial pressure.
- The main site of CSF absorption is thought to be the arachnoid granulations (arachnoid villi) of the lateral lacunae and superior sagittal sinus. Davson et al. showed that absorption of CSF depends on a pressure gradient between the subarachnoid space

Fig. 2 Normal ATECO MR Venogram showing exquisite demonstration of venous structures

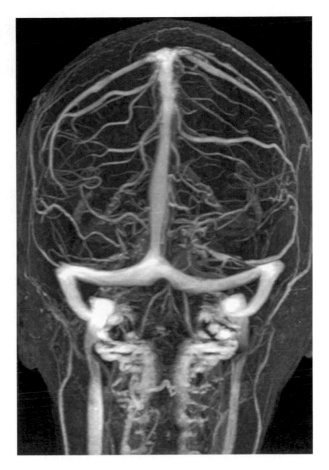

and the venous sinus of approximately 3 mmHg in health. Thus when venous pressure rises, CSF pressure must also rise in order for CSF absorption to continue.

- Bateman first proposed that a disordered positive biofeedback mechanism may be present in BIH where elevated CSF pressure compresses the venous sinuses, leading to further venous hypertension and further elevation of CSF pressure.
- Bateman and others have also shown that cerebral blood flow is increased in many patients with BIH, and decreases after treatment, raising the possibility that an additional disordered biofeedback loop may be operating leading to increased CSF formation.
- If venous sinus narrowing is identified in a patient with persistent symptoms of BIH despite medical management, and venous sinus stenting is being considered, the patient should proceed to DRCVM in order to assess the functional significance of the stenosis identified.

Fig. 3 Abnormal ATECO MR Venogram showing right transverse sinus stenosis (*arrow*) and atretic left transverse sinus (*arrowheads*)

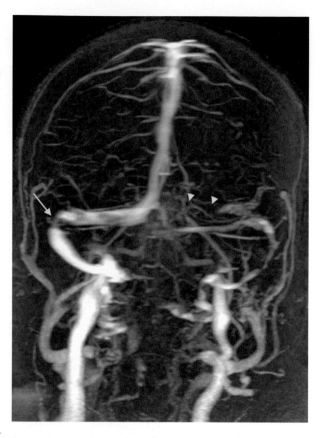

Indications for Treatment, Management Alternatives

- Any patient with symptoms should be offered medical management initially, with surgical or endovascular therapies reserved for nonresponders.
- The goal of treatment is to preserve vision and manage headache.

Medical Management

- Patients with BIH are typically managed with drugs that decrease the rate of CSF formation such as acetazolamide and topiramide (and occasionally furosemide), and are usually advised to lose weight (with the aim of decreasing central venous pressure).
- Lumbar puncture with 20–30 ml CSF drainage typically produces immediate relief of symptoms, and this relief may last far longer than the amount of time required for the body to replace the volume of CSF withdrawn.
- Repeated lumbar punctures may be required.

Conventional Surgical Management

- If not satisfactorily managed, patients may be considered for CSF diversion techniques such as optic nerve sheath fenestration, lumboperitoneal shunting or ventriculoperitoneal shunting, or methods aiming to increase the compliance of the cranial cavity such as subtemporal decompression.
- Shunt procedures are frequently associated with technical failures (blockage, kinking, disconnection, or dislodgement) resulting in a need for shunt revision in ≥30 % of patients per year.

Endovascular Therapy, Venous Sinus Stenting

- Patients who fulfill diagnostic criteria for BIH and are not satisfactorily managed by medical therapies can be considered for suitability for endovascular treatment as an alternative to surgical CSF-diversion therapies.
- Higgins et al. reported the first case in 2002, and since then small case series have been reported, prior to the series of 52 cases reported by Ahmed et al.
- Interest is growing in the literature but stenting remains a controversial therapeutic alternative and is not offered in all centers.

Evaluation Prior to Venous Sinus Stenting

- All patients with a venous sinus stenosis identified on MRV should have the functional significance of this stenosis evaluated with cerebral venography and pressure measurement studies prior to consideration for stenting.
- Some stenoses identified on MRV are not associated with elevated venous pressures or pressure gradients and should not be stented.

Direct Retrograde Cerebral Venography and Manometry

- This is an invasive procedure performed in an angiography suite.
- The study is usually an outpatient procedure performed under mild conscious sedation after fasting for 4–6 h.
- A femoral venous puncture is performed after administration of local anesthesia and a 6 French sheath placed in the common femoral vein.
- A 90-cm 6 French guiding catheter (e.g., Cordis Envoy Mod CBL) is placed through the IVC, right atrium, and SVC into the dominant internal jugular vein terminating just below the skull base.

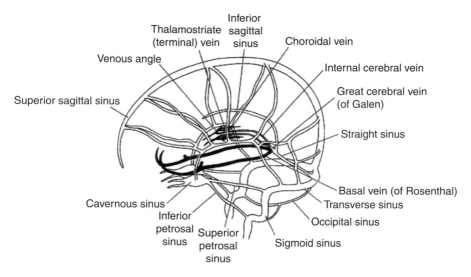

Fig. 4 Standardized pressure-recording form for DRCVM studies. *DRCVM* direct retrograde cerebral venography and manometry

- A jugular venogram is performed to exclude extracranial venous obstruction or stenosis.
- A large-caliber microcatheter (e.g., Boston Scientific Renegade Hi-Flo) is then manipulated over a 014″ guidewire (e.g., Boston Scientific Transend) through the jugular foramen, sigmoid, and transverse sinus and into the superior sagittal sinus.
- The catheter tip is placed as far anteriorly as the coronal suture.
- Venograms are then performed using hand injection with a high-pressure 3 cm³ syringe (e.g., Merit Medallion), obtaining right and left oblique frontal, lateral, and oblique lateral projections to demonstrate venous sinus stenoses.
- The importance of obtaining multiple oblique projections of the transverse sinuses cannot be overemphasized.
- Once adequate venograms have been performed, pressure measurements are obtained at multiple points during catheter pullback using an electronic manometer with the transducer zeroed to room air at the level of the patient's heart.
- Pressures are recorded on a standardized form (Fig. 4). Continuous recording of pressure waves on a paper chart is useful to recognize the presence of focal pressure gradients (Fig. 5) and mean pressures are annotated on images' multiple locations (Figs. 6 and 7).
- Adequate mean pressure measurements can be obtained despite the relatively small size of the catheter, which can damp systolic and diastolic fluctuations but does not affect mean pressure measurements.
- The transverse sinus receiving the dominant blood flow from the superior sagittal sinus should be studied.
- The most common site of stenosis is in the anterior transverse sinus. It is often helpful to study both transverse sinuses, and this can be done (depending on individual anatomy) either by passing the microcatheter from one transverse sinus to the other through the torcular or by a separate extracranial approach through the opposite internal jugular vein.

Fig. 5 Pressure trace recorded during catheter pullback across transverse sinus stenosis confirming sharp pressure gradient across stenosis

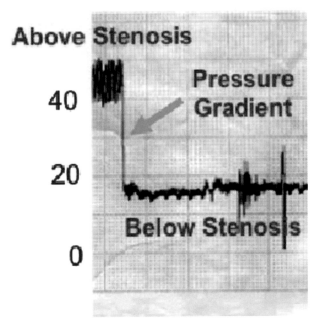

- Most patients tolerate the examination without difficulty. They should be told that they might hear a "scratching" sound in their ear during catheter manipulation.
- After completion of the examination, the catheters and sheath are removed with brief manual common femoral vein pressure for homeostasis.
- The patient is recovered for a period of 2–4 h and then discharged.

DRCVM Results

- Normal venogram, no stenosis, and normal venous pressure (≤16 mmHg)
- Abnormal venogram with stenosis but no pressure gradient
- Abnormal venogram with stenosis and elevated pressures and pressure gradient across stenosis ≤8 mmHg

Venous Stenoses (Figs. 8 and 9)

- Extrinsic long segment external compression.
- Intrinsic focal stenosis due to large arachnoid granulation.
- Intrinsic focal stenosis due to band structure partially occluding sinus.
- Combinations of the above.
- Extrinsic stenoses occur because the transverse sinus is collapsible due to extrinsic pressure.
- Patients with venous stenosis or occlusion due to venous sinus thrombosis are excluded by the diagnostic criteria for BIH (see above).

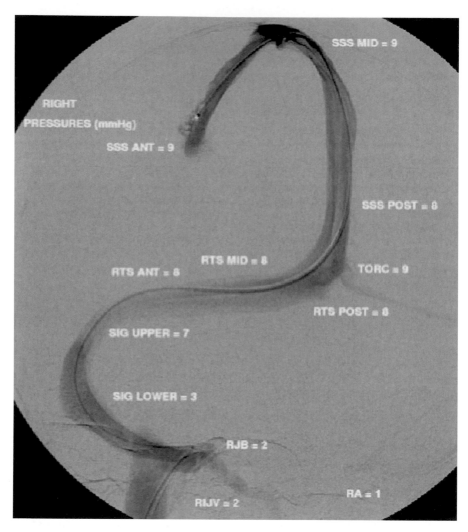

Fig. 6 Normal DRCVM study with normal pressures and no pressure gradient in patients with dominant right transverse sinus and atretic left transverse sinus. *DRCVM* direct retrograde cerebral venography and manometry

Indications for Venous Stenting

Symptoms of BIH unresponsive to medical therapy with:

- Threat to vision or uncontrolled headache
- Where a patient has an abnormal cerebral venogram and manometry study showing venous sinus stenosis and venous pressure gradient ≥8 mmHg
- Where CSF diversion surgery is not considered preferable.

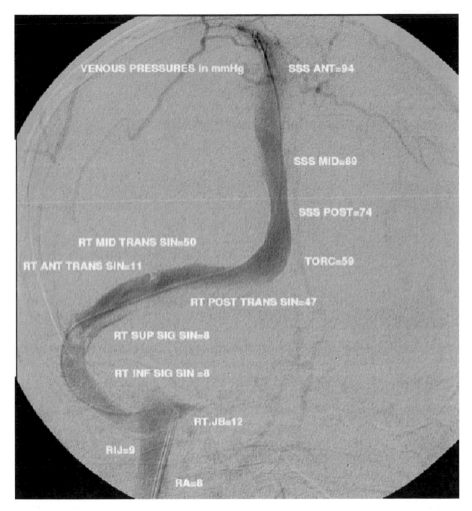

Fig. 7 Abnormal DRCVM study with markedly elevated pressures above and 36 mmHg gradient across; a right transverse sinus stenosis in patient with dominant right transverse sinus and atretic left transverse sinus. Pressure measurements are essential to distinguish normal from abnormal. *DRCVM* direct retrograde cerebral venography and manometry

Contraindications

Patients with:

- Venous sinus thrombosis
- Prothrombotic states
- Patients unable to take or respond to antiplatelet therapy

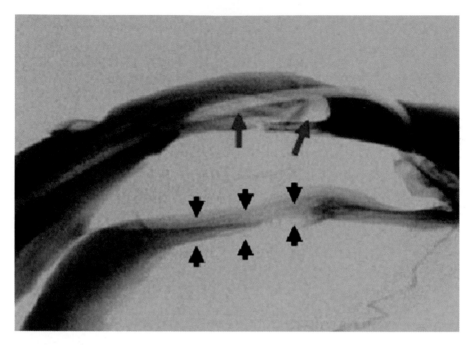

Fig. 8 Lateral oblique transverse sinus venogram showing intrinsic venous sinus stenosis on one side due to large arachnoid granulation and extrinsic sinus stenosis on contralateral side

Patient Preparation

- Consent for the procedure should include the remote possibility of need for urgent craniotomy for hemorrhage if guidewire perforation of a branch vein occurs inadvertently.
- The patient should also be warned that a unilateral frontal headache (different from their usual headache) on the side of the inserted stent is typically seen for 48–72 h after stenting due to stretching of the venous sinus by the stent and will be managed by analgesia.

Relevant Anatomy

Normal Anatomy

- The cerebral venous sinuses, particularly the transverse sinuses, have variable anatomy particularly in the region of the torcular Herophili.
- The superior sagittal sinus can drain into one or both transverse sinuses, and the deep veins draining to the straight sinus can also drain into one or both transverse sinuses, or have separate contralateral drainage from the superior sagittal sinus.
- Asymmetry in the size of the transverse sinuses is common, and one transverse sinus may be atretic or hypoplastic or not communicate with the torcular in normal asymptomatic patients.

Fig. 9 AP oblique transverse sinus venogram showing intrinsic venous sinus stenosis on *left side* due to bands partially obstructing transverse sinus with 17 mmHg gradient

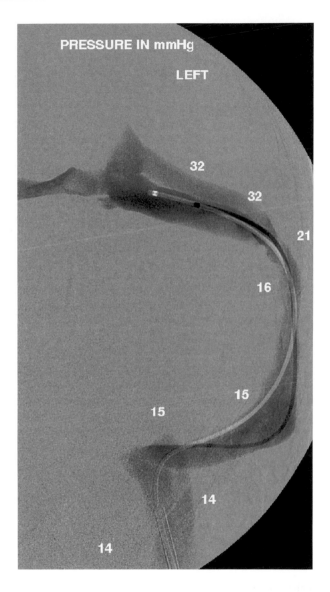

- It is generally only necessary to stent one transverse sinus when both are present and there are bilateral stenoses. The aim is to relieve the stenosis and normalize venous pressure. This can be achieved by unilateral stenting in almost every case.

Variant Anatomy

- Where there is significant asymmetry in the size of the transverse sinuses, the largest or dominant transverse sinus should be chosen for stenting, particularly the transverse sinus that has the most direct communication with the superior sagittal sinus.

Equipment

- 6 French 90 cm long guiding sheath with flexible tip (e.g., Cook Shuttle Flex) and continuous flush.
- 4 French 120 cm long hydrophilic catheter (e.g., Terumo Vertebral Glidecath).
- Exchange length 035″ guide wire (e.g., angle-tip Terumo Glidewire 300 or 260 cm Cook Rosen wire, rarely 300 cm Cook Amplatz Extra-Stiff).
- 035″ self-expanding 8 mm × 40 mm or 9 mm × 40 mm stent on 130 cm delivery system (e.g., Medtronic Complete SE stent). Occasionally smaller diameter 6 or 7 mm stents or longer 60 mm stents are required.
- 014″ self-expanding stents (e.g., Carotid Wallstent) are occasionally useful in the most difficult cases. If the Wallstent is used, care must be taken if there is a substantial discrepancy between the size of the venous sinus above and below the stenosis, due to the possibility of the stent slipping after deployment.
- Manometry equipment for post-stenting pressure measurement.

Pre-procedure Medications

- Premedication with aspirin 150 mg/day and clopidogrel 75 mg/day for 7 days. Check effectiveness with point-of-care platelet function test (e.g., VerifyNow) at time of procedure.

Procedure

Access

- Common femoral venous access allows successful stenting in >90 % of cases.
- Rarely need direct jugular venous puncture.
- A few cases described with direct access to sagittal sinus via a burr hole.

Venography

- Internal jugular venogram when sheath positioned.
- Venous sinus venograms when access gained to sinus to confirm exact site of lesion, assess size of sinus for appropriate stent, and exclude unintended placement of catheter in accessory parallel venous channel.

Intraprocedural Medications

- Heparin 5,000 U IV when sheath access gained, +1,000 U/h in longer procedures; monitor with ACT measurements
- Atropine 0.6 mg or glycopyrrolate 0.4 mg IV prior to stent deployment to prevent vagally mediated bradycardia seen in occasional patients

Assessing the Lesion

- The nature of the stenosis, i.e., intrinsic arachnoid granulation or extrinsic compression, should be known from the preoperative DRCVM study.
- Intrinsic stenoses such as giant arachnoid granulations or dural bands can be treated by localized stenting at the point of stenosis – typically use 40 mm stent.
- Extrinsic stenoses should be treated with longer stents as suggested by Bateman to prevent the rest of the transverse sinus later being compressed by extrinsic pressure, i.e., to interrupt an abnormal positive biofeedback loop by preventing secondary transverse sinus compression. If possible a 60 mm stent or two 40 mm stents inserted telescopically should be chosen to support as long a length of transverse sinus as possible.

Performing the Procedure

- Venous sinus stenting must be performed under general anesthesia. Mean arterial pressure should be carefully maintained (in view of high intracranial pressure) to maintain cerebral perfusion.
- A 6 French 90 cm long flexible tip sheath is placed high into the internal jugular vein on the side of proposed stenting.
- A 4 French 120 cm hydrophilic-coated angle-tip catheter is then placed over a 035″ exchange wire across the stenosis and into the superior sagittal sinus.
- In most cases, the sheath can then be advanced over the 4 French catheter and Glidewire into the transverse sinus at the level of the stenosis (Fig. 10). Occasionally stiffer exchange guidewires such as the Rosen wire or Amplatz Extra-Stiff wire are required, but these wires can make the procedure more difficult when friction is increased in the tortuous sinus at the level of the jugular foramen.
- Once the sheath has been placed a sufficient distance into the transverse sinus, the 4 French catheter is removed over the exchange wire and the stent gently advanced through the sheath into the transverse sinus across the stenosis. The stent is deployed (Fig. 11). Balloon dilatation of the deployed stent is almost never necessary.
- After the stent has been deployed, the delivery system is removed over the exchange guidewire and the 4 French catheter placed through the stent into the superior sagittal sinus. A check venogram is then performed (Fig. 12) together with pressure measurements during catheter pullback.

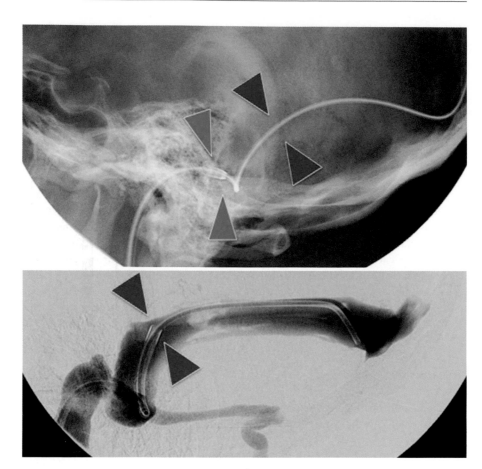

Fig. 10 Placement of flexible-tip 6 Fr sheath in transverse sinus prior to stenting. After 4 French catheter is placed distally, the sheath is gently advanced from the sigmoid sinus (*green arrowheads*) to the target location (*red arrowheads*)

Immediate Post-procedure Care

- The sheath is removed with manual hemostasis during emergence from anesthesia.
- The anesthesiologist must be warned that the patient has high intracranial pressure, which will not be immediately relieved by the procedure. Consequently hypoventilation and deliberate induction of hypercarbia (a standard anesthetic technique used to stimulate respiration, which raises intracranial pressure) must be avoided during the emergence phase from anesthesia. End-tidal pCO_2 monitoring is required.
- The patient is managed in the high-dependency unit without further heparin administration.
- Most patients can be discharged home after 48 h.

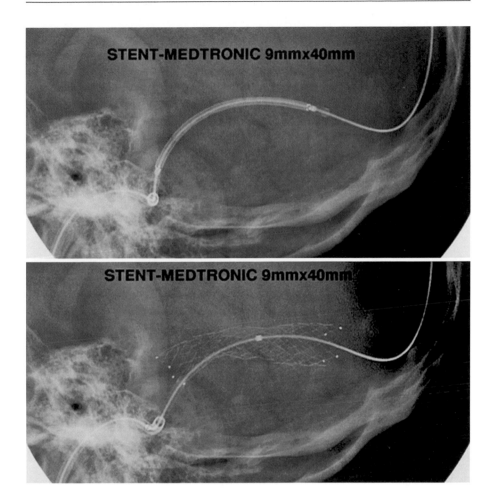

Fig. 11 9×40 mm self-expanding stent in right transverse sinus across stenosis before and after deployment

Follow-Up and Post-procedure Medications

- Clinical monitoring by neurologist and neuro-ophthalmologist particularly noting status of papilledema.
- Continue antiplatelet therapy with clopidogrel 75 mg/day for 3 months and aspirin 150 mg/day for 1 year.
- CT venogram only if symptomatic.
- Repeat lumbar puncture only if symptomatic and after clopidogrel therapy ceased.

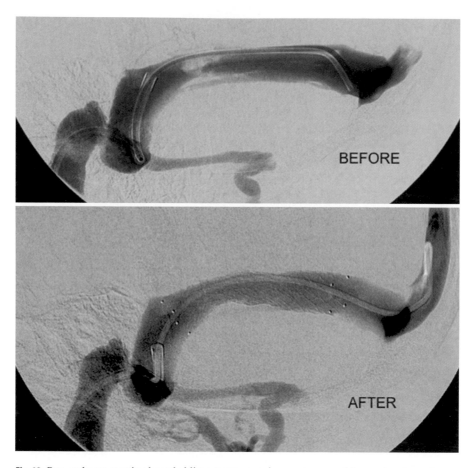

Fig. 12 Pre- and post-stenting lateral oblique transverse sinus venograms. Manometry showed pressure gradient was obliterated

Results

The paper by Ahmed et al. describes in detail our results in the largest series (52 patients) published to date. We have stented a further 18 patients since that paper was submitted, and combined results are tabulated in Table 3 and below:

- Stenting successfully undertaken in 100 % of patients (two patients on second attempt). Three patients required direct jugular venous puncture.
- Mean pressure gradient across the stenosis before stent placement was 20 mmHg and reduced to <1 mmHg immediately after stent placement.

Table 3 Clinical parameters before and after stenting

Clinical parameter (70 patients)	Before stent	After stent
Papilledema	58	0
Visual acuity loss	16	7
Visual field loss	37	10
Headache	60	9
Transient visual obscurations	25	0
Pulsatile tinnitus	30	0
Diplopia	6	0

- 6/52 patients of the original series required re-stenting (the majority was earlier in our experience when shorter stents were used) for recurrent extrinsic stenosis. 1/18 of the further series required re-stenting.
- After stent placement, nine patients still had some headache (seven required re-stenting) that resolved with time in five patients. One patient required four stents but now has normal CSF and venous pressures; another has normal venous pressures, with no gradient after one stent; and a third patient had normal venous pressures after one stent but required subtemporal decompression for resolution of headache
- After stent placement, no patient had visual obscurations, pulsatile tinnitus, or diplopia.

Alternative Treatments

CSF shunt diversion procedures (all of which have high complication and revision rates) remain the standard of care in many institutions for patients with BIH unresponsive to medical therapy.

Complications

In our series of 70 patients:

- No adverse effects seen from stenting across the entry point of the vein of Labbe into the transverse sinus.
- No patient has developed significant in-stent stenosis or late stent occlusion (Table 4).

Table 4 Results from the series by Parker et al. of 70 patients

Complication	Number
Ipsilateral frontal headache	Majority – all resolved within 1 week
Allergy to aspirin or clopidogrel	2
Transient hearing loss	2
Allergy to anesthetic muscle relaxant	1
Subdural hematoma due to guidewire perforation	1
Subdural hematoma due to fulminant BIH (contralateral side to stent)	1
Dural AV fistula adjacent to stent	1
Neointimal hyperplasia in stent (mild)	1
Uncontrolled rise in ICP during emergence from anesthesia causing death	1

Key Points

> Elevated CSF pressures can be evanescent in some patients with BIH, and consequently a single normal opening pressure at lumbar puncture does not exclude the diagnosis when other features are present. Continuous CSF pressure monitoring may be required to establish diagnosis in difficult cases.

> Papilledema can be absent in patients with BIH when there is secondary optic nerve atrophy.

> Some patients with BIH can present with symptoms of intracranial *hypotension*, including orthostatic headache, due to a CSF leak that has developed due to BIH.

> Abnormalities in the transverse sinuses are frequently underreported on MRV studies, due to an assumption that they are a normal variant or artifact.

> DRCVM studies should be performed with light conscious sedation only, to avoid the elevation of central venous pressure that occurs under general anesthesia with mechanical ventilation and therefore the potential to obscure a venous pressure gradient.

> Venograms during DRCVM must include oblique projections to adequately demonstrate venous stenoses.

> DRCVM pressure measurements should be continuously recorded during catheter pullback to allow pressure gradients to be recognized.

> Occasionally, false-negative DRCVM studies can be obtained when patient is partially controlled on medical therapy, and in this circumstance it may be necessary to repeat the study with the patient off medical therapy.

> Patients often complain of ipsilateral-referred pain to the frontal scalp after stenting, which is "different" to their usual headache and settles in 48–72 h.

> Rarely patients complain of persisting headache after stenting as a side effect of clopidogrel therapy.

> Some patients with long-standing BIH may develop secondary venous stenoses due to extrinsic venous sinus compression after successful stenting, as a result of persistent elevation of CSF pressure. We postulate that these patients may have arachnoid granulation dysfunction so that CSF drainage does not improve sufficiently after normalization of venous pressure. These patients may still require CSF diversion surgery.

Suggested Reading

1. Ahmed RM, Wilkinson M, Parker GD, et al. Transverse sinus stenting for idiopathic intracranial hypertension: a review of 52 patients and of model predictions. Am J Neuroradiol. 2011;32:1408–14.

2. Bateman GA. Idiopathic intracranial hypertension: priaprism of the brain? Medical Hypotheses. 2004;63:549–52.

3. Bateman GA. Stenoses in idiopathic intracranial hypertension: to stent or not to stent? Am J Neuroradiol. 2008;29:215.

4. Davson H, Hollingworth G, Segai M. The mechanism of drainage of the cerebrospinal fluid. Brain. 1970;93:665–78.

5. Degnan AJ, Levy LM. Pseudotumor cerebri: brief review of clinical syndrome and imaging findings. Am J Neuroradiol. 2011;32:1986–93.

6. Digre KB, Corbett JJ. Idiopathic intracranial hypertension (pseudotumor cerebri): a reappraisal. Neurologist. 2001;7:2–67.

7. Farb R, Vanek I, Scott J, Mikulis D, Willinsky R, Tomlinson G, terBrugge K. Idiopathic intracranial hypertension: the prevalence and morphology of sinovenous stenosis. Neurology. 2003a;60:1418–24.

8. Farb R, Scott J, Willinsky R, Montanera W, Wright G, terBrugge K. Intracranial venous system: gadolinium-enhanced three-dimensional MR venography with auto-triggered elliptic centric-ordered sequence – initial experience. Radiology. 2003b;226:203–9.

9. Friedman DI, Jacobson DM. Diagnostic criteria for idiopathic intracranial hypertension. Neurology. 2002;59:1492–5.

10. Higgins JN, Owler BK, Cousins C, et al. Venous sinus stenting for refractory benign intracranial hypertension. Lancet. 2002;359:228–30.

11. Osborn AG. Extracranial veins and dural venous sinuses. In: Osborn AG, editor. Diagnostic cerebral angiography. 2nd ed. Philadelphia: Lippincott Williams and Wilkins; 1999. p. 195–216.

12. Owler BK, Parker GD, Halmagyi GM, Johnston IH, Besser M, Pickard JD, Higgins JN. Cranial venous outflow obstruction and pseudotumor cerebri syndrome. Adv Tech Stand Neurosurg. 2005;30:108–74.

13. Scott JN, Farb RI. Imaging and anatomy of the normal intracranial venous system. Neuroimaging Clin N Am. 2003;13:1–12.

14. Wang VY, Barbaro NM, Lawton MT, et al. Complications of lumboperitoneal shunts. Neurosurgery. 2007;60:1045–8.

Inferior Petrosal Venous Sinus Sampling

Andrew Shawyer and Matthew Mattson

Abstract

Cushing's syndrome (CS) is most commonly due to exogenous glucocorticoid administration. The most common endogenous cause of CS (70–80 %) is an adrenocorticotropic hormone (ACTH)-secreting pituitary adenoma (Cushing's disease) for which the treatment of choice is surgical excision. Confirming the diagnosis of a pituitary source and excluding ectopic sources of ACTH using biochemical testing and cross-sectional imaging are often challenging.

Keywords

Cushing's syndrome • Exogenous glucocorticoid administration • Adrenocorticotropic hormone-secreting pituitary adenoma • Pituitary adenoma • Adenoma • Cushing's disease • Surgery • Ectopic source • Biochemical testing • Cross-sectional imaging • Bilateral interior petrosal sinus sampling • Peripheral venous sampling • Corticotropin-releasing hormone • Sensitivity • Specificity • Diagnosis

Introduction

Cushing's syndrome (CS) is most commonly due to exogenous glucocorticoid administration. The most common endogenous cause of CS (70–80 %) is an adrenocorticotropic hormone (ACTH)-secreting pituitary adenoma (Cushing's disease) for which the

A. Shawyer, BSc, MBBS, FRCR
Department of Interventional Radiology, Barts and the Royal London, London, UK

M. Mattson, MD, MRCP, FRCR (✉)
Department of Radiology, Barts and the London NHS Trust, London, UK
e-mail: matthew.matson@bartsandthelondon.nhs.uk

K. Murphy, F. Robertson (eds.), *Interventional Neuroradiology,*
Techniques in Interventional Radiology,
DOI 10.1007/978-1-4471-4582-0_17, © Springer-Verlag London 2014

treatment of choice is surgical excision. Confirming the diagnosis of a pituitary source and excluding ectopic sources of ACTH using biochemical testing and cross-sectional imaging are often challenging.

Bilateral inferior petrosal sinus sampling (BIPSS) with simultaneous peripheral venous sampling is performed before and after the administration of corticotropin-releasing hormone (CRH). This allows an IPS/peripheral ratio of plasma ACTH to be calculated and the source of the ACTH determined.

This technique is both highly sensitive (96 %) and specific (100 %) for diagnosing a pituitary cause for Cushing's syndrome.

Clinical Features

The clinical features of Cushing's syndrome are variable and differ widely in severity. They include:

- Central weight gain
- Proximal muscle weakness
- Hyperhidrosis
- Hypertension
- Hyperglycemia
- Moon facies
- Thinning of the skin
- Telangiectasia

Diagnostic Evaluation

- Often complex due to nonspecific clinical features and atypical biochemical features such as episodic hypercortisolism.
- Initially hypercortisolism is confirmed (urinary free cortisol, late-night salivary cortisol, low-dose dexamethasone suppression test).
- Once CS is confirmed, plasma ACTH levels are obtained. Low ACTH levels suggest an adrenal cause, and abdominal imaging is performed.
- High ACTH levels indicating an ACTH-dependent cause may be due to a pituitary source or an ectopic source (carcinoid/neuroendocrine tumors, pheochromocytoma, gastrinoma, medullary thyroid carcinoma, pancreatic carcinoma).
- High-dose dexamethasone testing, CRH stimulation tests, and fine-cut pituitary gadolinium-enhanced MRI are used to try to distinguish between pituitary and ectopic sources but may often give equivocal or ambiguous results.

Indications

Once a diagnosis of ACTH-dependent CS has been made, BIPPS is the gold standard to distinguish between pituitary and ectopic sources of ACTH. There is variation in the use of BIPSS between institutions, some reserving it for cases where noninvasive tests are equivocal and others performing it in all patients with ACTH-dependent CS.

Contraindications

Renal insufficiency is a relative contraindication.

Relevant Anatomy

Normal

A detailed knowledge of normal and variant pituitary venous drainage anatomy is essential to safely perform BIPSS. Venous drainage from the network of veins overlying the anterior pituitary passes through the intercavernous and cavernous sinuses into the inferior petrosal sinus. The inferior petrosal sinus (IPS) then drains into the internal jugular vein, typically at the level of the inferior margin of the jugular foramen (Fig. 1). Although there is communication between the cavernous sinuses, normal physiological venous drainage is unilateral necessitating bilateral sampling and allowing the source of ACTH to be isolated to one side.

Aberrant

There is considerable variation in both the anatomical positions of the junctions between each venous segment and their morphology. A variety of classifications of IPS anatomy have been proposed. Procedurally the key factors determining accurate catheter positioning are the position of the junction of the IPS into the internal jugular vein, its morphology (plexus or single vein), and the presence and position of the anterior condylar vein. Three basic patterns of venous anatomy (Types A–C) have been described, all with separate variants (Fig. 2).

The pattern of venous drainage differs between the two sides in up to 40 % of patients necessitating pre-sampling venous angiography. For example, in Type C anatomy, IPS sampling would lead to false-negative results as pituitary venous drainage is via the vertebral venous plexus.

Fig. 1 A detailed knowledge of normal and variant pituitary venous drainage anatomy. DSA venogram with catheter tips bilaterally in the inferior petrosal sinuses (*black arrowhead*). Internal jugular vein (*blue arrowhead*) and cavernous sinus (*white arrowhead*)

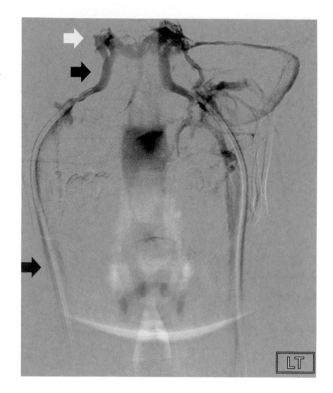

Equipment

- Catheters: MPA and microcatheter

Pre-procedure Medications

- Performed either under conscious sedation or without sedation or systemic analgesia.
- Pediatric BIPSS may require general anesthesia.

Procedure

Access

Review any relevant previous pre-procedural imaging.

- Femoral venous access.
- Two 6 or 7-French sheaths in the femoral vein. These can be unilateral, but in children/ smaller veins a bilateral technique used.

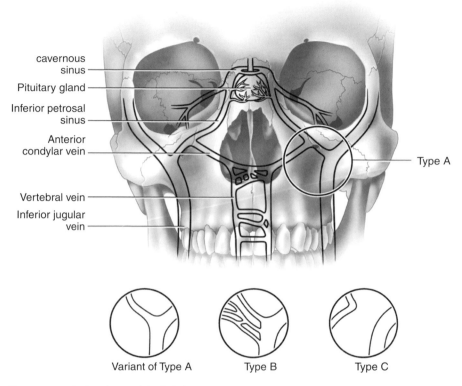

cavernous sinus

Pituitary gland

Inferior petrosal sinus

Anterior condylar vein

Type A

Vertebral vein

Inferior jugular vein

Variant of Type A   Type B   Type C

Fig. 2 Anatomical variants of the inferior petrosal sinus (IPS). *Type A* – venous drainage into the internal jugular vein is via a single inferior petrosal sinus (anterior condylar vein may or may not be in communication). *Type B* – drainage via a plexus of smaller vessels. *Type C* – IPS drains into the vertebral venous plexus via the anterior condylar vein

- The sheaths should be oversized by 1 French relative to the catheter used to allow peripheral venous sampling.

Intraprocedural Medications

- 3,000 IU of heparin following sheath insertion.
- CRH is given peripherally intraprocedurally. Human CRH should be used for BIPPS rather than alternatives such as ovine CRH that may interact with heparin to cause hypotension.

Performing the Procedure

- MPA 2 catheters positioned in the low internal jugular veins bilaterally. Venous sample taken over 60 s concurrently from both jugular veins and one femoral sheath.

- Both catheters positioned high in the internal jugular veins, further sample obtained over 60 s with peripheral sample.
- Catheter or micro-catheter used to access IPSS bilaterally. Venous angiogram to delineate IPS, cavernous, and intercavernous anatomy.
- Venogram should demonstrate both ipsilateral IPS filling and reflux into the contralateral system. Samples taken as described above.
- Peripheral administration of CRH (100 μg).
- Repeated sampling from both IPSS at 4–5 and 9–10 min post CRH.
- Following final sampling all samples are transported in an ice bath for immediate laboratory analysis.
- A diagnosis of a pituitary source for ACTH-dependent Cushing's syndrome can be made if the ratio of IPS to peripheral (IPS/P) ACTH level is >2 at baseline or >3 following CRH.

Potential Difficulties

- Crossing the left internal jugular valve – The angle between the innominate and left internal jugular combined with presence of a valve can make this difficult. A head-hunter (or similar) catheter can be useful as well as trying to cross the valve at different phases of respiration. If this fails, the procedure can easily be done via a low, direct puncture of the left internal jugular vein.
- Inferior petrosal sinus catheterization – Although this is more challenging in type B anatomy, with experience, this is often one of the more straightforward parts of the procedure. In the setting of the rare type C anatomy (approximately 1 %), adequate sampling can usually be achieved via the ipsilateral vertebral vein.

Alternative Techniques

- Some centers use desmopressin as an alternative to CRH.
- High jugular sampling is technically easier than BIPSS, with fewer complications. It has a similar specificity but slightly reduced sensitivity to BIPSS, 83 % vs 96 %.
- Cavernous sinus sampling has been proposed as an alternative technique to aid in tumor lateralization. This is more invasive and technically more challenging than BIPSS. Given the increased potential risk of neurological complications and the lack of consensus in the literature regarding the increased reliability of this technique, its use is currently not routine.

Complications

BIPSS is a safe procedure with serious complications being very rare when performed by experienced interventional radiologists.

Puncture Site Complications

- Groin hematoma 2–3 %
- Lower limb deep vein thrombosis 1 %

Procedural Complications

- Transient otalgia 1–2 %
- Transient 6th cranial nerve palsy 1 %
- Stroke <0.5 % but may be fatal

Key Points

> Noninvasive diagnostic tests often fail to exclude an ectopic source of ACTH in Cushing's syndrome.

> BIPSS with CRH administration can confirm or exclude a pituitary source for ACTH-dependent CS.

> BIPSS is technically challenging, and an awareness of anatomical variants is vital.

> BIPSS has a very high sensitivity and specificity with few complications.

Suggested Reading

1. Boscaro M, Arnaldi G. Approach to the patient with possible Cushing's syndrome. J Clin Endocrinol Metab. 2009;94:3121–31.
2. Deipolyi A, Karaosmanoğlu A, Habito C, Brannan S, Wicky S, Hirsch J, Oklu R. The role of bilateral inferior petrosal sinus sampling in the diagnostic evaluation of Cushing syndrome. Diagn Interv Radiol. 2012;18(1):132–8.
3. Doppman JL, Nieman LK, Chang R, et al. Selective venous sampling from the cavernous sinuses is not a more reliable technique than sampling from the inferior petrosal sampling in Cushing's syndrome. J Clin Endocrinol Metab. 1995;80:2485–9.
4. Ilias I, Chang R, Pacak K, et al. Jugular venous sampling: an alternative to petrosal sinus sampling for the diagnostic evaluation of adrenocorticotropic hormone-dependent Cushing's syndrome. J Clin Endocrinol Metab. 2004;89:3795–800.
5. Newell-Price J, Trainer P, Besser M, Grossman A. The diagnosis and differential diagnosis of Cushing's syndrome and pseudo-Cushing's states. Endocr Rev. 1998;19:647 72.

Intracranial Venous Thrombolysis/Mechanical Thrombectomy

Wilhelm Kuker and Lucy A. Matthews

Abstract

Thrombotic occlusions of the intracranial dural sinuses and veins are potentially life-threatening conditions occurring in all age groups. Predisposing factors are, among others, dehydration, clotting disorders, pregnancy, metabolic disorders, and smoking. The wider availability of noninvasive imaging techniques has led to an increasing pickup rate for this condition and an earlier diagnosis. This in turn has led to a reassessment of the risk of death or severe disability as initially fatal cases were mainly diagnosed postmortem.

Keywords

Intracranial venous thrombolysis • Mechanical thrombectomy thrombotic occlusion • Intracranial dural sinus • Intracranial dural veins • Life-threatening • Predisposing factors • Dehydration • Clotting disorders • Pregnancy • Metabolic disease • Smoking • Noninvasive imaging • Early diagnosis • Mortality • Severe disability

W. Kuker, MD, PhD, FRCR (✉) • L.A. Matthews, BMBS, MRCP
Department of Neuroradiology, John Radcliffe Hopsital, Oxford, UK
e-mail: wilhelm.kueker@orh.nhs.uk

K. Murphy, F. Robertson (eds.), *Interventional Neuroradiology,*
Techniques in Interventional Radiology,
DOI 10.1007/978-1-4471-4582-0_18, © Springer-Verlag London 2014

Introduction

- Cerebral venous thrombosis (CVT) is defined as thrombotic occlusion of the intracranial dural sinuses and veins and can occur in all age groups with potentially life-threatening consequences.
- Incidence of CVT:
  - Adult 0.22 per 100,000 per year
  - Pediatric 0.67 per 100,000 per year
- Mean presentation age is 39 years with 3 to 1 female predominance.
- Predisposing factors include dehydration, congenital and acquired coagulation disorders, pregnancy, metabolic disorders, and smoking.
- Increased awareness and availability of reliable imaging techniques has led to earlier diagnosis and more effective treatment.
- In the acute CVT, treatment aims to reverse the underlying cause, control seizures, and manage intracranial hypertension.
- Systemic anticoagulation (IV heparin followed by warfarin) has been shown to improve outcome, probably by preventing propagation of thrombus, allowing endogenous thrombolytic mechanisms to restore venous drainage pathways.
- Recent data suggests better outcomes with low-molecular-weight over unfractionated heparin.
- Among 624 patients in the ISCVT trial, the 30-day mortality was 3.4 % and mortality at end of follow-up was 8.8 %. 5.1 % of the patients were left dependent (modified Rankin scale >2).
- Despite these advances, medical treatment alone is insufficient in a minority.
- Endovascular strategies have been developed to disrupt or remove clot material and/or deliver local thrombolytic agents at the site of occlusion.
- Endovascular treatment results have been mixed, often because treatment has only been attempted late in the clinical course when medical treatment has failed and often where intracerebral hemorrhage has already occurred.
- Outcome data on thrombolysis in CVT is scant.
- A prospective study published in 2008 reported 20 patients of whom 14 had hemorrhagic infarcts, and 12 were comatose with 5 coning pre-thrombolysis. In spite of these unfavorable odds, 12 patients (60 %) made a full recovery or were left with minor disability. 6 patients died.

Diagnostic Evaluation

Clinical

Presenting features include headache, seizure, papilledema, focal neurological deficits, and impaired consciousness.

One or more risk factors are found in >85 % and include:

- Congenital or acquired prothrombotic disorder
- Head and neck infections
- Pregnancy or oral contraceptive pill
- Systemic infection, inflammation, or malignancy
- Connective tissue disorders

Laboratory

Full blood workup including thrombophilia screening
Exclusion of underlying septic, inflammatory and malignant processes, where appropriate

Imaging

CT Pre- and Post-intravenous Contrast (and/or CT Venogram)

- Usually reliable.
- Intravenous thrombus is hyperdense in the acute phase and expands the sinus, becoming hypodense over following weeks.
- Contrast demonstrates a filling defect "delta sign."
- May demonstrate parenchymal edema and hemorrhage.

MRI/MRV (+/– Gadolinium)

- All sequences are prone to artifact and can be confusing with both false positive and negative results, but usually experienced interpretation of all sequences in conjunction allows accurate detection and localization of clot (if in doubt do a CT).
- Superior to CT for demonstrating early parenchymal changes.

Indications

- Proven CVT with referable clinical deterioration despite >24 h of anticoagulation
- CVT with significant clinical impairment, i.e., coma due to deep cerebral venous thrombosis unlikely to respond to systemic anticoagulation
- Absolute contraindication to anticoagulation, i.e., active bleeding

Contraindications

- None

(Presence of parenchymal hematoma is NOT a contraindication to anticoagulant or locally delivered thrombolytic agents unless massive and likely to require surgical intervention.)

Patient Preparation

- Appropriate consent should be obtained documenting specific risks of procedure including cerebral venous hemorrhage and pulmonary embolus.
- Patient should be maintained well hydrated with intravenous fluid infusions, and anticoagulant therapy need not be stopped for the endovascular intervention.

Relevant Anatomy

- Location and extent of the thrombus as well as any patient-specific anatomical variants can be determined on noninvasive imaging. A careful assessment will allow therapeutic plan. The operator must therefore be familiar with the superficial and deep venous anatomy and its variants.
- The superficial cerebral structures drain into the superficial venous system, predominantly via the superior sagittal sinus into one or other transverse venous sinus at the torcula.
- The deep cerebral structures drain into the deep venous system-basal veins/vein of Galen, internal cerebral veins, and inferior sagittal sinus which drain via the straight sinus usually into the other transverse venous sinus.
- Usually there is communication between the deep and superficial systems at the torcula, but this connection can be very small and difficult to catheterize.
- Transverse sinuses are often unequal in size and one side may indeed be hypoplastic and difficult/dangerous to catheterize.
- A hypoplastic transverse sinus can usually be distinguished from a functionally collapsed one by the size of its bony groove on cross-sectional imaging (small groove equals true hypoplastic sinus).
- The internal jugular vein can sometimes be difficult to access retrogradely from the cava due to tortuosity, stenosis, or the presence of valves. Direct US-guided jugular vein puncture in the neck may be necessary.

Equipment

There are many strategies – the operator should have several at disposal, as a combined technique may be necessary. Equipment to be considered should include:

- Large caliber 6 F or greater guide catheter or long arterial sheath to allow stable working platform in proximal veins and big lumen for potential thrombectomy
- Coaxial distal access catheter (i.e., distal access catheter 038–057, Concentric Medical)
- Large microcatheter for access distal to clot (size 21 or larger)
- Soft-tipped 14 microwire for distal access
- Thrombectomy device, e.g., large syringe for suction, Penumbra suction device, or mechanical recanalization device, i.e., Solitaire FR stent
- Thrombolytic agent; tissue plasminogen activator (tPA) – dose according to locally agreed protocols (authors use up to maximum 0.9 mg /kg delivered as 20 % bolus followed by slow infusion)

Pre-procedure Medications

- None

Procedure

Access

- *4 F or 5 F arterial sheath* and operator's favored cerebral angiography catheter
- *Uni/bilateral 6 F venous sheath* depending on strategy [authors use 6 F guide catheter or long vascular sheath (e.g., Cook shuttle)]

Angiography

Cerebral Arteriography

- Will give a global picture of venous anatomy, drainage patterns, and current venous clot status (not obtainable from retrograde venography alone)
- Therefore performed initially

Retrograde Venography

- Guide catheter to the jugular bulb will support microcatheter or distal access catheter to pass into the intracranial venous system.
- Soft wire can be passed through soft sinus thrombus safely, but care must be taken to not pass inadvertently into fragile small cortical venous channels.
- Once into the target vein, contrast can be gently injected.

Treatment Plan and Technique

- Insufficient data to suggest optimal technique.
- Treatment centers around *clot disruption* to restore flow and increase clot surface area and to allow *delivery of rTPA* locally.
- A perfect venographic result is rarely possible or necessarily desirable.

Clot Disruption/Removal

- Various devices have been used including:
  - Mechanical disruption with catheter and wire
  - Suction thrombectomy with large catheter and 50 ml syringe or Penumbra device
  - Clot retrieval with "stroke" device, i.e., Solitaire stent-FR device

Local Thrombolysis

- Recombinant tissue plasmin activator (rTPA)
  - Ideally delivered upstream of clot so drug is maximally exposed to thrombus.
  - Optimal dosage unclear.
  - Authors use limit of maximum total rTPA dose of 0.9 mg/kg body weight.
  - Sometimes an rTPA bolus followed by infusion over several hours via a retained venous catheter is appropriate (i.e., with partial mechanical recanalization)
    - Bolus: 10–20 % total dose
    - Infusion: 0.1 mg/kg/h up to total dose of 0.9 mg/kg

Immediate Post-procedure Care

- Dependent on pre-procedural state (usually poor mandating intensive care with considerable support)
- Specific care if retained venous catheter – to ensure appropriate drug delivery and enable easy repeat venography to assess efficacy

Complications

- Parenchymal or subarachnoid hemorrhage – venous trauma or hemorrhagic transformation of venous ischemic brain
- Pulmonary embolus

Follow-Up and Post-procedure Medications

- Ongoing anticoagulation usually indicated.
- Correct timing to resume after rTPA is unclear after procedure.
- Usually IV heparin is used for the first few days as its effects are more easily reversed than low-molecular-weight heparin.
- Imaging:
  - Repeat direct venography if catheter retained.
  - MRI to evaluate evolution of parenchymal changes.
  - MR/CT venography to follow vessel abnormalities.

Key Points

> CVT may be missed unless it is suspected.
> CVT is usually best managed with systemic anticoagulation.
> Endovascular intervention should be considered in those who deteriorate despite treatment (recognizing this subgroup early is very difficult).
> Bad looking scan and bad clinical state do not mean bad outcome.
> Endovascular goal is to restore venous flow and to deliver rTPA locally (by infusion if necessary).
> A perfect angiographic result is rarely achieved and may not be desirable.

Case Report

A 15-year-old girl presented with acute confusion and generalized seizure following a 10-day history of headache with vomiting. No relevant past medical history; she was not on oral contraceptives. On examination she was afebrile, BP 118/69, GCS 15, no papilledema, and no focal neurological signs. Unenhanced CT study showed normal brain parenchyma but hyperdense dural venous sinuses including the straight sinus (Fig. 1). The internal cerebral veins were not affected.

CVT was diagnosed, and low-molecular-weight heparin was started, but she continued to deteriorate to unconsciousness. Repeat CT study the next day showed progression of the sinus thrombus to involve the internal cerebral veins with bilateral thalamic edema (Fig. 2).

At this point she was referred for endovascular clot extraction and thrombolysis.

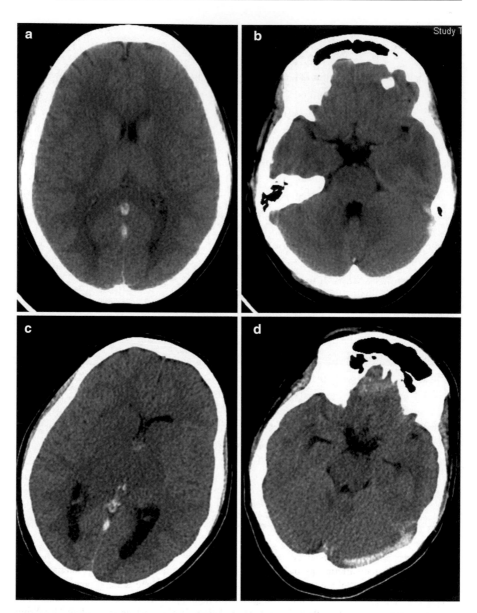

Fig. 1 Non-contrast-enhanced CT of the brain at presentation (**a, b**) and after clinical deterioration on the day of the angiography (**c, d**). (**a**) This non-contrast CT shows hyperdensity of the vein of Galen and the straight sinus consistent with thrombotic occlusion. Not the normal density of the superior sagittal sinus. There is no abnormality of the brain parenchyma, especially not of the thalami. (**b**) This CT at a more caudal location shows a hyperdense left sigmoid sinus and a normal right sigmoid. (**c**) This non-enhanced CT scan before and after the patient became unconscious shows prominent thalamic edema bilaterally. The low-density changes extend into the medial basal ganglia on the left. There is high density of the internal cerebral veins, the vein of Galen, and the straight sinus. (**d**) This slice shows now a large hyperdense thrombus in the left transverse sinus. As this clot propagation had occurred under intravenous heparin medication, the patient was referred for endovascular treatment with selective thrombolysis and clot aspiration

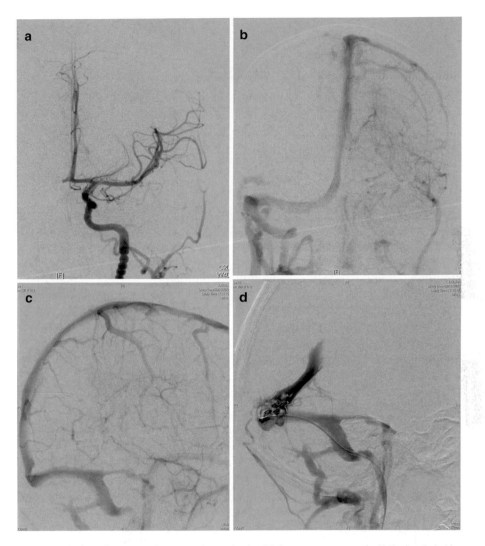

Fig. 2 Cerebral angiogram under general anesthesia. Right venous approach (6 F sheath in the femoral vein) and left arterial approach (5 F sheath in the femoral artery). (**a**) Left internal carotid artery injection, arterial phase, and anterior posterior projection. There is a conspicuous "string of pearls" appearance of the distal left ICA suggestive of homocystinuria. (**b**) The venous phase of the same injection does not show the left transverse and sigmoid sinus, which are occluded by thrombus. (**c**) The lateral view of the left ICA injection fails to demonstrate the straight sinus and the internal cerebral veins. Only one transverse and sigmoid sinus is visible. (**d**) A Vasco 35 microcatheter is seen in the confluens sinuum adjacent to a clot protruding from the straight sinus into the confluens. (**e**) The tip of the Vasco is now located at the junction of the vein of Galen and the straight sinus. Both structures are filled with thrombus. There is also partial filling of the inferior sagittal sinus. (**f**) Repeated injection of rTPA and aspiration has resulted in a substantial reduction of the clot with partial recanalization of the straight sinus. Several air bubbles can be seen in the inferior sagittal sinus. The vein of Galen is only partially recanalized. (**g**) After application of a total dose of 0.9 mg rTPA/kg body weight, there is a substantial recanalization of the straight sinus with some residual thrombus adjacent to the confluens sinuum. The procedure was terminated at this stage

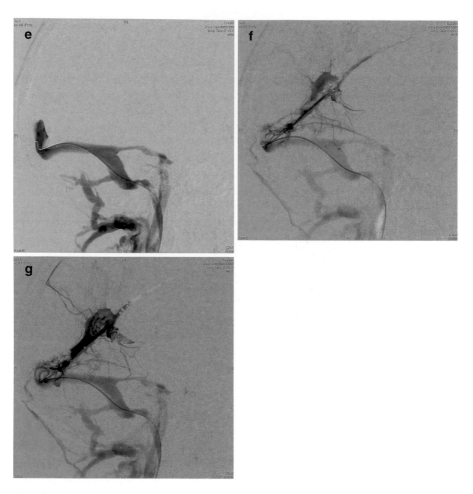

Fig. 2 (continued)

Under general anesthesia, diagnostic arteriography confirmed occlusion of the left transverse and sigmoid sinus, deep cerebral venous system, and straight sinus.

The angiogram also showed fibromuscular dysplasia in both internal carotid arteries.

From the pattern of deterioration, the primary treatment target was the straight sinus and internal cerebral venous system rather than the left transverse sinus. Via a 6 F femoral venous sheath, a 6 F Envoy guiding catheter was advanced into the right jugular bulb. A Vasco 35 microcatheter was then advanced through the right transverse sinus and into the occluded straight sinus over a Transcend 14 microwire. Local bolus injections of diluted rTPA were repeatedly made into the clot alternating with aspirations through the Vasco catheter, resulting in a significant reduction of the amount of thrombus in the straight sinus. The catheter was then advanced into the vein of Galen, and the process repeated. In total

0.9 mg/kg body weight of rTPA was used, most of which was re-aspirated during the procedure. At the end of the treatment, the straight sinus and vein of Galen were patent, while the internal cerebral veins and the left transverse sinus remained occluded. The patient remained intubated and sedated in intensive care under continuing intravenous heparin.

A CT study the next day showed a reduced thalamic edema and patent straight sinus, vein of Galen, and internal cerebral veins. She was extubated the same day and fully recovered with no residual deficit over the next weeks. Later factor VII deficiency and hyperhomocystinuria were identified as predisposing conditions for cerebral venous thrombosis.

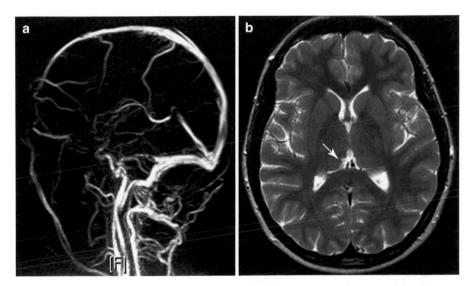

Fig. 3 Follow-up MRI and MRV after 3 months. (**a**) This sagittal maximum intensity projection of a 3D phase contrast MR venogram shows a patent straight sinus and vein of Galen with what appears a residual stenosis at the junction of these vessels. There is an asymmetry of the internal cerebral veins with the left larger than the right. (**b**) This T2-weighted MRI of the brain shows a very small residual defect of the right posterior and medial thalamus (*white arrow*)

Summary of Case

- 6 F catheter sheath right femoral vein
- 5 F catheter sheath left femoral artery
- 5 F diagnostic catheter for angiogram and then left in the carotid artery with flush
- 6 F guiding catheter in the internal jugular vein or jugular bulb with flush
- Vasco 35 or other flexible catheter placed into the sinus over soft guidewire
- Repeated injection of saline and rTPA into clot and aspiration of thrombotic material
- Total rTPA dosage not to exceed 0.9 mg/kg body weight

Recommended Reading

1. de Veber G, Andrew M, Adams C, Bjornson B, Booth F, Buckley DJ, Camfield CS, David M, Humphreys P, Langevin P, MacDonald EA, Gillett J, Meaney B, Shevell M, Sinclair DB, Yager J. Cerebral sinovenous thrombosis in children. N Engl J Med. 2001;345(6):417–23. doi:10.1056/NEJM200108093450604.
2. Ferro JM, Canhao P, Stam J, Bousser MG, Barinagarrementeria F. Prognosis of cerebral vein and dural sinus thrombosis: results of the International Study on Cerebral Vein and Dural Sinus Thrombosis (ISCVT). Stroke. 2004;35(3):664–70. doi:10.1161/01.STR.000011 7571.76197.26.
3. Stam J, Majoie CB, van Delden OM, van Lienden KP, Reekers JA. Endovascular thrombectomy and thrombolysis for severe cerebral sinus thrombosis: a prospective study. Stroke. 2008;39(5):1487–90. doi:10.1161/STROKEAHA.107.502658. STROKEAHA.107.502658 [pii].

Part VIII

Interventional Neuro-Oncology

Percutaneous Treatment of Venolymphatic Malformations, Extracranial Arteriovenous Malformations, and Tumors of the Head and Neck Using Particles, Alcohol, and Other Sclerosants

Jessica Spence and Ronit Agid

Abstract

Historically, craniofacial lesions have been treated surgically. The advent of image-guided endovascular techniques, however, enabled their application to the treatment of vascular malformations and tumors. Optimal treatment requires a multidisciplinary approach. This will be center specific and determined by available expertise and skills. Goals of treatment, nature of the lesion, and its associated angioarchitecture influence decisions regarding treatment planning. Venolymphatic malformations are typically treated by percutaneous sclerotherapy, with or without surgical adjunct. Different sclerosants are described in the literature, with bleomycin increasingly chosen because of its efficacy and favorable side effect.

Keywords

Percutaneous venolymphatic malformations • Extracranial AV malformations • Alcohol • Sclerosants • Extracranial arteriovenous malformations • Facial AVMs

J. Spence, MD
Department of Medical Imaging, Division of Neuroradiology, Toronto Western Hospital, Toronto, ON, Canada

R. Agid, MD, FRCPC (✉)
Department of Medical Imaging, Division of Neuroradiology, Toronto Western Hospital, University of Toronto, Toronto, ON, Canada

K. Murphy, F. Robertson (eds.), *Interventional Neuroradiology,*
Techniques in Interventional Radiology,
DOI 10.1007/978-1-4471-4582-0_19, © Springer-Verlag London 2014

Introduction

- Historically, craniofacial lesions have been treated surgically. The advent of image-guided endovascular techniques, however, enabled their application to the treatment of vascular malformations and tumors.
- Optimal treatment requires a multidisciplinary approach. This will be center specific and determined by available expertise and skills.
- Goals of treatment, nature of the lesion, and its associated angioarchitecture influence decisions regarding treatment planning.
- Venolymphatic malformations (VLMs) are typically treated by percutaneous sclerotherapy, with or without surgical adjunct (Fig. 1). Different sclerosants are described in the literature, with bleomycin increasingly chosen because of its efficacy and favorable side-effect profile.
- Extracranial arteriovenous malformations (facial AVMs) are generally treated by pre-operative embolization, followed by surgical resection. Typically, this is done transarterially, with percutaneous injection of embolic agents sometimes used as an adjunct (Figs. 2 and 3).
- Because of their hypervascularity, embolization of craniofacial tumors has become an established technique, either for curative, preoperative, or palliative management. Initially, transarterial approaches involving a variety of embolic agents were described. (Percutaneous treatment, alone or in conjunction with endovascular embolization, is increasingly preferred because of easier access and, as a result, more complete devascularization.)

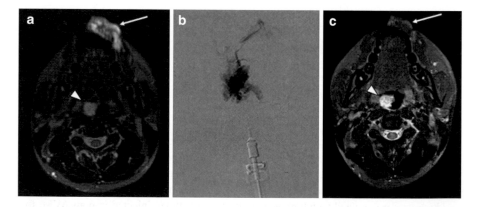

Fig. 1 Percutaneous sclerotherapy of facial venolymphatic malformation. A 25-year-old man presented with a left lower lip vascular malformation. Axial T2 fat sat MRI demonstrated a hyperintense lesion, consistent with a VLM (*arrow* **a**). Percutaneous sclerotherapy was performed using bleomycin. Throughout the procedure, each needle insertion was followed by phlebography to confirm location within the lesion and assess drainage (**b**). This was followed by injection of bleomycin under continuous subtraction fluoroscopy using the negative subtraction technique. A total of 3 sclerotherapy sessions was completed. Follow-up MRI performed several months after treatment demonstrates a significant reduction in size with a small area of residual hyperintensity (*arrow* **c**). This particular patient had multiple craniofacial VLMs, including one in the oropharynx (*arrow head* **a, c**), which was later treated with airway protection. *MRI* magnetic resonance imaging, *VLM* venolymphatic malformation

Using Embolic and Sclerosing Agents in the Treatment of Head and Neck Lesions

Selection of Approach and Choice of Embolic Agent

- Decisions regarding approach are contingent on the type of lesion and management goals. Definitive treatment will require a different modality than temporary diminishment of vascular supply (i.e., as for presurgical devascularization). This will inform the decision to use a liquid embolic, particles, or a sclerosant.
- Embolization is the intentional occlusion of vasculature using a foreign material (e.g., n-butyl cyanoacrylate (NBCA), ethylene vinyl alcohol copolymer (onyx), or polyvinyl alcohol (PVA) particles). Sclerotherapy, on the other hand, is the obliteration of a blood vessel using an agent (e.g., alcohol, bleomycin) that causes endothelial cell destruction and thrombosis through denaturation and cellular dehydration. There is no current consensus in the literature as to which agent/technique is ideal for a given clinical situation, with center-specific preferences and local expertise largely determining practice.
- Prior to selecting an embolic agent, it is important to consider why the embolization is being performed, whether temporary or permanent occlusion is required, the diameter of the vessel to be embolized, what is downstream from it, and the velocity of flow through this vessel.
- Whether performing percutaneous embolization or sclerotherapy, phlebography should always be completed as an initial step prior to treatment. This is important for complete visualization of the angioarchitecture of the lesion as well as its venous drainage.

Liquid Embolics

- These include the cyanoacrylate glues, most commonly NBCA and onyx. They are preferred clinically because of their low recanalization rates and are thus appropriate for permanent vessel occlusion (e.g., as in treatment of AVMs).
- Cyanoacrylate, or N--butyl-2-cyanoacrylate (NBCA), is a rapidly hardening liquid adhesive that polymerizes immediately on contact with blood or other ionic fluids. Polymerization causes an exothermic reaction that destroys the vessel wall.
- Because it hardens so quickly, controlling its final position can be difficult. As a result, safe use of this material requires extensive training and experience.
- Onyx is an ethylene vinyl alcohol copolymer dissolved in dimethyl sulfoxide (DMSO), which uses micronized tantalum as a contrast agent. When injected into an AVM, the DMSO dissipates, causing the copolymer to form a spongy occlusive cast in the artery. It propagates easily into vessels and has a consistency that makes it easier to resect than some cyanoacrylates used as embolic agents. Drawbacks include a need for slow injection, which results in a longer procedure with relatively increased radiation exposure for both patient and surgeon.
- Injection of any liquid embolic may result in opening of unexpected anastomoses and is thus associated with a risk of cerebral infarction, cranial nerve palsy, and cerebral hemorrhage.

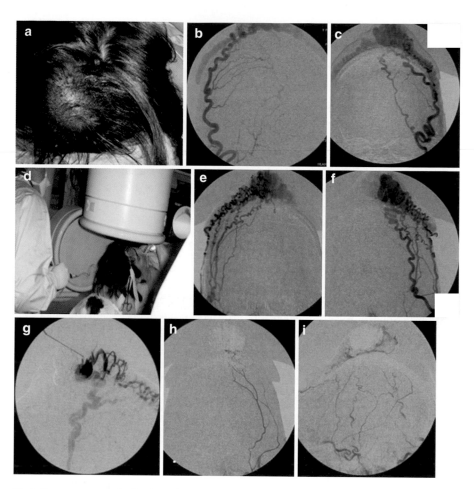

Fig. 2 Percutaneous embolization of scalp AVM with NBCA. Young women presented with progressive enlargement of a scalp AVM (**a**). Diagnostic angiogram showed bilateral supply this AVM from the external carotid arteries (**b, c, e, f**). AP views of right (**b**) and left (**c**) occipital artery and right (**e**) and left (**f**) distal external carotid artery are shown. These arteries were extremely torturous and it was unlikely to obtain an optimal distal positioning of microcatheter to cure the AVM via transarterial embolization. A tourniquet was applied to the patient's head around the nidus of the lesion and a butterfly needle was inserted into the nidus (**d**). Diagnostic phlebography was performed through each direct puncture prior to injection of glue (**g**). This was followed by percutaneous glue embolization which resulted in cure of AVM. Post-embolization angiogram of the left external carotid artery in AP (**h**) and lateral (**i**) projection shows no residual shunting. *NBCA* n-butyl cyanoacrylate, *AVM* arteriovenous malformation

Particles

- These are available in variable sizes (50–2,000 μm) and are relatively inexpensive. They cause a mild inflammatory response and nonpermanent occlusion, thus making them appropriate only for temporary embolotherapy. Typically, they are used for preoperative devascularization of tumors. They are also used to induce thrombosis in a vessel secondary to partial success of an earlier endovascular embolization procedure.

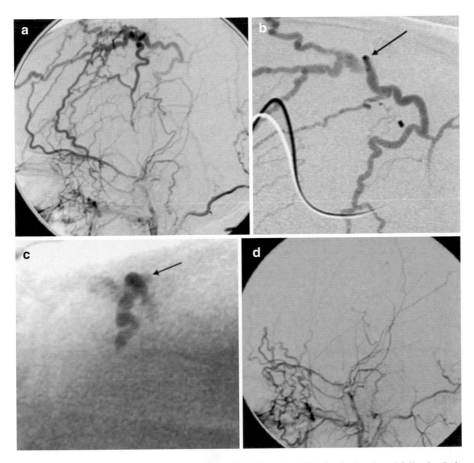

Fig. 3 Percutaneous embolization of iatrogenic AVF of the scalp. This fistula developed following hair transplantation. (**a**) Lateral angiogram of right ECA injection shows a single whole AVF supplied by tortuous branches of the superficial temporal artery and drains into several scalp veins. (**b**) Selective angiogram via direct percutaneous needle at the fistulous site showing the draining veins (*arrows* shows puncture site). (**c**) Image of the glue cast after embolization with NBCA through the percutaneous needle (*arrow* shows the puncture site). (**d**) Post-embolization angiogram of ECA shows complete cure of the AVF. *AVF* arteriovenous fistula, *NBCA* n-butyl cyanoacrylate, *ECA* external carotid artery

Drawbacks include recanalization, poor radiopacity, and the possibility of embolization to the arteries of lungs, brain, or cranial nerves.

Sclerosants

- All sclerosants work by causing damage to vascular endothelia through various mechanisms.
- Ethanol (absolute alcohol) is the most commonly used sclerosant. It has a direct toxic effect on vascular endothelia that activates the coagulation system and causes microaggregation of red blood cells. It damages capillary beds of healthy tissue (e.g., skin) and is usually associated with significant soft tissue swelling and pain on injection. As such, it is usually administered under general anesthesia.

- Most other commonly used sclerosants are alcohol derivatives, e.g., sodium tetradecyl sulfate (Sotradecol) and ethanolamine oleate. Use of these agents is both less painful and toxic then absolute alcohol. As a result, some lesions can be treated without general anesthesia.
- Recently, the off-label use of bleomycin – a cytotoxic antitumor agent – has been described. Its sclerosing effect on endothelial cells was originally applied to the treatment of venous malformations and hemangiomas. Since this initial report, a number of studies have been published, supporting both the treatment efficacy and relatively low complication rate.
- Regarding possible complications of sclerosants and safety measures (see chapter "Diagnostic Cerebral Angiography and Groin Access and Closure").

Delivery: Endovascular Versus Percutaneous

- Transarterial embolization is an established technique to devascularize lesions; results may be curative, preoperative, or palliative. However, endovascular embolization may be limited due to vessel tortuosity, vasospasm, atherosclerotic disease, or very small arterial feeders.
- Because of these limitations, there has been increasing use of percutaneous embolization (PTE) to devascularize head and neck lesions. Initially, this was applied to the treatment of VLMs (Figs. 1 and 2). More recently, this approach has been applied to the treatment of craniofacial AVMs (Figs. 2 and 3) and craniofacial tumors.
- PTE has allowed easy access to the lesion and overcomes the limitations of endovascular treatment. Though still an emerging modality, some authors have stated a preference for it, believing that PTE allows for a more complete devascularization of craniofacial lesions.

Indications for Intervention

Venolymphatic Malformations

- Pain, functional impairment (secondary to swelling or pain), or esthetic concerns.
- Absolute indications include lesions that threaten vital functions because of their location and mass effect (i.e., vision, airway compromise).

Facial AVMs

- Hemorrhagic events, pain, and ulceration.
- Treatment is absolutely indicated in cases associated with symptomatic congestive heart failure and where vital functions are threatened.
- Less commonly it may be provided for issues of cosmesis.
- Asymptomatic AVM should be observed unless possible to cure with minimal morbidity; embolization or incomplete excision may stimulate regrowth and increased symptoms.

Tumors of Head and Neck

- Preoperative embolization to reduce perioperative blood loss.
- Palliation of symptoms related to a growing tumor, including compression and destruction of adjacent structures.

Contraindications to Intervention

Absolute

- Known anaphylactic reaction to contrast or the intended embolic agent

Relative

- Inability to tolerate a general anesthetic.
- Kidney failure, which can be treated with prophylactic intravenous hydration and bicarbonate therapy plus oral dosing of N-acetyl cysteine.
- A high degree of risk associated with inherent post-procedural swelling due to lesion location, e.g., airway compromise. Swelling can be partially prevented by steroid administration at the end of the procedure and for several days thereafter. In extreme cases patients may require prophylactic tracheostomy prior to the procedure.

General Patient Preparation

- General anesthesia or conscious sedation is commonly used, although the decision of whether or not they are employed and the choice of one over the other are center specific.
- The procedure is performed under sterile conditions in an imaging suite that is adequately equipped for the modality chosen. The patient is positioned and draped in a sterile fashion that provides best access to the lesion.

Percutaneous Treatment of Venolymphatic Malformations of the Head and Neck

Clinical Features

- Venolymphatic malformations (VLMs) are rare with a prevalence of 1 % and an estimated incidence of 1–2 in 10,000 births. They represent, however, a common reason for referral to interventional radiology departments in vascular malformation centers.
- These congenital anomalies consist of "slow-flow" dysmorphic channels lined by flattened endothelium and a thin basement membrane.

- In VMs these channels are filled with venous blood and, in LMs, with lymphatic fluid.
- Historically, there have been issues with misdiagnosis and classification. In 1982 Mulliken and Glowacki developed a dichotomous classification system to which several subdivisions have since been proposed. The most clinically relevant does so on the basis of vascular dynamics, with arteriovenous malformations (AVMs) classified as high flow and venous malformations (VMs) as low flow. Although lymphatic malformations (LMs) are considered separately, most clinicians regard them as fitting in the same category as VMs because of both similar flow characteristics and treatment.
- Though present at birth, venolymphatic malformations (VLMs) may become clinically apparent at any time throughout the lifespan.

Diagnostic Evaluation

- VMs present in various ways, from a vague blue patch on the skin to a soft, compressible, nonpulsatile mass; 40 % of cases are found in the head and neck region.
- The most common symptoms include pain, compression of adjacent structures, and cosmetic deformity.
- Compressive symptoms relate to location of the lesion and compression of adjacent structures. In the oropharynx, they may cause dysphagia and airway compromise. Lesions located in and around the orbit may result in visual issues and impaired extraocular movements.
- Physical exam typically demonstrates a soft, compressible, blue-tinged mass that enlarges with dependent positioning or Valsalva.
- Confirmation of diagnosis with imaging is indicated in order to rule out other entities such as malignant solid tumors of the head and neck.
- Magnetic resonance (MR) imaging is largely recognized as the gold standard. The most useful sequence is fat saturated T2 weighting (Fig. 1). The classic MR appearance of VMs is that of a soft tissue mass that is hyperintense on T2-weighted images and hypointense on T1-weighted images. Multiple, rounded hypointense areas on T2 representing phleboliths, or intralesional calcifications, may be noted. Enhancement after intravenous (IV) administration of gadolinium will be noted, mostly peripherally.
- LMs have a similar appearance on MR, being hyperintense on T2 and hypointense on T1. These non-enhancing lesions appear as cysts containing fluid-fluid levels; phleboliths are not seen.
- Ultrasonography is frequently used as an initial imaging modality because of its low cost, widespread availability, and lack of ionizing radiation, a particular concern given the fact that lesions are often diagnosed in the pediatric population.
- The primary utility of ultrasound is to differentiate between high-flow (AVM) and low-flow (VM, LM) lesions and, if the latter, to distinguish LMs from VMs based on their cystic appearance.

Treatment

- Conservative management is advocated for those lesions that do not meet the threshold for intervention. It consists of reassurance, elevation of the involved area during sleep, and avoidance of activities associated with symptom exacerbation.
- Cessation of oral contraceptives may provide relief for those whose lesions are hormonally sensitive.
- When indicated, the treatment of choice is percutaneous sclerotherapy with or without surgical excision.
- Laser therapy has also been described in the literature.
- Multidisciplinary approaches are emphasized, such that combinations of sclerotherapy, surgery, and laser can be tailored to patient preferences and lesion anatomy.

Patient Preparation

- Patient's expectations regarding treatment outcome should be clearly established. Specifically, the patient should understand that sclerotherapy does not completely cure VLMs but rather leads to decrease in size. Clinical benefit is seen in 75–100 %, dependent on both the definition of response and sclerosant used.
- Patients should be warned about the post-procedural swelling inherent to treatment, particularly if alcohol is to be used as a sclerosant.
- Patients with tongue or intra-orbital lesions are more prone to post-procedural swelling and infection. Thus, they should be prophylactically treated with steroids and antibiotics for several days after the procedure. Strong consideration should also be given to the choice of bleomycin as sclerosant, as it is associated with less post-procedural swelling.

Treatment Techniques

Direct Percutaneous Sclerotherapy

- Sclerotherapy begins with the introduction of a needle into the lesion, whose location is usually apparent by palpation. Alternatively, US can be used for guidance.
- The needle is advanced until blood (for VMs) or lymphatic fluid (for LMs) is noted in the hub. This signifies intraluminal positioning of the needle.
- Small amount (1–2 cc) of low-osmolarity, water-soluble iodinated contrast material is injected for phlebography, which should be performed prior to sclerotherapy.
- Phlebography verifies needle location and provides information regarding flow characteristics and drainage of the lesion. This is important to ensure there is no outflow to critical structures (e.g., cavernous sinus) and is of particular importance when using alcohol.
- If the VLM drains to risky areas, these should be blocked by external compression and phlebography repeated to ensure its effectiveness.

- Slow injection of sclerosant is then performed under digital subtraction angiography at a rate of one image every 2 s. The sclerosant injected into the lesion gradually replaces the previously injected contrast, pushing it towards the periphery of the lesion or into the draining veins of the VM. It appears as negative contrast (white) on DSA (Figs. 1 and 4).
- This "negative subtraction" technique (Fig. 4) eliminates the need to premix the sclerosant with a contrast agent. As well, it allows real-time visualization of the sclerosant as it is injected into the VLM, while preserving its high concentration and potency as a sclerosing agent.
- During injection of the sclerosant, the patient should be carefully monitored to assess for extravasation. Signs that may indicate chemical toxicity or ischemia to the skin include overly rapid efflux of sclerosant into the venous outflow, resistance to injection, or skin blanching. The presence of any of these should prompt immediate cessation of injection.
- Typically 1–3 cc of sclerosant will be injected to each "pocket" of the malformation.
- The procedure is repeated using multiple needle insertions, each followed by phlebography and sclerosant injection. This continues until the maximal dose is administered or when no blood return is noted, indicating that the VLM "pocket" is adequately treated.
- According to our experience a total of 10 cc of alcohol per session or up to 15 mg of bleomycin per session is the recommended dose.
- After the final injection all needles are removed. Light compression should be applied for several minutes until oozing at the puncture site stops.

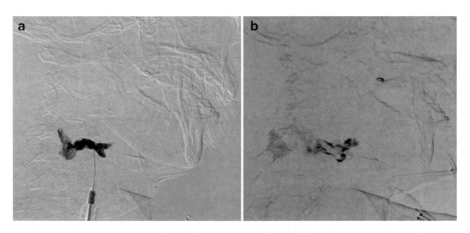

Fig. 4 Negative subtraction technique for sclerotherapy of VLM in the right neck: (**a**) RAO view of phlebography prior to sclerotherapy – contrast was injected into one of the pockets of the VLM. (**b**) Bleomycin injection under DSA into the region previously injected with contrast. Unopacified bleomycin is seen as a central white shadow due to "negative subtraction," while the previously injected contrast is pushed to the periphery of the lesion and posteriorly towards other parts of the VLM in the neck. *VLM* venolymphatic malformations

Choice of Sclerosant

- There is no consensus as to choice of sclerosant, with no randomized trials available to date. Currently, clinician familiarity, availability of the agent and lesion morphology has the greatest influence.
- Alcohol (100 % ethyl alcohol) is most commonly used, owing to the fact that it is readily available, inexpensive, and effective. It is also associated with the highest rates of complications, including skin necrosis, nerve damage, and severe post-procedural swelling.
- Other alcohol-based sclerosants include detergents and sclerosing foams. These are milder than alcohol and have lower complication rates. Concordantly, they also have lower potency and are less effective.
- Aggressive sclerosants (e.g., alcohol), which cause significant post-procedural swelling, are not recommended for use on lesions proximal to the airway or orbit.
- As it produces only minimal swelling after sclerotherapy (as opposed to ethanol-based agents), bleomycin is especially recommended for treatment of vulnerable areas such as the periorbit or regions related to the airway (i.e., the tongue and parapharyngeal spaces).

Modifications to Sclerotherapy Technique

- The above-described negative subtraction technique (Fig. 4) is an elegant way to visualize the injected sclerosant without the need to mix and dilute it with contrast material prior to injection. This increases sclerosant concentration and thereby its therapeutic efficacy.
- The use of alcohol to sclerose the draining vein of the lesion prior to bleomycin instillation has been described. This increases the therapeutic dwell time of the bleomycin within the lesion and decreases the dose (and potential toxicity) of the alcohol.
- In recent years, sclerosants have begun to be administered in foam form, a technique that maximally displaces blood from the treated vessel being treated, remains undiluted, and persists within the vessel so as to maximize its sclerosant effect. The method of foam production first described by Tessari has become the dominant method.
- Puig et al. have described a double-needle technique where a second needle is positioned away from the initial sclerotherapy needle but still within the lesion. Sclerosant is injected through the first needle and, as intralesional pressure increases, the combination of contrast, blood, and sclerosant exits out of the second needle, following the path of least resistance. This technique allows for close monitoring of the path and sclerosant distribution of the sclerosant and avoids passage into the systemic circulation. Additionally, by dispersing intraluminal pressure, the second needle prevents extravasation into adjacent normal vessels and thus local tissue damage.

Post-procedure Management and Follow-Up

- The pain and swelling associated with the post-sclerotherapy period almost invariably necessitates prescription of analgesics or anti-inflammatory agents.
- Steroids are not routinely given, although stronger sclerosants, larger treatment areas, or proximity to vital structures may necessitate their use.
- There is no consensus in the literature as to length of hospital stay post-procedure. Typically, the patient can be discharged after recovery from anesthesia.
- Patients should be seen in follow-up 3–4 weeks subsequent to their procedure. This visit can be used to assess level of satisfaction and need for further therapy. Additional ultrasound examinations may also be performed to evaluate flow and regional involution to direct further therapy.
- Most lesions require more than one session of treatment. Should the lesion require additional sclerotherapy sessions, these should be spaced 6–8 weeks apart.
- Though some have recommended MR imaging as a means of evaluating treatment outcome, several recent papers have shown that it does not correlate with clinical outcomes for either peripheral or craniofacial VLMs.

Results of Sclerotherapy

- The efficacy of sclerotherapy has been evaluated by a number of different measures. These include qualitative measures, such as patient survey, clinician's review of before and after photographs, and documentation in the chart. No quantitative measures have been validated.
- Owing to the lack of standardized outcome measures, it is difficult to compare results of different studies. Nonetheless, depending on both the measure and sclerosant used, 75–100 % of patients receive some benefit from treatment according to reports in the literature.
- Two studies have compared sclerosants. The first, a nonrandomized examination of patients treated with sodium morrhuate and/or pingyangmycin found that outcomes were slightly better with pingyangmycin than sodium morrhuate and that results were best when the two sclerosants were combined. A second retrospective comparison of alcohol and bleomycin in matched lesions found that alcohol had a slightly higher success rate as compared to bleomycin, which usually requires a greater number of treatment sessions. Additionally, alcohol was found to have a higher complication rate and more inherent post-procedural swelling, and it was suggested that bleomycin treatment may be better tolerated.

Safety of Sclerotherapy

- Percutaneous sclerotherapy for VLM is a relatively safe procedure, provided certain guidelines are followed:
  - Doses of sclerosant should be limited to the maximal allowable dose per treatment session. According to our experience it is not recommended to inject more than 10 cc of alcohol per session and up to 15 mg of bleomycin per session.

— Consideration should be given to completing the sclerotherapy using lower doses over a greater number of sessions when treated VLMs in sensitive regions (e.g., orbit, parotid, tongue).

— Phlebography should always be used to assess drainage prior to sclerosant injection. If external compression is deemed necessary, effectiveness of compression should be confirmed by repeat phlebography.

— Steroids and antibiotics should be administered when treating sensitive locations (orbit, tongue) so as to prevent infection and regional swelling and its sequelae, as well as infection.

— When bleomycin is used, precautions should be taken to prevent skin hyperpigmentation (see section "Complications of Sclerotherapy").

Complications of Sclerotherapy

All Sclerosants

- Post-procedural swelling and pain. The degree to which this is an issue depends on the dose and the sclerosant used, with alcohol the most severe in this regard.
- Studies have found that the degree of post-procedure swelling correlates with treatment efficacy of alcohol-based sclerosants, and it is speculated to represent the degree of endothelial damage that has taken place.
- Other adverse effects are sclerosant-specific (see below).

Bleomycin

- Nausea, mouth dryness, and vomiting, which may last up to 48 h after sclerotherapy. This is treated with antiemetics and hydration (rarely IV fluids are needed).
- Skin hyperpigmentation, which is typically reversible but may persist. Hyperemia in treated regions, with local infusion of bleomycin, results in blood vessel microtrauma with even minor abrasion of the skin (e.g., removal of tape and EKG stickers). It may be prevented by securing the endotracheal tube by tying and not applying adhesives to the skin during treatment – particularly on the face. ECG leads should be left in place for several days post-procedure until hyperemia resolves. Additionally, trauma to the skin should be avoided (e.g., playing with house pets, sports) for 48 h following treatment.
- Pulmonary fibrosis is the major complication seen in cancer patients treated with systemic bleomycin. To date, no cases of pulmonary fibrosis have been reported in the literature secondary to its use as a sclerotherapy agent. This is likely because, as opposed to patients treated systemically, sclerotherapy does not result in substantial amount of bleomycin in the bloodstream. As well, both the per session and cumulative doses used for sclerotherapy (<15 mg and <120 mg, respectively) (1–6, 43, 48–49) are well below the systemic dose of 200–450 mg recognized in the cancer literature to be associated with an increased risk of pulmonary fibrosis.

Alcohol

- Alcohol is widely recognized to be associated with the highest complication rates of all sclerosants, with some reporting rates as high as 50 %. These are related to tissue extravasation with resultant ischemia and are best prevented by careful periprocedural monitoring and the use of lower doses.
- If large amounts of absolute alcohol enter the systemic circulation, toxic effects can occur. These include central nervous system (CNS) depression, hemolysis, and cardiac arrest. Slow, careful delivery, using occlusion of venous outflow systems through manual compression, tourniquet control, or balloon occlusion may decrease alcohol washout from the lesion and reduce acute systemic toxicity. According to literature ethanol 1 cc/kg is the maximum amount that can be injected during a single session. However, according to our experience it is not recommended to inject more than 10 cc per session.
- Facial nerve palsy is commonly reported when treating lesions in the region of the parotid gland with alcohol. It is typically transient although may be permanent.
- Other complications include skin ulceration and venous thrombosis.

Alcohol Derivatives

- These have a similar adverse effect profile to alcohol, although they are less frequent and tend to occur at higher doses.

Percutaneous Treatment of Extracranial Arteriovenous Malformations (Facial AVMs)

Clinical Features

- Arteriovenous malformations (AVM) represent direct communications between an artery and a vein with or without an intervening nidal component that occurs as a result of turbulent flow. They are most commonly found intracranially, with the most common extracranial sites being the cheek, ear, nose, and forehead in order of frequency.
- Although mostly congenital in nature, facial AVMs are not typically detected until later in childhood after additional growth or vascular engorgement occurs.
- Clinically, they present as a pulsatile mass and cause asymmetry, pain, pressure, dental malalignment, or hemorrhage.
- Given that AVMs are rarely located extracranially, clinicians evaluating patients with craniofacial AVM should have a high index of suspicion for the possibility of an underlying craniofacial arteriovenous metameric syndrome (CAMS). These patients should be evaluated for the presence of intracranial AVMs.

- Craniofacial arteriovenous fistulas (AVF), while extremely rare, are seen (Fig. 3). These differ from other craniofacial high-flow lesions in that they are single, whole fistulas. They are fed by branches of the external carotid artery and may be congenital, spontaneously developing or traumatic in origin. The congenital type is present at birth and grows with time. Spontaneously developing lesions may represent undetected congenital lesions or an underlying predisposition due to fibromuscular disease such as neurofibromatosis type I (NFI) or Ehlers-Danlos type IV (ED IV). While they may be of the traumatic type, posttraumatic and iatrogenic lesions should lead to consideration of the presence of these disorders.

Diagnostic Evaluation

- Diagnosis is initially made through history and physical exam, which demonstrates the pathognomonic finding of pulsatile mass that produces a bruit.
- Multiple imaging modalities have been used to confirm the diagnosis, including ultrasound, CT, MRI, MR angiogram, and digital subtraction angiography (DSA).
- MRI is useful to determine the extent of the lesion and plan treatment. T2-weighted sequences with contrast and fat suppression are necessary for adequate assessment. The appearance of AVM on MRI is that of tortuous and dilated feeding arteries and draining veins, which enhance and contain flow voids.
- Cerebral digital subtraction angiography (DSA) represents the gold standard in delineating the lesion and providing an accurate map of the arterial and venous channels involved. Study information is integral in planning both surgical and endovascular treatment (Figs. 2 and 3).

Treatment

- Asymptomatic facial AVMs should be observed unless they can be completely removed and cured with minimal morbidity. Embolization or incomplete excision of an asymptomatic lesion may stimulate it to enlarge and become symptomatic.
- AVMs not reaching the threshold for intervention (see indications for treatment) may be managed conservatively. Application of hydrated petroleum may prevent desiccation and subsequent ulceration of superficial AVMs. Compression garments for extremity lesions may reduce pain and swelling but can also exacerbate symptoms.
- Because estrogen is proangiogenic and may stimulate progression, progesterone-only oral contraceptives are recommended for women of childbearing age with AVM.
- Treatment options are diverse and include surgical excision, transarterial and/or transvenous embolization, injection of sclerosant into the nidus, and electrothrombosis. These methods have been used either independently or in combination, with embolization followed by surgical resection most commonly reported.
- Recently, the pharmacologic use of marimastat, a broad-spectrum matrix metalloproteinase inhibitor, has been described for the treatment of aggressively enlarging AVMs that cause significant functional impairment.

- Embolization alone is usually not curative, and most lesions will recur. Consequently, it is most commonly used preoperatively to reduce blood loss during resection or for palliation of symptomatic, unresectable lesions. Excision should be performed 24–72 h after embolization, before recanalization and angiogenesis restores blood flow to the lesion. This is of particular importance if particulate agents (e.g., PVA) are used.
- The aim of endovascular treatment is to disconnect the fistulous connection between the arterial and venous components of the malformation. It is important not to perform proximal ligation, as this is both ineffective in treating the AVM and eliminates access to the lesion for future intervention. In particular, ligation of the external carotid artery may lead to recruitment of collateral circulation from the internal carotid, the vertebral, and the contralateral vessel systems.
- The approach to embolization is primarily via transarterial injection of liquid embolic material (i.e., NBCA or onyx) or PVA particles.
- The direct percutaneous approach alone is preferred when superselective catheterization of all the pedicles is not possible transarterially because of lesion angioarchitecture.
- Typically, percutaneous treatment is performed as an adjunct to endovascular treatment. Generally, liquid adhesives are used for PTE to complete devascularization after partial transarterial disconnection.
- Craniofacial AVF are typically treated via transarterial liquid embolization. Direct percutaneous injection of glue is possible (as with the rest of the facial AVMs) if intra-arterial access is an issue (Fig. 3).

Patient Preparation

- When the goal of treatment is palliation, the patient and family are consulted prior to treatment and should understand that cure will not be achieved and that the lesion is likely to re-expand in the future, possibly requiring additional embolizations.

Treatment Techniques

- Initial steps of treatment are similar to PTE of VLM described above.
- When liquid adhesives are used, the glue is injected into the vascular channels (AVM nidus or fistulous connection).
- When sclerosant or antiangiogenetic agents are used, the drug is injected around the malformation into the surrounding connective tissues.
- In both percutaneous techniques a tourniquet is first placed around the injection site to prevent distal embolization of embolic material (Fig. 2). In the case of liquid adhesives, the tourniquet is placed around the "nidus" or fistulous connection of the facial AVM to be injected.
- Initial results of the use of a circular ring compression device during PTE with glue suggest that the device provides a safe glue injection route as well as effective compression of multiple venous drainage routes, thus avoiding inadvertent distal migration.

Modifications to Embolization Technique

- As part of a multidisciplinary preoperative approach, percutaneous injection of the sclerosing agents OK-432 (streptococcal pyrogenic exotoxin A) and pingyangmycin (bleomycin A5) into the connective tissues surrounding the AVM has been used to decrease blood supply and divide the lesion into compartments with considerably reduced flow.

Safety Measures During Treatment

- When using liquid adhesives, tourniquets should only be removed after the injected agent hardens and cannot migrate distally.
- When using sclerosants in the treatment of these high-flow lesions, there is danger that the agent may escape into the systemic circulation. To prevent this, pre-procedural phlebography should be completed, the maximal injected dose (see chapter "Diagnostic Cerebral Angiography and Groin Access and Closure") should not be exceeded, and compression should be maintained for several minutes after injection.

Post-procedure Management and Follow-Up

- Unlike sclerotherapy for slow-flow malformations, posttreatment edema after facial AVM embolization is rare, unless ethanol sclerotherapy is used.
- Except for small lesions, most patients are observed overnight in the hospital.
- If swelling is a significant concern, dexamethasone can be administered perioperatively followed by a 1-week oral corticosteroid taper.
- If airway or orbital lesions are embolized, concerns about post-procedural edema may necessitate closer monitoring in an ICU setting.

Treatment Outcomes

- Whether percutaneous embolization, sclerotherapy, or injection of antiangiogenetic agents is used, nearly all lesions will eventually recur after treatment if they are not surgically resected. Most studies suggest that multiple embolizations do not lower the rate of recurrence although newer embolic agents may offer more lasting results.
- Despite the high likelihood of re-expansion, embolization can effectively palliate a facial AVM by reducing its size, slowing expansion, and alleviating pain and bleeding. When used preoperatively, embolization can decrease operating room time and perioperative blood loss.

Complications of Treatment

- The most frequent complication of embolization is ulceration, which is more common for superficial lesions. Wounds are allowed to heal secondarily with local wound care.
- Distal migration of liquid embolic material can cause ischemic injury to uninvolved tissues. Neurointerventionalists treating these lesions need to be especially vigilant, as the significant sump effect of the nidus may cause normal arteries, arising from nidal feeders and leading to vital structures, to be angiographically occult. This may, as a result, lead to nontarget sclerosant embolization and significant morbidity. Prevention entails a detailed pre-procedural cerebral angiogram and a complete understanding of lesional and regional vascular anatomy prior to embolization. Additionally, tourniquets should not be removed until time is allowed for the liquid adhesive to completely harden.

Percutaneous Treatment of Head and Neck Tumors

Clinical Features

- The vascular nature of many craniofacial neoplasms has historically presented a challenge for surgical management, as profuse perioperative bleeding was frequently encountered. Advances in superselective angiography have enabled high success rates of preoperative devascularization, which has been shown to reduce operating room time and mean blood loss and has allowed for surgical resection of tumors previously felt to be inoperable.
- Palliative embolization for hemorrhage, pain, or growth has also been reported.
- The tumors for which this procedure is most frequently used include paragangliomas and juvenile nasopharyngeal angiofibromas (JNAs).
- Embolization is typically performed through transarterial injection of particles and/or liquid embolics such as NBCA or onyx.
- More recently, a percutaneous approach has been used, either alone or in combination.
- Because of its success, several centers report PTE as their primary approach because of its increased applicability and success in achieving complete devascularization.

Diagnostic Evaluation

- Tumor extent and topography should be initially evaluated via CT or MR examination.
- According to tumor location, a detailed cerebral angiogram should be performed. This includes selective injections of the common, internal, and external carotid branches, vertebral arteries, as well as sometimes the thyrocervical and costocervical trunks of the subclavian artery. In lesions suspected to have bilateral supply, contralateral arteries should be visualized.

- Once the main arterial supply is identified, it should be injected superselectively by microcatheter so as to check for dangerous anastomoses between the internal/external carotid or vertebral artery systems. It should be kept in mind that these dangerous anastomoses might not appear on the diagnostic angiogram and remain "potential." They might open during transarterial or percutaneous injection of embolization material when intra-arterial pressure increases. Thus a detailed understanding of the regional vascular anatomy is needed prior to performing these procedures so one can identify migration of embolic material through such an anastomosis.
- Angiographic results are used to determine the preferred treatment approach, embolic material and appropriate angiographic projections required for monitoring embolic material migration.

Patient Preparation

- It is recommended that these procedures be performed under general anesthesia with airway protection, particularly if the tumor is located in this region.

Treatment Technique

- A 20- or 22-gauge spinal needle is inserted into the lesion. Needle positioning can be considered correct if reflux of blood into the hub is slow but continuous.
- As with PTE of other craniofacial lesions, diagnostic phlebography is performed prior to injection of the embolic agent. This allows assessment of reflux, venous drainage, and potential for extravasation. It also allows the interventionalist to determine which vascular compartment of the tumor will be filled with liquid adhesive.
- Injection of the embolic agent is performed using negative roadmapping. The procedure is stopped after complete devascularization is achieved or if there is high risk of intracranial reflux.
- To allow direct puncture of skull base lesions, infrazygomatic, transnasal, transpalatal, or transoral approaches are often used.
- If critical anastomoses are detected or present, the anastomotic connection can be occluded using coils or a balloon to prevent migration of the embolic agent. A common scenario would be placement of a balloon at the cavernous segment of the internal carotid artery to protect it during percutaneous injection of liquid embolic into a nasopharyngeal tumor.

Modifications to Treatment

- A transnasal approach to juvenile nasopharyngeal angiofibroma using endoscopic guidance has been described.

Safety Measures During Treatment

- A detailed understanding of the anatomy of the external carotid artery (ECA) is essential for performing safe and effective embolization of craniofacial tumors – whether transarterial or percutaneous – because of the many anatomic variations, territorial anastomoses, and collateral supplies found in this region.
- As mentioned, occult anastomoses may reveal themselves as regional blood flow changes occur during the embolization.

Post-procedure Management and Follow-Up

- As in the preoperative treatment of craniofacial AVM, embolization is usually performed 24–72 h prior to surgical resection.
- Patients undergoing palliative embolization are usually observed for 12 h prior to discharge.

Treatment Outcomes

- A percutaneous approach by using liquid embolic material such as cyanoacrylate glue has been shown to be safe and effective in obliterating the vasculature in a number of different hypervascular head and neck lesions.

Complications of Treatment

- Dangerous anastomoses may open periprocedurally secondary to changes in pressure within the arteries and in the regional blood flow. As a result, embolic material may penetrate another arterial territory resulting in stroke.
- Continuous angiographic guidance, operator vigilance, and careful selection of an embolic agent that can be controlled are all important for prevention of this serious complication.

Key Points

> Neurointerventional treatment of craniofacial lesions requires a multidisciplinary approach.

> Percutaneous embolization and sclerotherapy are emerging treatment modalities for craniofacial lesions that overcome access difficulties associated with endovascular treatment.

> These may be used in isolation or in conjunction with any combination of endovascular embolization, surgery, radiotherapy, and laser therapy.

> Phlebography should always be completed prior to any percutaneous technique.

> Venolymphatic malformations (VLMs) are congenital, low-flow lesions that present clinically through the life span.

> Diagnostic standard is magnetic resonance imaging (MRI), with fat saturated T2 weighting the preferred sequence.

> When indicated, treatment of choice is percutaneous sclerotherapy with or without surgical excision.

> Arteriovenous malformations (AVMs) are direct communications between an artery and vein with or without an intervening nidal component.

> Digital subtraction angiography (DSA) is the diagnostic gold standard, though MRI is frequently used.

> Treatment options for extracranial AVMs include surgery, endovascular and percutaneous techniques, and electrothrombosis. These may be used alone or in combination with embolization followed by surgical resection most commonly reported.

> Because of their hypervascularity, craniofacial neoplasms are associated with profuse perioperative bleeding. Recently, preoperative devascularization using transarterial or percutaneous embolization has been shown to reduce blood loss and has allowed for resection of tumors previously felt to be inoperable.

Acknowledgements We would like to thank Karel G terBrugge for his advice during the writing of this manuscript.

Suggested Reading

1. Abud DG, Mounayer C, Benndorf G, et al. Intratumoral injection of cyanoacrylate glue in head and neck paragangliomas. AJNR Am J Neuroradiol. 2004;25(9):1457–62.
2. Agid R, Burvin R, Gomori J. Sclerotherapy for venous malformations using a "negative subtraction" technique. Neuroradiology. 2006;48:127–9.
3. Ayad M, Eskioglu E, Mericle RA. Onyx: a unique neuroembolic agent. Expert Rev Med Devices. 2006;3(6):705–15.
4. Aziz-Sultan MA, Moftakhar R, Quintero Wolfe S, et al. Endoscopically assisted intratumoral embolization of juvenile nasopharyngeal angiofibroma using Onyx. J Neurosurg Pediatr. 2011;7:600–3.
5. Berenguer B, Burrows PE, Zurakowski D, Mulliken JB. Sclerotherapy of craniofacial venous malformations: complications and results. Plast Reconstr Surg. 1999;104:1–11.
6. Berenstein A, Lasjaunias P, ter Brugge KG, editors. Surgical neuroangiography. Clinical and endovascular treatment aspects in adults, vol. 2.1. 2nd ed. New York: Springer; 2004a. p. 201–26.
7. Berenstein A, Lasjaunias P, ter Brugge KG, editors. Surgical neuroangiography. Clinical and endovascular treatment aspects in adults, vol. 2.2. 2nd ed. New York: Springer; 2004b. p. 359–88.
8. Blum R. A clinical review of Bleomycin: a new anti-neoplastic agent. Cancer. 1973;31: 903–14.
9. Buckmiller LM. Update on hemangiomas and vascular malformations. Curr Opin Otolaryngol Head Neck Surg. 2004;12(6):476–87.
10. Burrows PE, Mulliken JB, Fishman SJ, et al. Pharmacological treatment of a diffuse arteriovenous malformation of the upper extremity in a child. J Craniofac Surg. 2009;20:S1–6.
11. Cabrera J, Cabrera JJ, Garcia-Olmedo MA, et al. Treatment of venous malformations with sclerosant in microfoam form. Arch Dermatol. 2003;139(11):1409–16.
12. Carneiro SC, Batista LL, Vasconcelos BC, et al. Massive oral hemorrhage due to mandibular arteriovenous malformation treated with percutaneous approach: a case report. J Oral Maxillofac Surg. 2009;67:2525–8.
13. Casasco A, Houdart E, Biondi A, et al. Major complications of percutaneous embolization of skull-base tumors. AJNR Am J Neuroradiol. 1999;20:179–81.
14. Chaloupka JC, Mangla S, Huddle DC, et al. Evolving experience with direct puncture therapeutic embolization for adjunctive and palliative management of head and neck hypervascular neoplasms. Laryngoscope. 1999;109(11):1864–72.
15. Chen Y, Li Y, Zhu Q, et al. Fluoroscopic intralesional injection with pingyangmycin lipiodol emulsion for the treatment of orbital venous malformations. AJR Am J Roentgenol. 2008;190(4):966–71.
16. Chen WL, Ye JT, Xu LF, et al. A multidisciplinary approach to treating maxillofacial arteriovenous malformations in children. Oral Surg Oral Med Oral Pathol Oral Radiol Endod. 2009;108:41–7.
17. Deng W, Huang D, Chen S, et al. Management of high-flow arteriovenous malformation in the maxillofacial region. J Craniofac Surg. 2010;21:916–9.
18. Do YS, Yakes WF, Shin SW, et al. Ethanol embolization of arteriovenous malformations: interim results. Radiology. 2005;235:674–82.
19. Donnelly LF, Bisset GS, Adams DM. Marked acute tissue swelling following percutaneous sclerosis of low-flow vascular malformations: a predictor of both prolonged recovery and therapeutic effect. Pediatr Radiol. 2000;30(6):415–9.
20. Dubois J, Soulez G, Oliva VL, et al. Soft-tissue venous malformations in adult patients: imaging and therapeutic issues. Radiographics. 2001;21:1519–31.
21. Fisher-Jeffes ND, Domingo Z, Madden M, et al. Arteriovenous malformations of the scalp. Neurosurgery. 1995;36:656–60.

22. Geibprasert S, Pongpech S, Armstrong D, et al. Dangerous extracranial-intracranial anastomoses and supply to the cranial nerves: vessels the neurointerventionalist needs to know. AJNR Am J Neuroradiol. 2009;30:1459–68.

23. Gemmete JJ, Ansari SA, McHugh J, et al. Embolization of vascular tumors of the head and neck. Neuroimaging Clin N Am. 2009;19:181–98.

24. Gemmete JJ, Chaudhary N, Pandey A, et al. Usefulness of percutaneously injected ethylene-vinyl alcohol copolymer in conjunction with standard endovascular embolization techniques for preoperative devascularization of hypervascular head and neck tumors: technique, initial experience, and correlation with surgical observations. AJNR Am J Neuroradiol. 2010; 31:961–6.

25. Greene AK, Orbach DB. Management of arteriovenous malformations. Clin Plast Surg. 2011;38:95–106.

26. Gruber A, Bavinzski G, Killer M, et al. Preoperative embolization of hypervascular skull base tumors. Minim Invasive Neurosurg. 2000;43(2):62–71.

27. Gupta AK, Purkayastha S, Bodhey NK, et al. Preoperative embolization of hypervascular head and neck tumours. Australas Radiol. 2007;51:446–52.

28. Han MH, Seong SO, Kim HD. Craniofacial arteriovenous malformation: preoperative embolization with direct puncture and injection of n-butyl cyanoacrylate. Radiology. 1999;211: 661–6.

29. Hyder SM, Huang JC, Nawaz Z, et al. Regulation of vascular endothelial growth factor expression by estrogens and progestins. Environ Health Perspect. 2000;108:785–90.

30. Hyodoh H, Hori M, Akiba H, et al. Peripheral vascular malformations: imaging, treatment approaches, and therapeutic issues. Radiographics. 2005;25:S159–71.

31. Ionescu G, Mabeta P, Dippenaar N, et al. Bleomycin plasma spill-over levels in paediatric patients undergoing intralesional injection for the treatment of haemangiomas. S Afr Med J. 2008;98:539–40.

32. Jackson IT, Carreno R, Potparic Z, et al. Hemangiomas, vascular malformations, and lympho-venous malformations: classification and methods of treatment. Plast Reconstr Surg. 1993;91:1216–30.

33. Jin Y, Lin X, Li W, Hu X, Ma G, Wang W. Sclerotherapy after embolization of draining vein: a safe treatment for venous malformations. J Vasc Surg. 2008;47:1292–9.

34. Kluba S, Meiss A, Prey N, et al. Arteriovenous malformation of the mandible: life-threatening manifestation during tooth extraction. Mund Kiefer Gesichtschir. 2007;11:107–13.

35. Klurfan P, TerBrugge KG, Tan K, Simons ME. Interventional vascular radiology in musculo-skeletal lesions. In: Baert L, Knauth M, Sartor K, editors. Imaging in percutaneous musculo-skeletal interventions. Berlin: Springer; 2009. p. 369–70.

36. Kohout MP, Hansen M, Pribaz JJ, Mulliken JB. Arteriovenous malformations of the head and neck: natural history and management. Plast Reconstr Surg. 1998;102:643–54.

37. Konez O, Burrows PE. Magnetic resonance of vascular anomalies. Magn Reson Imaging Clin N Am. 2002;10:363–88.

38. Krishnamoorty T, Gupta AK, Rajan JE, et al. Stroke from delayed embolization of polymer-ized glue following percutaneous direct injection of a carotid body tumor. Korean J Radiol. 2007;8:249–53.

39. Lee BB, Bergan JJ. Advanced management of congenital vascular malformations: a multidis-ciplinary approach. Cardiovasc Surg. 2002;10:523–33.

40. Lee CH, Chen SG. Direct percutaneous ethanol instillation for treatment of venous malforma-tions in the face and neck. Br J Plast Surg. 2005;58(8):1073–8.

41. Lee BB, Do YS, Byun HS, Choo IW, Kim DI, Huh SH. Advanced management of venous malformation with ethanol sclerotherapy: mid-term results. J Vasc Surg. 2003;37:533–8.

42. Legiehn GM, Heran MK. Venous malformations: classification, development, diagnosis, and interventional radiologic management. Radiol Clin North Am. 2008;46:545–97.

43. Liu AS, Mulliken JB, Zurakowski D, et al. Extracranial arteriovenous malformations: natural progression and recurrence after treatment. Plast Reconstr Surg. 2010;125:1185–94.
44. McClinton MA. Tumors and aneurysms of the upper extremity. Hand Clin. 1993;9:151–69.
45. Muir T, Kirsten M, Fourie P, Dippenaar N, Ionescu GO. Intralesional bleomycin injection (IBI) treatment for haemangiomas and congenital vascular malformations. Pediatr Surg Int. 2004;19:766–73.
46. Mulliken JB, Glowacki J. Hemangiomas and vascular malformations in infants and children: a classification based on endothelial characteristics. Plast Reconstr Surg. 1982;69:412–20.
47. Norris JS, Valiante TA, Wallace MC, et al. A simple relationship between radiological arteriovenous malformation hemodynamics and clinical presentation: a prospective, blinded analysis of 31 cases. J Neurosurg. 1999;90:673–9.
48. Puig S, Aref H, Brunelle F. Double-needle sclerotherapy of lymphangiomas and venous angiomas in children: a simple technique to prevent complications. AJR Am J Roentgenol. 2003;180(5):1399–401.
49. Puig S, Cassati B, Staudenherz A, et al. Vascular low-flow malformations in children: current concepts for classification, diagnosis and therapy. Eur J Radiol. 2005;53(1):35–45.
50. Quadros RS, Gallas S, Delcourt C, et al. Preoperative embolization of a cervicodorsal paraganglioma by direct percutaneous injection of onyx and endovascular delivery of particles. AJNR Am J Neuroradiol. 2006;27(9):1907–9.
51. Ryu CW, Whang SM, Suh DC, et al. Percutaneous direct puncture glue embolization of high-flow craniofacial arteriovenous lesions: a new circular ring compression device with a beveled edge. AJNR Am J Neuroradiol. 2007;28:528–30.
52. Sainsbury DCG, Kessell G, Guhan A, et al. Unexpected hyperpigmentation following intralesional bleomycin injection. J Plast Reconstr Aesthet Surg. 2009;62:e497–9.
53. Sainsbury DCG, Kessell G, Fall AJ, et al. Intralesional bleomycin injection treatment for vascular birthmarks: a 5-Year experience at a single United Kingdom Unit. Plast Reconstr Surg. 2011;127:2031–44.
54. Schere K, Waner M. Nd:YAG lasers (1,064 nm) in the treatment of venous malformations of the face and neck: challenges and benefits. Lasers Med Sci. 2007;22:119–26.
55. Siu WW, Weill A, Gariepy JL, et al. Arteriovenous malformation of the mandible: embolization and direct injection therapy. J Vasc Interv Radiol. 2001;12:1095–8.
56. Smith TP. Embolization in the external carotid artery. J Vasc Interv Radiol. 2006;17(12): 1897–912.
57. Spence J, Krings T, ter Brugge KG, et al. Percutaneous sclerotherapy for facial venous malformations: subjective clinical and objective MR imaging follow-up results. AJNR Am J Neuroradiol. 2010;31(5):955–60.
58. Spence J, Krings T, ter Brugge KG, et al. Percutaneous treatment of facial venous malformations: a matched comparison of alcohol and bleomycin sclerotherapy. Head Neck. 2011; 33(1):125–30.
59. Starke RM, Komotar RJ, Otten ML, et al. Adjuvant embolization with N-butyl cyanoacrylate in the treatment of cerebral arteriovenous malformations: outcomes, complications, and predictors of neurologic deficits. Stroke. 2009;40(8):2783–90.
60. Tan KT, Kirby J, Rajan D, et al. Percutaneous sodium tetradecyl sulfate sclerotherapy for peripheral venous vascular malformations: a single centre experience. J Vasc Interv Radiol. 2007;18:343–51.
61. Tessari L. Nouvelle technique d'obtention de la sclera-mousse. Phlebologie. 2000;53: 129–33.
62. Tikkakoski T, Luotonen J, Leinonen S, et al. Preoperative embolization in the management of neck paragangliomas. Laryngoscope. 1997;107(6):821–6.

63. Türkbey B, Peynircioğlu B, Arat A, et al. Percutaneous management of peripheral vascular malformations: a single center experience. Diagn Interv Radiol. 2011. doi:10.4261/1305-3825.DIR.3808-10.0.
64. Vikkula M, Boon LM, Mulliken JB. Molecular genetics of vascular malformations. Matrix Biol. 2001;20(5–6):327–35.
65. Willems PW, Farb RI, Agid R. Endovascular treatment of epistaxis. AJNR Am J Neuroradiol. 2009;30(9):1637–45.
66. Wu IC, Orbach DB. Neurointerventional management of high-flow vascular malformations of the head and neck. Neuroimaging Clin N Am. 2009;19:219–40.
67. Wu JK, Bisdorff A, Gelbert F, Enjolras O, Burrows PE, Mulliken JB. Auricular arteriovenous malformation: evaluation, management, and outcome. Plast Reconstr Surg. 2005;115:985–95.
68. Yi B, Jun J, Xing-Xing H, et al. Sclerotherapy of microcystic lymphatic malformations in oral and facial regions. J Oral Maxillofac Surg. 2009;67(2):251–6.
69. Young AE. Arteriovenous malformations. In: Mulliken JB, Young AE, editors. Vascular birthmarks: hemangiomas and malformations. Philadelphia: WB Saunders; 1988. p. 228–45.
70. Zhao JH, Zhang WF, Zhao YF. Sclerotherapy of oral and facial venous malformations with use of pingyangmycin and/or sodium morrhuate. Int J Oral Maxillofac Surg. 2004;33:463–6.
71. Zhi K, Wen Y, Li L, Ren W. The role of intralesional pingyangmycin in the treatment of venous malformations of the facial and maxillary region. Int J Pediatr Otorhinolaryngol. 2008;72:593–7.

Retinoblastoma Intra-arterial Chemotherapy

Edward D. Greenberg, Y. Pierre Gobin, Brian P. Marr, Scott E. Brodie,
Ira J. Dunkel, and David H. Abramson

Abstract

Retinoblastoma is the most common intraocular tumor of childhood with an average age at diagnosis is 18 months. First-line intra-arterial chemotherapy is very promising for intraocular retinoblastoma and may be superior to intravenous chemotherapy or external beam radiotherapy. Intra-arterial chemotherapy is associated with tolerable systemic toxicity.

Keywords

Retinoblastoma • Intraocular tumor • Childhood tumor • Intra-arterial chemotherapy • Intravenous chemotherapy • External beam radiotherapy • Systemic toxicity • Family history • Sporadic • Retina • Vitreous seeding • Subretinal fluid

E.D. Greenberg, MD (✉)
Division of Interventional Neuroradiology, Department of Neurosurgery,
New York Presbyterian Hospital-Weill Cornell Medical Center, New York, NY, USA
e-mail: edward.greenberg.98@alumni.brown.edu

Y.P. Gobin, MD
Department of Neurosurgery, Weill Cornell Medical College
of New York Presbyterian Hospital, New York, NY, USA

B.P. Marr, MD
Ophthalmic Oncology Service, Memorial Sloan-Kettering Cancer Center, New York, NY, USA

S.E. Brodie, MD, PhD
Department of Ophthalmology, Mount Sinai Hospital, New York, NY, USA

I.J. Dunkel, MD
Department of Pediatrics, Memorial Sloan-Kettering Cancer Center, New York, NY, USA

D.H. Abramson, MD
Department of Surgery, Memorial Sloan-Kettering Cancer Center, New York, NY, USA

K. Murphy, F. Robertson (eds.), *Interventional Neuroradiology,*
Techniques in Interventional Radiology,
DOI 10.1007/978-1-4471-4582-0_20, © Springer-Verlag London 2014

Clinical Features

- Retinoblastoma is the most common intraocular tumor of childhood.
- Average age at diagnosis is 18 months.
- 90 % sporadic and 10 % family history.
- RB1 gene mutation, 60 % somatic, and 40 % germinal.
- Reese-Ellsworth classification of extent of disease ranges from group Ia to Vb, with Va representing tumors involving over half the retina and Vb with vitreous seeding.
- International Classification for Intraocular Retinoblastoma, groups A–E, based on the chance of cure without the need for enucleation or external beam radiotherapy (EBRT) given current treatment options.
  - Group A includes small tumors (<3 mm) confined to the retina and located further than 3 mm from the foveola and 1.5 mm from the optic disk.
  - Group B includes all other tumors confined to the retina not in Group A with tumor-associated subretinal fluid less than 3 mm from the tumor and no subretinal seeding.
  - Group C includes discrete local disease with minimal subretinal or vitreous seeding. Subretinal fluid may involve up to one-fourth of the retina, local fine vitreous seeding may be present close to discrete tumor, and local subretinal seeding must be less than 3 mm from the tumor.
  - Group D includes diffuse disease with significant vitreous or subretinal seeding.
  - Group E includes the presence of any one or more of the following poor prognostic features: tumor touching the lens, tumor anterior to the anterior vitreous face involving the ciliary body or anterior segment, diffuse infiltrating retinoblastoma, neovascular glaucoma, opaque media from hemorrhage, tumor necrosis with aseptic orbital cellulitis, and phthisis bulbi.

Diagnostic Evaluation

- Leukocoria and strabismus are the most common presenting signs on standard ophthalmologic examination.
- Brain/orbital magnetic resonance imaging (MRI) for diagnosis and detection of extraocular spread as well as associated pineal or suprasellar tumors. Pre-procedure ophthalmologic examination under anesthesia, which may include indirect ophthalmoscopy, fundus photography, ophthalmic ultrasonography, and electroretinography.

Indications

- Patients with advanced intraocular retinoblastoma that cannot be treated with focal treatment (laser ablation, cryocoagulation, or radioactive plaque) without compromising vision.

Contraindications

- Patients who have a disease that can be adequately treated with focal treatment alone.
- Advanced intraocular disease at risk for extraocular or metastatic disease.
- Extraocular disease.
- Metastatic disease or trilateral disease.

Anatomy

- The ophthalmic artery arises from the anterior aspect of the internal carotid artery, medial to the anterior clinoid process.
- Ophthalmic artery branches can be grouped into the following: (1) ocular group (central retinal artery and ciliary arteries), (2) orbital group (lacrimal artery and arteries to the extraocular muscles), and (3) extra-orbital group (ethmoidal arteries, palpebral arteries, dural arteries, and terminal branches including the supratrochlear branch).
- A common normal anatomic variant is a middle meningeal origin of the ophthalmic artery.

Equipment

- Access: 4 French Micropuncture Introducer Set (Cook Medical, Bloomington, IN) and 5 French sheath (AVANTI + Introducer; Cordis, Bridgewater, NJ).
- Catheters/wires: Marathon microcatheter, Mirage 0.008 microwire (ev3, Irvine, CA), Magic 1.5 microcatheter (Balt, Montmorency, France), 5 French Envoy guiding catheter (Codman, Raynham, MA), and standard 0.035″ guidewire.
- Balloon: 4 × 7 mm HyperForm balloon catheter (ev3, Irvine, CA).

Chemotherapeutic Agents

- Melphalan, topotecan hydrochloride, and carboplatin.
- Chemotherapeutic dose is based on empirical evidence balancing efficacy and toxicity allowing for a standard, age-based dose for standard ophthalmic artery angioanatomy (Table 1).
- The standardized dose is customized to the specific angioanatomy of the patient and can be increased by up to 50 % if large extraocular branches arising from the ophthalmic artery are present, as seen by angiography or if a previous treatment did not result in sufficient tumor reduction.

Table 1 Current drug dosages according to age

Drug	Drug dosage, mg			
	3–6 months	6–12 months	1–3 years	=/more than 3 years
Melphalan	2.5	3	4	5
Topotecan	0.3	0.3	0.3	0.4
Carboplatin	Not tested	30	30	30

From Pierre Gobin Y, Dunkel IJ, Marr BP, Brodie SE, Abramson DH. Intra-arterial chemotherapy for the management of retinoblastoma: four-year experience. Arch Ophthalmol. 2011;129(6): 732–7

Dose is increased if the ophthalmic artery has large extraocular branches or if there is insufficient tumor reduction from the previous cycle. Dose is increased if there was previous treatment with intravenous chemotherapy and radiation (especially if recent), if the microcatheter is in "wedge flow" in the ophthalmic artery, if there is an inflammatory reaction after the previous cycle, if there is a decreased amplitude in electroretinogram after the previous cycle, if parents noted vision decrease (not reliable in young children), and/or if bilateral treatment is planned and the total (body) dose of melphalan would exceed 0.5 mg/kg

- The dose is generally decreased if the patient has undergone recent intravenous chemotherapy and/or radiation treatment, if the microcatheter is in "wedge flow" within the ophthalmic artery, if there was an exuberant inflammatory reaction prior to treatment, if there was a decrease in electroretinogram amplitude or in visual acuity as a result of prior treatment, if there was severe myelosuppression as a result of prior treatment, or if the total dose of melphalan would exceed 0.5 mg/kg.

Medications

- No routine pain medications or antibiotics are administered pre- or post-procedure.
- Patients may require standard antiemetics postanesthesia, such as ondansetron.

Procedure

General Considerations

- General endotracheal anesthesia.
- A nasal decongestant (oxymetazoline hydrochloride, 0.05 %) is sprayed in the nostril on the treatment side to reduce the diversion of drug into the nasal circulation.
- The fluoroscopy equipment is calibrated to a low-dose pediatric protocol to limit radiation dose.

Access

- The right or left femoral artery is punctured using a 4 French Micropuncture® Introducer Set (Cook Medical, Bloomington, IN) including a 21G needle, 0.018″ wire, and 4 French dilator.
- After puncturing the artery and advancing the wire coaxially, the needle is exchanged out over the wire for the 4 French dilator that is directly connected to a continuous heparinized saline flush (1,000 U heparin/1 L NS) using a Y hemostasis valve.
- The right and left groins are alternatively punctured for patients undergoing multiple consecutive procedures.

Angiography

- A blood sample for measurement of an activated clotting time (ACT) is sent, and a standard dose of heparin (70 IU/kg) is administered.
- Much of the procedural can be performed using digital subtraction fluoroscopy as opposed to digital subtraction angiography, thus significantly decreasing the radiation dose.
- In most cases, a straight microcatheter, such as the Marathon microcatheter (ev3, Irvine, California) or a Magic 1.5 microcatheter (Balt, Montmorency, France) is advanced over a Mirage 0.008 microwire (ev3, Irvine, California) through the abdominal and thoracic aorta, into the cavernous internal carotid artery. Angiography is then performed in order to visualize the angioanatomy and to determine whether selective catheterization of the ophthalmic artery is appropriate. In cases where the ophthalmic artery is too small or arises at an acute angle from the internal carotid artery, alternative techniques are used (see below).

Treatment Plan and Techniques

Direct Catheterization Technique

- Assuming the ophthalmic artery is deemed appropriate, the microcatheter is positioned at the ostium of the ophthalmic artery, using fluoroscopic guidance and roadmap technique.
- Selective angiography of the ophthalmic artery is performed with particular attention paid to the anterograde flow of contrast within the ophthalmic artery and the presence of a choroid blush (Fig. 1).
- The chemotherapy drug(s) are diluted with saline to obtain a volume of 20–30 cm³ of solution that is injected manually by repeated small bolus (pulsatile injection) at a rate of 1 mL/min.

Fig. 1 Lateral projection of an ophthalmic artery angiogram performed prior to chemotherapy infusion using the direct catheterization method. The tip of the microcatheter is at the ostium of the ophthalmic artery. Note the normal anterograde flow and normal choroid blush

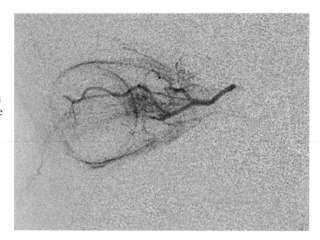

Fig. 2 Lateral projection of an ophthalmic artery angiogram performed prior to chemotherapy infusion using the middle meningeal catheterization technique. The tip of the microcatheter is within the orbital branch of the middle meningeal artery. Note normal choroid blush

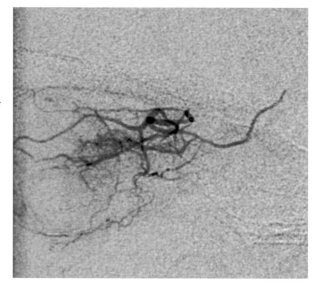

Middle Meningeal Technique

- If the direct catheterization technique is not possible, the middle meningeal technique may be utilized.
- Using fluoroscopic guidance and roadmap technique, the ipsilateral middle meningeal artery is catheterized, and a selective angiogram is performed in order to determine whether the orbital branch of the middle meningeal artery is of sufficient size to allow for catheterization and selective infusion of the chemotherapeutic agents. Again, particular attention is paid to flow within the ophthalmic artery as well as the presence of a choroid blush (Fig. 2).
- The chemotherapy drug(s) are diluted and infused as above, at a pulsatile injection at a rate of 1 cm^3/min.

Fig. 3 Lateral projection of an internal carotid angiogram with a 4×7 mm HyperForm balloon (ev3, Irvine, CA) inflated above the level of the ophthalmic artery. Note the normal anterograde flow within the ophthalmic artery with no flow past the inflated balloon

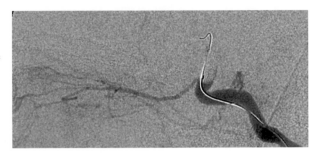

Balloon Technique

- In cases not amenable to the direct infusion technique, and without a well-developed orbital branch of the middle meningeal artery, one can consider using the balloon technique, which consists of placement of a temporary balloon to occlude the internal carotid artery above the origin of the ophthalmic artery and chemotherapeutic infusion into the internal carotid artery below the balloon.
- In order to use the balloon technique, the 4 French dilator is exchanged out for a 5 French sheath, which is then connected to a continuous heparinized saline flush.
- A 5 French guide catheter, such as a 5 French Envoy guiding catheter (Codman, Raynham, MA), is then advanced over a standard 0.035″ guidewire into the ipsilateral internal carotid artery.
- A 4×7 mm HyperForm balloon catheter (ev3, Irvine, CA) is then advanced over its microwire via the guide catheter and positioned within the internal carotid artery, just distal to the origin of the ophthalmic artery.
- The balloon is inflated, and angiography is performed via the guide catheter to confirm occlusion of the internal carotid artery and flow into the ophthalmic artery (Fig. 3).
- A chemotherapeutic agent is then infused via the guide catheter with the balloon inflated. The balloon is not kept inflated for more than 4 min at a time for the infusion.
- Regardless of which technique is ultimately utilized, a post chemotherapy angiogram is performed of the ipsilateral internal carotid artery at the conclusion of the infusion in order to exclude arterial injury or significant vasospasm and to confirm presence of the choroid blush.
- At the conclusion of the procedure, the catheters are removed, an ACT is measured, and the 4 French dilator or groin sheath is removed.
- Hemostasis is achieved with manual compression.

Choice of Chemotherapeutic Agents

- Melphalan is almost always administered given its short half-life, excellent chemotherapeutic effect, and low toxicity profile when administered intra-arterially.
- Topotecan is added for treating difficult tumors with vitreous seeding.
- Carboplatin can be used if the above agents are not successful or if bilateral treatment is required and the corresponding dose of melphalan would be too high (greater than 0.5 mg/kg).

Follow-Up

- Postanesthesia recovery unit for 5 h before being discharged home.
- Counseling of the parents regarding fever and neutropenia and other possible acute side effects.
- Complete blood cell count with platelets and absolute neutrophil count 7–10 days after the procedure.
- Decisions regarding the number of sessions are not standardized but are based on the findings of the examinations under anesthesia, which can also be performed at 3–4-week intervals.
- Intra-arterial chemotherapy sessions can be repeated every 3–4 weeks.
- Posttreatment of tumors with focal therapy can be performed if indicated.

Alternative Therapies

- Focal treatments such as laser ablation or cryotherapy are effective only on small tumors without extensive vitreous seeds.
- Advanced tumors have historically required tumor reduction with intravenous chemotherapy, EBRT, or both, in order to avoid enucleation. However, in our center, intra-arterial chemotherapy has largely replaced intravenous chemotherapy and EBRT.
- EBRT is still used as second-line treatment after the failure of intra-arterial chemotherapy.

Specific Complications

- Femoral artery puncture site complications such as hematoma and vascular injury.
- Allergic reactions to contrast material.
- Intra-procedural bronchospasm, bradycardia, and hypotension, typically occurring when the microcatheter reaches the cavernous carotid or ophthalmic arteries, effectively treated with IV epinephrine bitartrate.
- Ocular complications include temporary periocular edema and redness, transient red discoloration of the skin in the mesial frontal area (in the cutaneous territory of the ophthalmic artery), and temporary thinning or loss of eyelashes along the medial third of the upper eyelid. Avascular retinopathy is a dose-related, toxic arteriopathy seen after multiple infusion of chemotherapy drugs at high doses, especially if the eye had already been compromised by EBRT.
- Neutropenia (and less frequently, anemia and/or thrombocytopenia).

Key Points

> First-line IA chemotherapy is very promising for intraocular retinoblastoma and may be superior to intravenous chemotherapy or EBRT.
> Intra-arterial chemotherapy is associated with tolerable systemic toxicity.

Suggested Reading

1. Abramson DH, Dunkel IJ, Brodie SE, Kim JW, Gobin YP. A phase I/II study of direct intraarterial (ophthalmic artery) chemotherapy with melphalan for intraocular retinoblastoma initial results. Ophthalmology. 2008;115(8):1398–404, 1404.e1.
2. Abramson DH, Dunkel IJ, Brodie SE, Marr B, Gobin YP. Superselective ophthalmic artery chemotherapy as primary treatment for retinoblastoma (chemosurgery). Ophthalmology. 2010a;117(8):1623–9.
3. Abramson DH, Dunkel IJ, Brodie SE, Marr B, Gobin YP. Bilateral superselective ophthalmic artery chemotherapy for bilateral retinoblastoma: tandem therapy. Arch Ophthalmol. 2010b;128(3):370–2.
4. Gobin YP, Dunkel IJ, Marr BP, Brodie SE, Abramson DH. Intra-arterial chemotherapy for the management of retinoblastoma: four-year experience. Arch Ophthalmol. 2011;129(6):732–7.
5. Graeber CP, Gobin YP, Marr BP, et al. Histopathologic findings of eyes enucleated after treatment with chemosurgery for retinoblastoma. Open Ophthalmol J. 2011;5:1–5.
6. Marr B, Gobin PY, Dunkel IJ, Brodie SE, Abramson DH. Spontaneously resolving periocular erythema and ciliary madarosis following intra-arterial chemotherapy for retinoblastoma. Middle East Afr J Ophthalmol. 2010;17(3):207–9.
7. Patel M, Paulus YM, Gobin YP, et al. Intra-arterial and oral digoxin therapy for retinoblastoma. Ophthalmic Genet. 2011;32:147–50.
8. Schefler AC, Abramson DH. Retinoblastoma: what is new in 2007–2008. Curr Opin Ophthalmol. 2008;19(6):526–34.

Part IX

Spine Intervention

Vertebral Body Augmentation

Martin G. Radvany and Sudhir Kathuria

Abstract

The fundamental goal of vertebral augmentation procedures is to stabilize and improve compressive strength of vertebral body through the safe injection of a stabilizing material. This can be achieved by both vertebroplasty and kyphoplasty. Vertebral augmentation is a safe and effective, minimally invasive treatment primarily for patients suffering from back pain associated with a vertebral compression fracture caused by osteoporosis, tumor invasion, or hemangioma.

Keywords

Vertebral body augmentation • Compressive strength • Vertebral body • Stabilizing agent • Vertebroplasty • Kyphoplasty • Safety • Efficacy • Minimally invasive treatment • Back pain • Vertebral compression fracture • Osteoporosis • Tumor invasion • Hemangioma

Introduction

The fundamental goal of vertebral augmentation procedures is to stabilize and improve compressive strength of vertebral body through the safe injection of a stabilizing material. This can be achieved by both vertebroplasty and kyphoplasty. Vertebral augmentation is a

M.G. Radvany, MD (✉)
Division of Interventional Neuroradiology, The Johns Hopkins Hospital, Baltimore, MD, USA
e-mail: mradvan2@jhmi.edu

S. Kathuria, MD
Division of Interventional Neuroradiology, Department of Radiology,
The Johns Hopkins Hospital, Baltimore, MD, USA

K. Murphy, F. Robertson (eds.), *Interventional Neuroradiology,*
Techniques in Interventional Radiology,
DOI 10.1007/978-1-4471-4582-0_21, © Springer-Verlag London 2014

safe and effective, minimally invasive treatment primarily for patients suffering from back pain associated with a vertebral compression fracture caused by osteoporosis, tumor invasion, or hemangioma.

Types of Vertebral Augmentation

Vertebroplasty

This involves the injection of special bone cement inside the fractured vertebral body using a needle under image guidance generally X-ray or CT fluoroscopy.

Kyphoplasty

Kyphoplasty, in comparison to vertebroplasty, involves an additional step of creating a cavity inside the diseased vertebral body using balloon inflation or certain devices followed by injection of the bone cement in the cavity. Any additional proposed benefits of kyphoplasty such as height restoration and kyphotic angle reduction remain to be proven.

Clinical Features

Pain from compression fracture is generally acute in onset, worsens with weight bearing or motion, and is often partially relieved in recumbent position. The fracture-related pain is hypothesized to originate from nerve stimulation during micromotion at the fracture site.

Diagnostic Evaluation

- Clinical assessment.
- Perform a physical exam to confirm that pain and tenderness on palpation correlates with level of radiographic compression fracture.
- Document neurologic status to include lower extremity strength, sensation (i.e., light touch and/or pinprick), and proprioception.
- Evaluate heart, lungs, and airway, as required for sedation.
- Review medication list for any blood thinner (Coumadin) or antiplatelet agents that need to be stopped at an appropriate interval before the day of procedure.

- Laboratory.
- CBC.
- Platelet count: PTT/PT/INR.
- Imaging.
- MRI demonstrates a characteristic low signal on T1-weighted sequences and high signal on STIR and T2-weighted sequences in acute or subacute fractures.
- MRI has the advantage of demonstrating additional spine conditions which may contribute to the pain syndrome, in particular disc or other degenerative disease.
- Available plain films should be reviewed to evaluate level and degree of vertebral body compression. It can be difficult to determine the age of the fracture from single plain film with no prior comparison film.
- Nuclear medicine bone scan can help localize symptomatic levels in patients with contraindication to MRI such as a pacemaker or spinal instrumentation that compromises image quality. However, caution is recommended as bone scans may show increased uptake for as long as 12 months following a fracture.
- CT can identify fractures that are potential routes of cement extravasation. CT can also help determine which pedicle will be available for access if there is a fracture of the pedicle.

Indications for Intervention

Painful compression fracture secondary to:

- Osteoporosis.
- Malignancy such as myeloma, lymphoma, or metastases.
- Hemangioma.

Contraindications

Absolute

- Ongoing local or systemic infection.
- Retropulsed bone fragment resulting in compressive myelopathy.
- Spinal canal compromise secondary to tumor resulting in myelopathy.
- Uncorrectable coagulopathy.
- PT (INR) greater than 1.4× control.
- PTT greater than 1.3× normal.
- Platelets less than 50,000/uL.

Relative

- Radiculopathy in excess of vertebral pain, caused by a compressive syndrome. Occasionally, preoperative vertebroplasty or kyphoplasty can be performed before a spinal decompressive procedure.
- Asymptomatic retropulsion of a fracture fragment causing significant spinal canal compromise. Cement injection can potentially worsen the retropulsion and make it symptomatic.
- Asymptomatic tumor extension into the epidural space. In experienced hands, such cases can be safely done by combining plasma-mediated tumor ablation to create a cavity in tumor followed by judicious cement injection.

Anatomy

- Understand radiographic anatomy and localize important neural and vascular structures to avoid injury.
- Following routes for needle placement are available.
- Transpedicular – classic and most common route.
- Parapedicular (Transcostovertebral) – commonly used in thoracic.
- Posterolateral – lumbar only.
- Anterolateral – cervical only.
- Transoral – upper cervical especially C2.

Equipment

Image Guidance System

- X-ray fluoroscopy.
- Offers the advantage of multiple planes and direct imaging.
- Biplane system is ideal and saves procedure time and enables orthogonal visualization of cement injection.
  - High-quality single-plane unit that can rapidly move from the lateral to AP position can suffice.
- Disadvantage of poor soft tissue contrast.
- CT fluoroscopy (Fig. 1).
- Offers excellent soft tissue contrast, useful in cases that require precise needle placement or close monitoring of cement injection such as in hemangioma or malignancy.
- Disadvantage of only single-plane capability and delayed imaging.

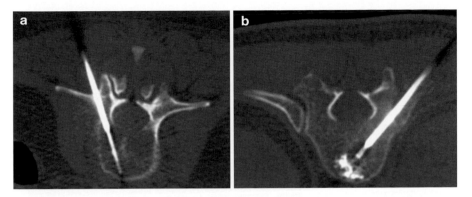

Fig. 1 CT-guided vertebroplasty. (**a**) Transpedicular needle placement in an L1 malignant compression fracture. (**b**) Extrapedicular approach used in the treatment of T11 painful hemangioma

Vertebroplasty Kit

- Needle size.
- Lumbar spine – 11 gauge or 13 gauge.
- Thoracic spine – 11 gauge or 13 gauge.
- Cervical spine – 15 gauge.
- Needle tip.
- Beveled tip – allows to steer needle while advancing in the bone.
- Diamond tip – does not slip off the pedicle so easier to penetrate the bone.
- Curved needle – can be advanced coaxially through outer straight needle and helps injecting cement in different desired parts of the bone that are otherwise difficult to reach by straight needle.

Procedure

- Patient preparation.
- Administer preprocedure antibiotics.
- Ancef, 1–2 g IV, 30 min before the procedure.
- Vancomycin 500 mg or clindamycin 600 mg substituted if patient is allergic to Ancef.
- Localize levels to be treated.
- Conscious sedation; selected cases under general anesthesia.
- Sterilize the skin (field) with iodinated scrub and place drapes.
- Anesthetize skin and periosteum with 1 % lidocaine.

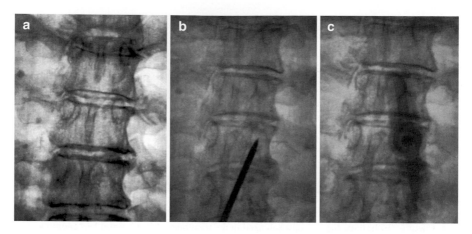

Fig. 2 Transpedicular needle placement. (**a**) AP image with image intensifier aligned perpendicular to pedicle with desired square adjacent end plate appearance. (**b**) Image with slightly lateral angle with excellent visualization of medial wall of pedicle. (**c**) Needle positioned as bull's eye for transpedicular placement through the center of pedicle

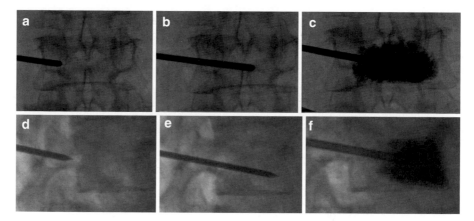

Fig. 3 Serial progression of the vertebroplasty needle through pedicle followed by cement injection as seen on AP images (**a–c**) in *upper panel* and corresponding lateral images (**d–f**) in the *lower panel*. Note that cement is injected with tip of the needle in anterior 1/3 of vertebral body

- Needle-placement technique (Fig. 2):
    - Align AP image intensifier perpendicular to pedicle with square adjacent end plate appearance. Craniocaudal and lateral angulation of the image intensifier are usually required.
    - Medial wall of pedicle must be well defined to prevent needle passage through spinal canal.
    - Lateral image intensifier should be angled so that posterior wall is clearly seen.
    - Tip of the needle in anterior one-third of vertebral body.
- Cement Injection (Fig. 3):
    - Several Food and Drug Administration (FDA)-approved PMMA-based cement and more recent biological (cortoss) material are available.

— Monitor cement injection under real-time fluoroscopy or visualize small quantities of 0.1–0.2 cc injection distribution before additional cement is introduced.
— Stop injection if any leakage outside of vertebral body or cement is seen in posterior one-fourth of vertebral body.

Immediate Post-procedure Care

Post-procedure

- Bed rest for 1 h after the procedure.
- Allow sitting up with assistance after 1 h.
- Monitor vital signs and perform neurologic examination.
- Record pain level and compare with baseline.

Discharge

- Return home keeping minimal activity for the next 24 h.
- Resume regular diet and medications.
- Procedure site is expected to be sore and tender up to 48 h.
- Notify physician if there is any neurologic dysfunction such as leg or arm weakness and/or urinary or bowel incontinence.
- Notify physician if there is increasing pain, fever, redness, swelling, or discharge from operative site.

Follow-Up Care

- Residual pain from additional sources such as degenerative disc or facet joint should be appropriately managed.
- Treatment of underlying disorder such as osteoporosis or malignancy is important to avoid additional fractures.

Results

Clinical success is defined as significant pain relief and/or improved mobility.

Success Rate

- Osteoporotic fractures 90 %.
- Metastatic disease 70–80 %.

Alternative Therapies

- Conservative management of fracture using rest, brace, and pain medications; longer recovery time.
- No other good surgical alternatives.

Complications

- Osteoporotic fractures 3 %; most are minor and transient.
- Metastatic disease 10 %; relative higher rate in malignancy is due to increased propensity of cement leakage.

Minor Complications

- Hemorrhage, infection, and nerve root irritation.
- Rib or vertebral posterior element fracture, small pneumothorax.
- Small asymptomatic cement embolization to the lungs via the paravertebral venous plexus.

Major Complications

- Spinal cord or nerve root injury or compression.
- Permanent complications requiring decompressive surgery occur in less than 1 % of cases.
- Most of these complications happen because of the use of poor imaging equipment. Portable C-arms are generally not adequate for this procedure.
- Death is rare but reported both in vertebroplasty and kyphoplasty.

Key Points

> Vertebral augmentation is a safe and effective, minimally invasive treatment for painful vertebral compression fracture caused by osteoporosis, tumor invasion, or hemangioma.
> Appropriate patient selection using clinical history, physical examination, and imaging evaluation is critical for success.
> Medial wall of pedicle must be well defined to prevent needle passage through spinal canal.
> Monitor cement injection under real-time fluoroscopy or visualize small quantities of 0.1–0.2 cc injection distribution before additional cement is introduced.
> Treatment of underlying disorder such as osteoporosis or malignancy is important to avoid additional fractures.

Suggested Reading

1. Fourney DR, Schomer DF, Nader R, et al. Percutaneous vertebroplasty and kyphoplasty for painful vertebral fractures in cancer patients. J Neurosurg Spine. 2003;98:21–30.
2. Gaitanis I, Hadjipavlou AG, Katonis PG, et al. Balloon kyphoplasty for the treatment of pathological vertebral compressive fractures. Eur Spine J. 2005;14:250–60.
3. Gangi A, Clark WA. Have recent vertebroplasty trials changed the indications for vertebroplasty? Cardiovasc Intervent Radiol. 2010;33:677–80.
4. Jensen ME, Evans AJ, Mathis JM, et al. Percutaneous polymethylmethacrylate vertebroplasty in the treatment of osteoporotic vertebral body compression fracture: technical aspects. AJNR Am J Neuroradiol. 1997;18:1897–904.
5. Kasperk C, Meeder PJ, Noldge G, et al. Vertebroplasty and kyphoplasty: inefficient treatments for degenerative spine disease. Exp Clin Endocrinol Diabetes. 2010;118:71–4.
6. Laredo JD, Hamze B. Complications of percutaneous vertebroplasty and their prevention. Skeletal Radiol. 2004;33:493–505.
7. Layton KF, Thielen KR, Koch CA, et al. Vertebroplasty, first 1000 levels of a single center: evaluation of the outcomes and complications. AJNR Am J Neuroradiol. 2007;28:683–9.
8. Mathis JM. Percutaneous vertebroplasty: complication avoidance and technique optimization. AJNR Am J Neuroradiol. 2003;24:1697–706.
9. Maynard AS, Jensen ME, Schweickert PA, et al. Value of bone scan imaging in predicting pain relief from percutaneous vertebroplasty in osteoporotic vertebral fractures. AJNR Am J Neuroradiol. 2000;21:1807–12.
10. Murphy KJ, Deramond H. Percutaneous vertebroplasty in benign and malignant disease. Neuroimaging Clin N Am. 2000;10:535–45.
11. Zoarski GH, Snow P, Olan WJ, et al. Percutaneous vertebroplasty for osteoporotic compression fractures: quantitative prospective evaluation of long-term outcomes. J Vasc Interv Radiol. 2002;13:139–48.

Disc Interventions: Oxygen-Ozone (O2-O3)

Gianluigi Guarnieri, Fabio Zeccolini, and Mario Muto

Abstract

Low back pain (LBP) is one of the most common spine diseases and causes of absence from work in developed countries. Around 80 % of adults suffer from low back pain during a lifetime, and 55 % are suffering from back pain associated with radicular syndrome. The most common cause of LBP with classical irradiation along the nerve root course is disc herniation with a natural history characterized by resolution of clinical symptoms in up to 60 % of cases by conservative medical treatment and bed rest for about 6 weeks and natural shrinkage of the disc herniation revealed by CT or MR within 8–9 months after the beginning of back pain. Surgery is considered the treatment of choice for extruded, migrated, and free fragment herniated disc, with a success rate in the short term around 85–90 %.

Keywords

Disc intervention • Oxygen-ozone • Low back pain • Spine disease • Radicular syndrome • Nerve root irritation • Disc herniation • Natural history • Clinical symptoms • Digital imaging • Surgery • Extruded herniated disc • Migrated herniated disc • Free fragment herniated disc • Failed back syndrome • Hypertrophic scar

Introduction

- Low back pain (LBP) is one of the most common spine diseases and causes of absence from work in developed countries. Around 80 % of adults suffer from low back pain during a lifetime, and 55 % are suffering from back pain associated with radicular syndrome.

G. Guarnieri, MD • F. Zeccolini, MD • M. Muto, MD (✉)
Department of Neuroradiology, AORN Cardarelli, Naples, Italy
e-mail: mutomar@tiscali.it

K. Murphy, F. Robertson (eds.), *Interventional Neuroradiology,*
Techniques in Interventional Radiology*,*
DOI 10.1007/978-1-4471-4582-0_22, © Springer-Verlag London 2014

- The most common cause of LBP with classical irradiation along the nerve root course is disc herniation with a natural history characterized by resolution of clinical symptoms in up to 60 % of cases by conservative medical treatment and bed rest for about 6 weeks and natural shrinkage of the disc herniation revealed by computed tomography (CT) or magnetic resonance (MR) within 8–9 months after the onset of back pain.
- Surgery is considered the treatment of choice for extruded, migrated, and free fragment herniated disc, with a short-term success rate of approximately 85–90 %, and then decreasing to around 80 % in the long term (more than 6 months) due to failed back syndrome (FBS) characterized by recurrent back pain and/or hypertrophic scar with severe symptoms in 15–20 % of patients.
- Recently minimally invasive techniques have been developed as "alternative" treatments to surgical intervention for patients affected by LBP due to a small or contained herniated disc, without any benefit from medical treatment, with an outcome that depends on the characteristics of hernia itself and on the chosen technique. These include:
  - Chemodiscolysis with chymopapain (*no longer used*).
  - Automated percutaneous lumbar discectomy by Onik (APLD).
  - Percutaneous laser disc decompression (PLDD).
  - Intradiscal electrothermal therapy (IDET).
  - Percutaneous coblation nucleoplasty.
  - Dekompressor percutaneous discectomy.
  - Chemodiscolysis with O2-O3 mixture with periradicular and periganglionic infiltration.
  - Jellified ethyl alcohol (*Discogel®*, *Gelscom*, *Hérouville-Saint-Clair*, *France*).
- All techniques can be performed under CT or fluoroscopic guidance in patient in prone position and under local anesthesia, offering good results with good patient compliance, low cost, and low rate of complications.
- Patients need a short period of hospitalization, all techniques can be performed on the day of surgery, and in case of failed treatment, all techniques can be reproduced one more time without preventing surgery at a later date.
- All procedures can be performed at cervical or lumbar level.
- The rationale of all percutaneous treatments is to reduce the intradiscal pressure in different ways, creating the space required to decompress retropulsion or mass affect of the disc.
- Background for a percutaneous disc treatment is:
  - A complete clinical evaluation: to distinguish radicular pain from articular facet syndrome or piriformis syndrome and to discern a discal origin from a vertebrogenic origin of pain.
  - Evaluation with diagnostic examinations [X-Ray, CT, MRI, electromyography (EMG)].
  - Do not treat patients in whom there is an urgent need for surgery (patients with cauda equina syndrome, patients with progressive foot drop, and patients with severe sciatica).

Pathogenesis of Low Back Pain

- The pathogenesis of LBP is multifactorial:
  1. A mechanical cause: the nerve root compression.
  2. Acute inflammatory factors.

Direct Mechanical Factors

- Direct compression of herniated disc on the dorsal root ganglion (extraforaminal herniation).
- Mechanical deformation of posterior longitudinal ligament and annulus with nociceptor stimulation of recurrent nerve of Luschka.

Indirect Mechanical Factors

- Ischemia due to compression on afferent arterioles and nerve bundle microcirculation (with associated anoxic demyelination of nerve fibers).
- Venous stasis.

Inflammatory Factors

- Cell-mediated inflammatory reaction to disc protrusion: Nucleus pulposus is formed by proteoglycans immunologically segregated after birth; a herniated fragment may trigger an inflammatory process with autoimmune cell-mediated response, led by macrophages.
- Bio-humoral immunological response, due to phospholipase A2 (inflammatory inductor) that produces prostaglandin (PGE2) and leucotrieni from arachidonic acid.
- Matrix metalloproteinase (MMP-1, MMP-2, MMP-3, MMP-9) that degrade discal tissue and increase inflammatory reaction.
- IL-1, IL-6, and TNF-alfa that cause matrix degradation.

General Selection Criteria: Indications and Contraindications

General Exclusion Criteria

- Extruded herniated disc.
- Free herniated fragment.
- Recent disc or vertebral infection.
- High arm deficit.

- Sphincter dysfunction.
- Extreme sciatica.
- Progressive neurological deficits of the involved body segment.
- Last three conditions are absolute indications for surgery.
- The best results are reported for small- and medium-sized herniations with a normal spinal canal, without disc calcifications.

Prognostic Factors for an Unsuccessful Outcome

- The presence of a calcified herniated disc.
- High-grade spinal stenosis.
- Small descending herniated disc in the lateral spinal recess.
- Failed back syndrome and recurrent disc herniation.

Inclusion Criteria

Clinical Criteria

- LBP and sciatica resistant to conservative medical therapy, physiotherapy, and other interventions for a period not shorter than 2–3 months.

Neurological Criteria

- Paresthesia or altered sensitivity over the dermatome involved, mild muscle weakness, and signs of root ganglion irritation.

Psychological Criteria

- A firm resolve on the part of the patient to recover with a commitment to cooperate and undergo subsequent physiotherapy with postural and motor rehabilitation.

Neuroradiological Criteria (CT, MRI)

- Small- and medium-sized herniated discs correlating with the patients' symptoms with or without degenerative disc-vertebra disease complicated by intervertebral disc changes (protrusion, herniation).
- Pain provoked by low-pressure contrast injection in the compromised disc during discography for IDET, nucleoplasty, and APLD techniques.
- Residual of surgical (micro)-discectomy with herniation recurrence and/or hypertrophic fibrous scarring.

The Choice of "Radiological Guide": CT or Fluoroscopy

- All techniques need a radiological specific support: CT or fluoroscopic guided (DSA, C-arm). The choice among any different techniques depends on personal preference and availability of a good-quality guidance and technology.
- Generally, all procedure can be performed under fluoroscopic guide or CT without any significant difference.
- The use of CT helps to identify the presence of bowel loops behind the muscle psoas, an absolute contraindication for any oblique approach to the disc.

Techniques

Minimally invasive percutaneous techniques of lumbar herniated disc introduced in clinical practice are:

- Automated percutaneous lumbar discectomy (APLD).
- Percutaneous laser disc decompression (PLDD).
- Intradiscal electrothermal therapy (IDET).
- Percutaneous coblation nucleoplasty.
- Dekompressor percutaneous discectomy.
- Chemodiscolysis with O2-O3 mixture with periradicular and periganglionic infiltration.
- Jellified ethyl alcohol (*Discogel®*).

Automated Percutaneous Lumbar Discectomy (APLD)

- It uses an instrument called a "nucleotom" composed by a pneumatic pump working with air compressed, connected to an "aspirating-cutting" probe with an external diameter of 2 mm. The probe is introduced in the disc through a needle of 2.5 mm diameter under fluoroscopic guidance. The nucleus pulposus is aspirated through a lateral window of the probe while a blade, that moves coaxial in the probe, destroys it and allows it to be drained outside.
- The indications are all types and locations of protrusion or herniated disc without extrusion or free fragment.The success is about 70–80 % with good results; if the exclusion criteria are not considered, the success rate drops down to 49.4 %.
- When the procedure is not performed correctly, it may damage nerve roots or dura tissue. The greatest complication that has been reported of this procedure is "cauda equina syndrome" characterized by saddle anesthesia of perineal region, retention or urine/fecal incontinence, and bilateral hyposthenia.

Percutaneous Laser Disc Decompression (PLDD)

- Consists of introducing a soft flexible needle (0.8 mm calibre) inside the nucleus pulposus of the herniated disc, under fluoroscopic guidance.
- After confirming the correct position of the needle, a thin optical fiber is introduced, which is connected to a Nd-YAG laser, a special laser who works with a solid energy source, the yttrium-aluminum-garnet crystal addicted with neodymium (YAG – yttrium, aluminum, and garnet).
- The action is based on the idea that the vertebral disc is a closed hydraulic system composed by the nucleus pulposus, made of water, surrounded by the fibrous annulus. An increasing water content of nucleus pulposus causes a disproportionate increase of intradiscal pressure. By vaporizing the nucleus pulposus, it leads to a reduction of intradiscal pressure and it facilitates a relocation of the extruded nucleus pulposus into its original position.
- The laser vaporizes water in the nucleus pulposus, allowing a decompression of disc pressure and nerve root with resolution of symptoms.
- It can be performed under CT or fluoroscopic guidance.
- If the hernia is contained, it is possible to perform PLDD under fluoroscopic guide releasing laser energy at the vertebral disc's center and in the posterior portion.
- If the disc herniation is not contained but still connected to intervertebral disc, it is better to perform the decompression or procedure under CT to better assess the connection of disc and hernia portion. In this way the laser energy can be released in multiple locations of the herniated disc, obtaining a better vaporization and a higher retraction of the hernia with resultant root decompression and resolution of symptoms.
- The outcomes reported are success rates between 75 and 87 % of cases with an immediate reduction of back pain in 48 % cases.
- Septic and aseptic discitis is the most common complication, with an average of recurrence of 0–1.2 % of cases. Septic discitis is caused by introduction of microorganisms during positioning of the needle into the disc. A sterile technique is required.
- Aseptic discitis is caused by the action of laser itself on the disc and on the adjacent vertebral plate.
- Uncommon complications such as intestinal perforation, cauda equina syndrome, and nerve root lesion with consequent impairments have been reported.

Intradiscal Electrothermal Therapy (IDET)

- It acts on the posterior aspect of the fibrous annulus, unlike other techniques in which the action is on the nucleus pulposus.
- Under fluoroscopic guidance, a trocar is introduced in the intervertebral disc; then an electrothermic flexible catheter is introduced between the nucleus pulposus and annulus. The tip of the catheter has a resistor that, once placed near the posterior margin of the annulus, is warmed at 90° for 16–17 min and then removed (Fig. 1a–e).
- Warming of the fibrous annulus reduces the symptoms and stabilizes the discal lesion through the reorganization of the collagen fibers, the strengthening of the disc, the lesion of ring fissures, and ablation of pain receptors.

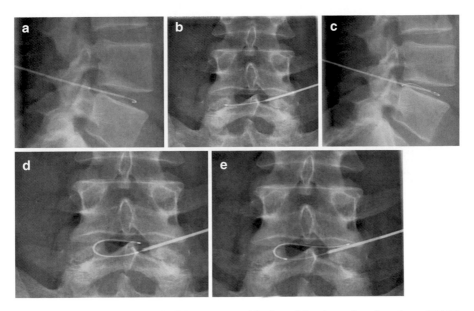

Fig. 1 (a–e) Fluoroscopic control of the correct positioning of the electrothermic catheter (IDET) in the L4–L5 disc using the posterolateral approach

- It is indicated for the treatment of bulging disc or contained herniated disc without root compression symptoms and resistance to pharmacological therapy and physiotherapy for more than 6 months.
- To obtain a better evaluation of contained hernia, disc compression, or disc pressure, a previous discography may be needed.
- The complication rate is 0.8 % with high frequency of osteonecrosis post-IDET.
- The success rate is between 40 and 71 % of cases.

Percutaneous Coblation Nucleoplasty

- This technique is performed with low temperatures (50–70°) differently from traditional radiofrequency that uses high temperatures (150–200°), obtaining the same results in a shorter time (2–3″ versus 15–17″).
- Under fluoroscopic guidance, a thermic coagulator (Perc-D coblation Probe) is introduced into the nucleus pulposus; then a bipolar current is applied on the extremity of the electrode, producing a radiofrequency field that breaks collagen bonds. It creates inside the nucleus "an ionic plasma" containing simple molecules and ionized gas such as O_2, H_2, and NO that will be removed through the needle used to introduce the electrode. The warmth produced does not exceed 70°, and it has a limited diffusion of 2 mm, creating a canal of thermic lesion in the nucleus pulposus. By a manual 360° rotation of the probe for 6 times, without any other movements of in-outside, the system creates six canals of thermic lesion with a rapid dehydration of the nucleus and reduction of disc volume of

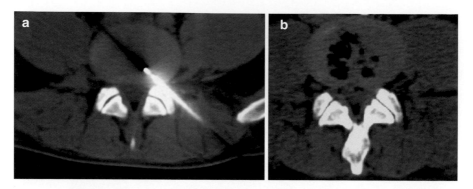

Fig. 2 (**a**) Coblation nucleoplasty at level L4–L5 under CT control using the posterolateral approach in a patient in the prone position; (**b**) posttreatment control LL and AP fluoroscopic control of the correct position of the needle at the C5–C6 level

about 10–20 %. The following contraction of the collagen fibers allows the reduction of the protruded portion with decompression of the compressed root (Fig. 2a–b).

- Essential condition is the integrity of the fibrous annulus; otherwise, the mechanism of retraction cannot happen. Best indication is the symptomatic herniated but not extruded disc.
- Results obtained from control trials report the resolution of pain symptoms in 70–80 % of cases with duration of pain relief for at least 6 months.
- The risk of complications is very low. Principal complications are discitis, anterior disc perforation caused by probe, and cauda equina syndrome.

Dekompressor Percutaneous Discectomy

- The aim of this technique is to remove the nucleus pulposus.
- A discogram is suggested.
- The dekompressor probe (*Stryker, Kalamazoo, MI, USA*) is introduced through the coaxial 17 gauge trocar into the nucleus pulposus. The trocar can be curved manually if the access is difficult, especially when the herniated disc is at level L5–S1. After switching on the rotating engine, the probe is moved forward and backward, removing and removing tissue (Fig. 3a–d).
- The procedure is complete when there is no more material to extract or when the radiologist feels obtaining a satisfactory decompression.
- The lumbar percutaneous discectomy dekompressor can be performed under CT or fluoroscopic guidance, without technique limitations; however, if it is performed by fluoroscopic guidance with the patient in the prone position, a posterolateral approach is needed to arrive into the disc using the lateral foramen as the landmark.
- The location of the hernia is the most important parameter for the efficacy of therapy. The indications are central or posterolateral and foraminal or extraforaminal herniated disc. The reduction of symptoms is over 70 in 79 % of foraminal posterolateral or extraforaminal hernia.

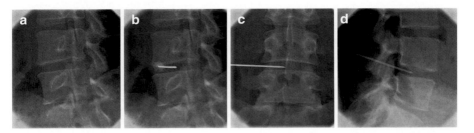

Fig. 3 (**a–d**) Dekompressor percutaneous discectomy at level L4–L5 in patient in the prone position and under fluoroscopic guidance with oblique tube orientation using the posterolateral approach

- This technique offers many advantages:
  - The calibre of the probe is only 16G (1.5 mm), reducing the risk of damage to the longitudinal posterior ligament and the annulus.
  - The probe and the trocar can be curved manually in case of difficult approach.
  - The probe rotation system allows the nucleus aspiration not only in case of central or paracentral herniation but also in case of foraminal and extraforaminal herniated disc without root damage.
- Removing 3 cm of disc material resulted in a significant pressure decrease on the peripheral disc portion, resolving the disc-radicular conflict.
- Success is achieved in 70–79 % of cases.
- Three cases of broken probe have been reported.

Chemodiscolysis with O2-O3 Mixture with Periradicular and Periganglionic Infiltration

- Ozone is an unstable, colorless, irritating gas, with a thorny smell, oxidative power, and antiseptic, disinfectant, and antiviral properties. It is prepared and used in real time, transforming a small percentage of O2 to O3 by special generators. The mixture O2-O3 is injected in the intradiscal space and in the foramen: 3–4 mL in the disc and 10 mL in the foramen. The administrated dose for treating the disc is 30–40 μm/mL, and it is resulted to be the best concentration to dehydrate the nucleus and to reduce the inflammation.
- The rationale is that the pain is due to mechanical compression on the root with associated inflammatory changes in periganglionic and periradicular spaces.
- With the patient in the prone position, the technique is usually performed under CT for better evaluation of gas distribution into the disc or periganglionic space.
- The technique can be performed also by fluoroscopic guidance with control of the intradiscal or canal gas distribution.
- A needle is inserted in the nucleus pulposus (18–20 gauge calibre and 7–10 cm length) by oblique paravertebral approach using as target the specific articular facet (Fig. 4a–c). Sometimes, especially at the L5–S1 level, when the "classic" oblique approach might

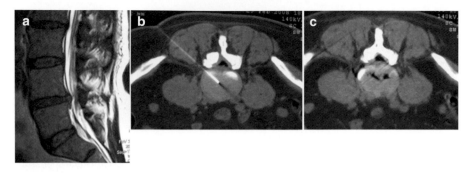

Fig. 4 (**a**) Sagittal T2W MRI shows a herniated disc at level L4–L5; (**b**) axial T2W MRI shows right posterolateral herniated disc L4–L5; (**c**) axial CT at level L4–L5 in a patient in the prone position; the needle is inserted in the nucleus pulposus L4–L5 by the posterolateral approach, with gas distribution into the disc and right periganglionic space

be difficult for anatomical reasons, a further needle inclination of 30° is necessary in the craniocaudal direction, to reach the specific disc space, or a translaminar medial approach should be performed without fear of crossing the dural sac to reach the vertebral disc (Figs. 5a–d and 6a–c).

- The needle is placed in the center of the disc and the gas mixture is slowly injected in the nucleus pulposus, then into the epidural and intraforaminal space with a local anti-inflammatory effect.
- Extruded herniated disc or free herniated fragments are contraindications.
- Discography is not needed because it adds no diagnostic information necessary for the treatment and may affect the impact of the ozone gas.
- The oxygen-ozone mechanisms of action have been investigated and include:
  - Anti-inflammatory effect due to oxidative action on the chemical pain mediators.
  - Improvement of capillary blood perfusion and the resolution of venous stasis with better tissue oxygenation and reduction of the root edema.
  - Direct action, through oxygenation process, on the bounds of nucleus pulposus mucopolysaccharides filled with water with secondary disc dehydration.
- No damage is reported if the O2-O3 goes into the CSF or subarachnoid space.
- The success rate is reported in 70–80 % of cases.
- No early or late neurological or infectious complications have been reported following O2-O3 injection.
- A recent meta-analysis about the effectiveness and safety of ozone treatments for herniated lumbar discs shows that pain and function outcomes are similar to the outcomes for lumbar discs treated with surgical discectomy, but the complication rate is much lower (<0.1 %) and the recovery time is significantly shorter.

Jellified Ethyl Alcohol (Discogel®)

- It is formed by a sterile viscous solution containing 96 % pure ethyl alcohol (a cellulose derivative product) added to a radiopaque element – *tungsten* – that when injected into the vertebral disc at the cervical or lumbar level produces a local necrosis of the *nucleus*

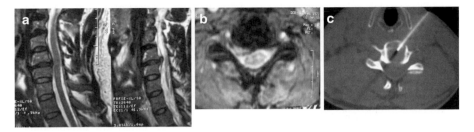

Fig. 5 (**a**) Sagittal T2W MRI shows a herniated disc at level L5–S1; (**b**) axial T2W MRI shows left posterolateral herniated disc at L5–S1; (**c**) axial CT at level L5–S1 in a patient in the prone position; the needle is inserted into the nucleus pulposus L5–S1 by left translaminar approach

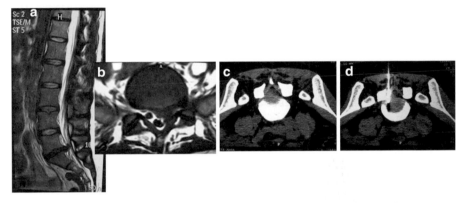

Fig. 6 (**a**, **b**) Sagittal and axial T2W show a herniated disc at level C5–C6; (**c** and **d**) axial CT at level C5–C6 in a patient in the supine position; the needle is inserted into the nucleus pulposus by anterolateral approach with manual dislocation of the carotid axis

pulposus. Its action is mechanical via dehydration of the turgescent and protruding disc, which is compressing the peripheral nerves of the cord, causing extreme pain.

- After asepsis and local anesthesia, the product is injected into the *nucleus pulposus* under CT or fluoroscopic guide with post-lateral approach for thoracic or lumbar level and anterolateral approach at for the cervical level.
- Preferably the disc is punctured using a small needle of:
  - 18 gauge for thoracic and lumbar discs, so as to reach the central region of the intraspinal space.
  - 20 gauge for cervical disc.
- The quantity of jellified ethyl alcohol injected varies between 0.2 and 0.8 mL, according to the dimension of the disc and extent of the hernia.
- It is recommended to use:
  - 0.2 mL of jellified ethyl alcohol for cervical discs.
  - 0.3–0.5 mL of jellified ethyl alcohol for thoracic discs.
  - 0.6–0.8 mL of jellified ethyl alcohol for lumbar discs.
- At the onset of the injection, the patient may experience a transitional scalding sensation in the region of injection which disappears in the course of injection. To minimize this risk, the product must be injected very slowly. Once the product has been injected, the needle is left 2 min before being withdrawn.

- The viscosity of jellified ethyl alcohol depends on the temperature. Avoid an administration of the product warmed up above room temperature, because gel becomes more liquid and is below optimum viscosity. To increase its viscosity, jellified ethyl alcohol can be refrigerated just prior to injection.
- It is not indicated in pregnant woman and in patients known to be allergic to one of the components and patients in severe depression or any other conditions making the interpretation of pain difficult.
- Experimental study on pigs performed injecting Discogel intradiscal, intraforaminal, epidural, and intramuscular elements demonstrated that Discogel does not produce any changes in contact with nervous system structures or muscular tissue. In fact no tissual alteration was found but only some inflammatory elements like lymphomonocyte cells and venous stasis with same granular material colored black by hematoxylin-eosin method (the tungsten) in paravertebral tissue in the muscular and connective tissue. The success rate is between 89 and 91 % of cases without any minor or major complications.

Which Percutaneous Disc Treatment Do You Choose?

- Clinical and diagnostic imaging selection criteria are very important to avoid an overtreatment.
- Surgical indications have been previously underlined and should always be respected also to exclude medicolegal problems.
- Our first choice is always intradiscal-intraforaminal CT-guided oxygen-ozone injection; this is related to its ease of use, reproducibility, rate of success, rate of complications, as well as cost-relatedness.
- In case of failure of this technique, we go usually over with a different technique in which if low back pain is prevalent on radicular pain, we suggest nucleoplasty while if radiculopathy is prevalent on low back pain, we suggest Discogel.

Key Points

> Minimally invasive techniques can be a valuable alternative to traditional surgery with low cost, low risk of complications, ease of use, and reproducibility without preventing the surgery in a later date, in case of failure.

> All techniques can be performed under CT or fluoroscopy guidance, in patient in prone position and under local anesthesia and requiring a short period of hospitalization.

> All procedures can be performed at cervical or lumbar level.

> The rationale of all percutaneous treatments is to reduce the intradiscal pressure by creating the space required to retropulsion or digestion of the disc.

> Surgery remains indicated in emergency cases of neurological deficit or severe low back pain.

Suggested Reading

1. Agarwal S. Ho:YAG laser-assisted lumbar disc decompression: a minimally invasive procedure under local anesthesia. Neurol India. 2003;51:35–8.
2. Amoretti N, Huchot F, Flory P, Brunner P, et al. Percutaneous nucleotomy: preliminary communication on a decompression probe (dekompressor) in percutaneous discectomy. Ten case reports. Clin Imaging. 2005;29:98–101.
3. Amoretti N, Davida P, Grimaud A, et al. Clinical follow-up of 50 patients treated by percutaneous lumbar discectomy. Clin Imaging. 2006;30:242–4.
4. Andersson G, Totta M, et al. Meta-analysis of the efficacy and safety of intradiscal electrothermal therapy (IDET). Pain Med. 2006;7(4):308–16.
5. Andreula C. Lumbar herniated disk and degenerative changes. Interventional spinal treatment with chemiodiscolysis with nucleoptesis with O2-O3 and perigangliar infiltration in 150 cases. Riv Neuroradiol. 2002;14:81–8.
6. Andreula C. Interventional spinal procedures. Riv Neuroradiol. 2005;18:71–4.
7. Andreula CF, Simonetti L, De Santis F, Agati R, Ricci R, Leonardi M. Minimally invasive oxygen-ozone therapy for lumbar disk herniation. AJNR Am J Neuroradiol. 2003;24:996–1000.
8. Andreula C, Muto M, Leonardi M. Interventional spinal procedures. Eur J Radiol. 2004;50:112–9.
9. Bocci V. Ossigeno-ozonoterapia. Comprensione dei meccanismi di azione e possibilità terapeutiche. Milano: Ambrosiana; 2000.
10. Bonaldi G, Baruzzi F, et al. Plasma radio-frequency–based diskectomy for treatment of cervical herniated nucleus pulposus: feasibility, safety, and preliminary clinical results. AJNR Am J Neuroradiol. 2006;27:2104–11.
11. Bonetti M, Cotticelli B, et al. Oxygen-ozone therapy versus epidural steroid injection. Riv Neuroradiol. 2000;13:203–6.
12. Bonetti M, Leonardi M, et al. Intraforaminal O2-O3 versus periradicular steroidal infiltrations in lower back pain: randomized controlled trial. AJNR Am J Neuroradiol. 2005;26: 996–1000.
13. Bossaco SJ, Bossaco DN, Berman AT, et al. Functional results of percutaneous laser discectomy. Am J Orthop. 1996;25:825–8.
14. Boswell MV, Shah RV, Everett CR, Sehgal N, et al. Interventional techniques in the management of chronic spinal pain: evidence-based practice guidelines. Pain Physician. 2005;8(1): 1–47.
15. Bush K, Cowan N, Katz DE, Gishen P. The natural history of sciatica associated with disc pathology. A prospective study with clinical and independent radiologic follow-up. Spine. 1992;17(10):1205–12.
16. Choy DS. Percutaneous laser disc decompression (PLDD): twelve years experience with 752 procedures in 518 patients. J Clin Laser Med Surg. 1998;16:325–31.
17. Choy DSJ, et al. Percutaneous laser disc decompression: a new therapeutic modality. Spine. 1992;17:949–56.
18. D'Erme M, Scarchilli A, et al. Ozone therapy in lumbar sciatic pain. Radiol Med. 1999; 95:21–4.
19. Domsky R, Goldberg ME, Hirsh RA, et al. Critical failure of a percutaneous discectomy probe requiring surgical removal during disc decompression. Reg Anesth Pain Med. 2006;31(2):177–9.
20. Eckel TS. Intradiscal electrothermal therapy. In: Williams AL, Murtagh FR, editors. Handbook of diagnostic and therapeutic spine procedures. St. Louis: Mosby; 2002. p. 229–44.

21. Gallucci M, Splendiani A, Masciocchi C. Spine and spinal cord: neuroradiological functional anatomy. Riv Neuroradiol. 1997;11:293–304.

22. Gallucci M, Limbucci N, Masciocchi C, et al. Sciatica: treatment with intradiscal and intraforaminal injections of steroid and oxygen-ozone versus steroid only. Radiology. 2007;242: 907–17.

23. Gangi A, Dietemann JL, Mortazavi R, Pfleger D, et al. CT-guided interventional procedures for pain management in the lumbosacral spine. Radiographics. 1998a;18(3):621–33.

24. Gangi A, Guth S, Dietemann J-L, et al. Interventional radiology with laser in bone and joint. Radiol Clin North Am. 1998b;36:547–56.

25. Gibson JNA, Grant IC, Waddell G. Surgery for lumbar disc prolapse (Cochrane Review). In: The cochrane library, vol. 2. Oxford: Update Software; 2003.

26. Guarnieri G, De Dominicis G, Muto M. Intradiscal and intramuscular injection of discogel® – radiopaque gelified ethanol:pathological evaluation. Neuroradiol J. 2010;23:249–52.

27. Gupta AK, Bodhey NK, Jayasree RS, Kapilamoorthy TR, et al. Percutaneous laser disc decompression: clinical experience at SCTIMST and long term follow up. Neurol India. 2006;54(2):164–7.

28. Hammon W. Percutaneous lumbar nucleotomy. West Neuro Soc. 1989;635.

29. Hellinger J. Technical aspects of the percutaneous cervical and lumbar laser-disc decompression and nucleotomy. Neurol Res. 1999;21:99–102.

30. Hijikata S, et al. Percutaneous nucleotomy. A new concept technique and 12 years experience. Clin Orthop Relat Res. 1989;238:9–23.

31. Iliakis E, et al. Ozone treatment in low back pain. Orthopaedics. 1995;1:29–33.

32. Kelekis AD, Somon T, Yilmaz H, Bize P, Brountzos EN, et al. Interventional spine procedures. Eur J Radiol. 2005;55(3):362–83.

33. Kenneth M, Robert E. Percutaneous lumbar discectomy: clinical response in an initial cohort of fifty consecutive patients with chronic radicular pain. Pain Pract. 2004;4:19–27.

34. Leonardi M, Barbara C, et al. Percutaneous treatment of lumbar herniated disk with intradiscal injection of ozone mixture. Riv Neuroradiol. 2001;14:51–3.

35. Long DM. Decision making in lumbar disc disease. Clin Neurosurg. 1991;39:36–51.

36. Mathews RS. In: Savitz MH et al., editors. The practice of minimally invasive spine technique. 1st ed. Lima: CCS; 2000. p. 97–100.

37. Muto M. Alterazioni indotte da infiltrazioni intradiscali e intramuscolari di ossigeno-ozono:studio anatomo-patologico. Risultati preliminari. Riv Italiana di Ossigeno-Ozonoterapia. 2004;3:7–13.

38. Muto M, Avella F. Percutaneous treatment of herniated lumbar disk by intradiscal oxygen-ozone injection. Interv Neuroradiol. 1998;4:279–86.

39. Muto M, De Maria G, Izzo R, Fucci G, et al. Nondiscal lumbar radiculopathy:combined approach by CT and MR. Riv Neuroradiol. 1997;10:165–73.

40. Muto M, Andreula C, Leonardi M. Treatment of herniated lumbar disc by intradiscal and intraforaminal oxygen-ozone injection. J Neuroradiol. 2004;31(3):183–9.

41. Nerubay J, Caspi I, Levinkopf M. Percutaneous carbon dioxide laser nucleolysis with 2- to 5-year follow-up. Clin Orthop. 1997;337:45–8.

42. Ohnmeiss DD, Guyer RD, Hochschuler SH. Laser disc decompression: the importance of proper patient selection. Spine. 1994;19:2054–8.

43. Onik G, Helms CA, Ginsburg L, et al. Percutaneous lumbar discectomy using a new aspiration probe. AJNR Am J Neuroradiol. 1985;6:290–6.

44. Onik G, Mooney V, Maroon JC, Wiltse L, et al. Automated percutaneous discectomy: a prospective multi-institutional study. Neurosurgery. 1990;26(2):228–32.

45. Onik G, Maroon J, Jackson R. Cauda equina syndrome secondary to an improperly placed nucleotome probe. Neurosurgery. 1992;30(3):412–4.

46. Pauza KJ, Howell S, Dreyfuss P. A randomized, placebo-controlled trial of intradiscal electro-thermal therapy for the treatment of discogenic low back pain. Spine. 2004;4:27–35.

47. Saal JA, Saal JS. Intradiscal electrothermal treatment for chronic discogenic low back pain: a prospective outcome study with minimum 1-year follow-up. Spine. 2000;25:2622–7.

48. Saal JA, Saal JS. Intradiscal electrothermal treatment for chronic discogenic low back pain: prospective outcome study with a minimum 2-year follow-up. Spine. 2002a;27:966–74.

49. Saal JA, Saal JS. Intradiscal electrothermal treatment for chronic discogenic low back pain. Clin Sports Med. 2002b;21:167–87.

50. Sharps L. Percutaneous disc decompression using nucleoplasty. Pain Physician. 2002;5(2):121–6.

51. Singh V, Piryani C, Liao K. Percutaneous disc decompression using coblation in the treatment of chronic discogenic pain. Pain Physician. 2002;5:250–9.

52. Steppan J, Meaders T, Muto M, Murphy KJ. The effectiveness and safety of ozone treatments for herniated lumbar disc. J Vasc Interv Radiol. 2010;21:534–48.

53. Takeno K, Kobayashi S, Yonezawa T, Hayakawa K, et al. Salvage operation for persistent low back pain and sciatica induced by percutaneous laser disc decompression performed at out-side institution: correlation of magnetic resonance imaging and intraoperative and pathologi-cal findings. Photomed Laser Surg. 2006;24(3):414–23.

54. Theron J. "Jellified alcohol". Presented at the ESNR XXXIII Congress, Cracow, Poland; Sept 18–21, 2008 (personal oral communication).

55. Theron J, Guimaraens L, Casasco A, Sola T, Cuellar H. Percutaneous treatment of lumbar intervertebral disk hernias with radiopaque gelified ethanol: a preliminary study. J Spinal Disord Tech. 2007;20(7):526–32.

56. Theron J, Cuellar H, Sola T, et al. Percutaneous treatment of cervical disk hernias using geli-fied ethanol. AJNR Am J Neuroradiol. 2010;31:1454–6.

57. Tian JL, et al. Changes of CSF and spinal path-morphology after high concentration ozone injection into the subarachnoid space: an experimental study in pigs. AJNR Am J Neuroradiol. 2007;28:1051–4.

58. Turgut M. Extensive damage to the end-plates as a complication of laser discectomy: an experimental study using an animal model. Acta Neurochir (Wien). 2007;139:404–10.

59. Von Tulder MW, Koes BW, Bouter LM. Conservative treatment of acute and chronic non-specific low back pain. Spine. 1997;22:2128–56.

60. Wilco CP, van Houwelingen HC, Brand R, et al. Surgery versus prolonged conservative treat-ment for sciatica for the Leiden-The Hague Spine Intervention Prognostic Study Group. N Engl J Med. 2007;35622:2245–56.

Percutaneous Spinal Injections: Nerve Epidural and Neural Foraminal/Facet Joint Injections

Gianluigi Guarnieri, Roberto Izzo, and Mario Muto

Abstract

Low back pain (LBP) and neck pain (NP) are the most common spine diseases and the cause of absence from work in developed countries. Around 80 % of adults suffer from back pain or low back pain during a lifetime. Fifty-five percent suffer from radicular pain, of these 44 % in the cervical region, 15 % thoracic, and 66 % lumbar level. Most symptoms revolve spontaneously within few days or weeks with medical/conservative therapy, while about one-third of patients progress to chronic pain. The causes of chronic LBP or NP include vertebral body pathology, vertebral disc disease, spinal stenosis, nerve entrapment syndrome, and facet joint disease. The diagnosis of LBP or NP is difficult and should be done by a multidisciplinary team including clinical evaluation, imaging (CT, MRI, EMG), and multi-specialist approach (radiologist, neuroradiologist, neurosurgeons, and neurologist).

Keywords

Low back pain • Neck pain • Spine disease • Radicular pain • Cervical pain • Lumbar pain • Conservative therapy • Chronic pain • Vertebral body pathology • Vertebral disc disease • Spinal stenosis • Nerve entrapment syndrome • Facet joint disease • Diagnosis • Multidisciplinary approach • Diagnostic imaging • Percutaneous spinal analgesic injection • Epidural space • Foraminal space • Facet joints • Complications

G. Guarnieri, MD • R. Izzo, MD • M. Muto, MD (✉)
Department of Neuroradiology, AORN Cardarelli, Naples, Italy
e-mail: mutomar@tiscali.it

K. Murphy, F. Robertson (eds.), *Interventional Neuroradiology*,
Techniques in Interventional Radiology,
DOI 10.1007/978-1-4471-4582-0_23, © Springer-Verlag London 2014

Introduction

- Low back pain (LBP) and neck pain (NP) are the most common spine diseases and the cause of absence from work in developed countries. Around 80 % of adults suffer from back pain or low back pain during a lifetime; 55 % suffer from radicular pain, and of these 44 % are in the cervical region, 15 % in the thoracic region, and 66 % at the lumbar level.
- Most symptoms revolve spontaneously within a few days or weeks with medical/conservative therapy, while about one-third of patients progress to chronic pain.
- The causes of chronic LBP or NP include:
  - Vertebral body pathology.
  - Vertebral disc disease.
  - Spinal stenosis.
  - Nerve entrapment syndrome.
  - Facet joint disease (FJD).
- The diagnosis of LBP or NP is difficult and should be done by a multidisciplinary team including clinical evaluation, imaging [computed tomography (CT), magnetic resonance imaging (MRI), electromyography (EMG)], and multi-specialist approach (radiologist, neuroradiologist, neurosurgeons, and neurologist).
- Many mini-invasive spinal procedures have been developed for the management of this disease including percutaneous spinal analgesic injections in the epidural space or foraminal space and into facet joints with good results and with low complication rates (approximately 1 %).
- For the *pathogenesis* of LBP or NP.
- All procedures require a rigorous sterile approach.

Perineural, Epidural, and Foraminal Pain Injections

- This technique can be performed under CT, CT fluoroscopy, or fluoroscopic guidance (DSA or C-arm) with the patient in the prone position and with local skin anesthesia.
- The intention is to inject 1–2 cc of analgesic drug (Depo-Medrol 20–40 mg or Solu-Medrol 20 mg steroid drug) in a selective way at the specific level correlated by the patient's clinical status to obtain an analgesic effect.
- Local anesthetic must never be injected into the cervical spine because of the risk of cervical epidural block or intrathecal injection with resultant cardiorespiratory arrest.

General Inclusion, Exclusion, and Contraindication Criteria

- Low back pain with or without radicular symptoms with an MR examination if there is evidence of degenerative disc disease or herniated disc, refractory to 2–3 weeks of medical therapy.

- At the cervical region, we suggest treating only patients with clinical signs of radiculopathy and herniated disc. There is no correlation between clinical symptoms and herniated disc dimension.
- Patients with edematous nerve roots with inflammatory reaction due to degenerative disc disease. These can be seen on MRI.

Exclusion Criteria

- Extruded herniated disc.
- Free or sequestered herniated fragment.
- Recent disc or vertebral infection/discitis.
- Cord or conus compression.
- Progressive neurologic deficits of the involved cervical or lumbar root.

General Contraindication to Steroid Therapy

- Uncontrolled hypertension.
- Glaucoma.
- Gastric ulcers.

Procedures

- Intravenous access is always required for emergency in case of a vagal reaction with hypotension.
- If fluoroscopic guidance is used, it is important to perform a CT scan prior to the procedure to exclude a retro-psoas loop bowel. CT fluoroscopy is the best guidance, but there is a potential higher radiation dose exposure to the patient.
- The technique is performed by the postero-oblique approach with a 17–20-gauge (for thoracic or lumbar level) or 19–21-gauge (for cervical level) Chiba needle to get to epidural, perigangliar, or foraminal space for lumbar or thoracic level, while for cervical level, a posterior or anterolateral approach with manual dislocation of carotid axis is requested (Fig. 1a).
- For epidural injection, the needle is advanced into the epidural space by dorsal, oblique (20–30° caudal and lateral to the midline), and paramedian approach up to the superior margin of the spinal lamina, just subjacent to the interlaminar gap; then the needle can be pushed over the lamina, through the ligamentum flavum into the dorsal epidural space at the midline.
- For foraminal injection, a lateral angle greater than that used for the interlaminar technique, generally 35–45° from the midline, is used.
- The drug will be injected slowly to avoid reflux near the needle.

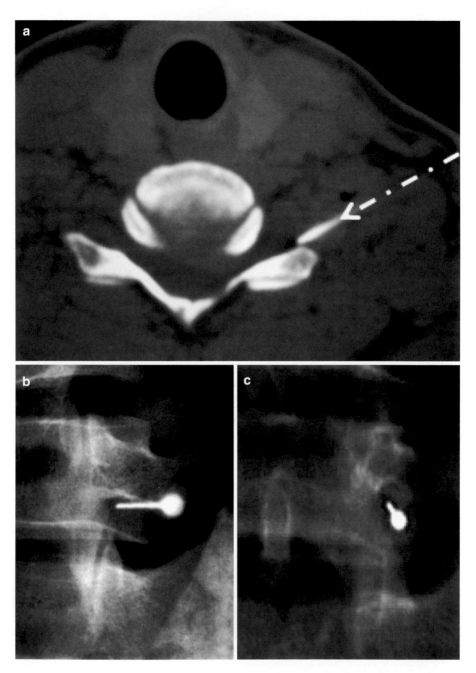

Fig. 1 (**a**) Patient affected by left posterolateral herniated disc at level C5–C6: scheme of anterolateral approach to foraminal space; (**b**) Fluoroscopic-guided needle placed into left foraminal at level C6–C7 with oblique tube orientation. (**c**) Fluoroscopic-guided needle placed into right foraminal at level L5–S1 in patient in prone position

- An injection of oxygen-ozone therapy (10 mL of 30 µg/mL at lumbar area and 3–4 mL at cervical area) can be performed after steroid injection to increase the anti-inflammatory and analgesic action.
- At lumbar level, it is suggested to add a local anesthetic (just 1 cc of lidocaine 1 %), while this is never performed at the cervical level to prevent epidural diffusion with respiratory distress.
- Patients do not require hospitalization and can be mobilized after the procedure without need of any other medical treatment.
- Good outcome short-term results up to a rate of 40–65 % are achieved while the results at long-term follow-up are lower.

Epidural Injection

- Epidural injection of corticosteroids with or without anesthetic drug is another therapy option commonly used in managing chronic spinal pain. Targets are patients suffering from back or neck pain with or without radiculopathy.
- All patients must be studied by CT and/or MRI before the treatment to clearly evaluate the pathology.
- The technique can be performed with the patient in the prone position by three different approaches:
  - The *transforaminal approach* is target specific and requires the smallest volume to reach the primary site of pathology, specifically, the anterolateral epidural space as well as the dorsal root ganglion (Fig. 1b–c).
  - The *interlaminar entry* can be directed more closely to the assumed site of pathology, requiring less volume than the caudal route (Fig. 2).

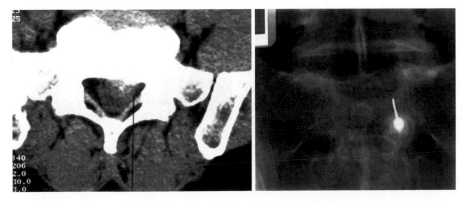

Fig. 2 CT scheme of translaminar approach; fluoroscopic-guided needle placed into right epidural space by translaminar approach at level L5–S1 in patient in prone position

- — The *caudal entry* is relatively easily achieved with minimal risk of inadvertent dural puncture, but requires a relatively high volume (10–20 mL) of injectate to reach the site of pathology.
- The mechanism of action of epidurally administered steroid with or without local anesthetic injections is well understood. The achieved neural blockade alters or interrupts nociceptive input, reflex mechanisms of the afferent fibers, self-sustaining activity of the neurons, and the pattern of central neuronal activities. Conversely, the local anesthetic interrupts the pain-spasm cycle, and reverberating nociceptor transmission, the corticosteroids reduce inflammation by inhibiting either the synthesis or release of a number of pro-inflammatory mediators and by causing a reversible local anesthetic effect.
- A radiopaque marker is used to identify the skin entry point and a sterile fashion is recommended.
- For the epidural approach, with the patient in the prone position under fluoroscopic or CT guidance, a 22-gauge spinal needle is advanced into the epidural space via a dorsal, oblique paramedian approach. The puncture site is typically 2–4 cm from the midline and 2–3 cm caudal to the intended point of entry into the dorsal epidural space.
- An 18-gauge venipuncture needle is placed from a puncture site 2–3 cm from the midline and without caudal offset over the desired interlaminar gap. An epidural needle with a blunt tip and side hole is then passed through the introducer needle to the midline dorsal epidural space. After the needle is placed, contrast material can be injected for epidurography, followed by therapeutic injection.
- For *transforaminal epidural injection*, the patient is placed in the prone position on the fluoroscopy/CT table. The skin is marked with the C-arm/CT tube oriented posterolaterally approximately 308–458 and with craniocaudal angulation to profile the caudal undersurface of the pedicle above the target foramen. For sacral foramen (S1 or S2) injections, a dorsal approach from directly above the appropriate foramen is used, and the same injection technique is employed.
- For *caudal (sacral hiatus) epidural injection*, the patient is place in the prone position, so the sacral hiatus can be palpated and visualized fluoroscopically. A fenestrated drape is placed and a 22-gauge spinal needle is advanced ventrally and rostrally at the midline to the sacral hiatus.
- For *cervical and thoracic epidural injection*, the patient is always placed in the prone position and the skin is marked 1–2 cm from the midline, slightly caudal to the interlaminar gap. The C-arm fluoroscopic axis is angled 108–158 off midline and caudal for this alignment. After sterile preparation and draping, 1–3 mL of 1–2 % lidocaine is injected subcutaneously for local anesthesia. The skin is then punctured and an epidural needle is advanced to the dorsal midline epidural space and just 2–5 mL of steroid can be injected. Anesthetic agent is not injected into the cervical epidural space to avoid the risk of respiratory suppression resulting from high cervical anesthesia.
- For lower thoracic injections (T7 to T8 or below), 3–5 mL of 1 % lidocaine can be injected after instillation of the steroid suspension.

Facet Joint Analgesic Injection

- The facet joints [zygapophyseal or z-joints (FJ)] are paired synovial joints at the posterior aspect of the spinal column. Each joint consists of the articulation between adjacent superior and inferior articular processes arising from adjacent vertebrae. They make a tripod support for each spinal level with the intervertebral disc.
- Approximately 30 % of patients affected by LBP, 55 % by NP, and 40 % with thoracic pain experience chronic spinal pain due to facet syndrome.
- Causes of facet syndrome include trauma, arthritis, inflammatory, and especially degeneration.
- FJ is manifested as axial low back or neck pain or headache; axial pain of thoracic level is less common.
- Symptoms are nonspecific and overlap with other diseases (cerviogenic headache, shoulder, or scapular pain).
- Clinical investigations include:
  - Pain aggravated by palpation of paraspinal muscles, standing, spinal extension, and facet joint loading with rotation with ameliorated by sitting and flexing the spine.
  - Morning pain and stiffness.
  - Occasional improvement with anti-inflammatory drugs.
- Diagnosis is done by exclusion criteria ruling out other causes of LBP or NP like vertebral body fracture, herniated disc, spinal stenosis, spondylolisthesis, and nerve entrapment.
- Imaging is not specific or sensitive. Degeneration and hypertrophy facet finding or accumulation of fluid in the joint capsule or MRI enhancement locally about facet joint can suggest FJ.
- In acute pain, medical conservative therapy is suggested, but if it fails after 6–12 weeks, an FJ syndrome can be considered.
- If there is pain relief after administration of local anesthetic directly into the joint capsule, a diagnosis of FJ syndrome can be made.
- The technique consists of injection of steroid drugs (1 cc of Depo-Medrol 20–40 mq) plus 1 cc lidocaine 1 % directly into facet joint with antalgic long effect under CT or fluoroscopic guidance and the patient in the prone position with an 18–20- or 22-gauge Chiba needle.
- A radiopaque marker is used to identify the skin entry point and a sterile fashion is recommended.
- The orientation of the needle rides on the orientation of each joint. The cervical facet joints are typically oriented in an oblique coronal plane angled superior to inferior in a posterior direction. The thoracic facet joints are nearly vertical and coronal in orientation. The superior lumbar facet joints are oriented in a nearly sagittal plane.
- CT guidance is easier than fluoroscopy to identify the correct orientation to approach to facet joint.
- For the cervical level, patient is in the prone position and the chest elevated with neck flexed; the technique is performed with the posterior or posterolateral approach, under

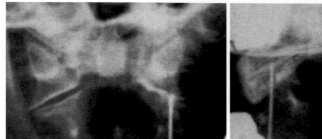
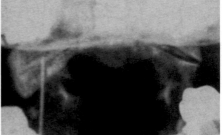

Fig. 3 Fluoroscopic-guided facet joint infiltration at level C1–C2 in patient in prone position.

Fig. 4 Fluoroscopic-guided left facet joint infiltration at level L4–L5 in patient in prone position

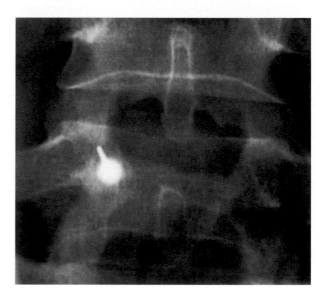

CT or fluoroscopic guidance. If fluoroscopic guidance is preferred, the tube may be angled in a craniocaudal direction to identify the lateral masses and FJ (Fig. 3).

- Once the needle is placed into the joint capsule, an arthrography may be performed with intra-articular injection of 0.2–0.5 of contrast drug that will be aspirated before steroid, plus anesthetic drug injection.
- Thoracic FJ level is rare and infrequently requested, but the technique performed is similar to that at the cervical level.
- For the lumbar level, the patient is in the prone position; a different angulation of the tube can be requested in order to view the joint along the imaging plane, parallel to the articular surfaces of the articular process (Figs. 4 and 5a–b).
- Steroid drugs and 1 % lidocaine can be injected directly into the joint capsule with or without arthrography anterior to or in the periradicular space.
- General contraindications include:
  - Systemic infection.
  - Skin infection.

- — Coagulopathy.
- — Thrombocytopenia.
- — Antiplatelet therapy.
- Early good outcome is achieved after FJ analgesic injection with low rate (less than 1 %) of minor complications such as infection, abscess, facet capsule rupture, allergic reaction, and vasovagal response.
- Intra-articular injection of steroid may be used for longer acting anti-inflammatory activity, and there are reports of long-term effectiveness in pain management depending on exact pathological process in the joint.
- Facet joint steroid injections can be performed with radiologic guidance in compressive vertebral facet joint synovial cysts.

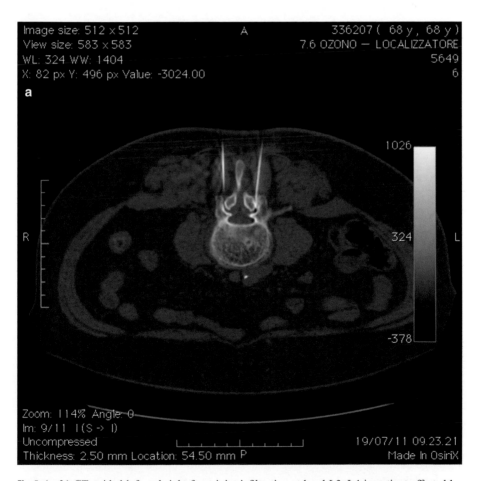

Fig. 5 (**a, b**) CT-guided left and right facet joint infiltration at level L3–L4 in patient affected by facet joint syndrome with good gas distribution into facet joint and paravertebral muscles

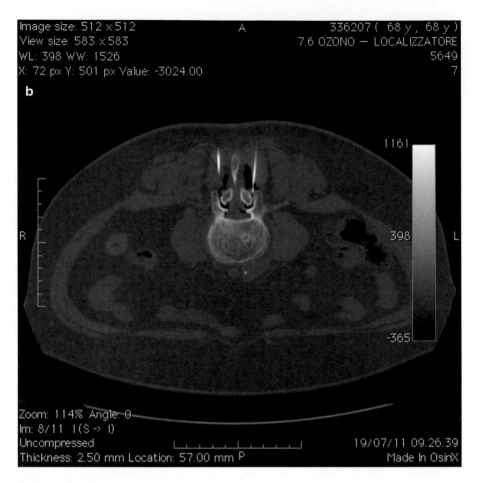

Fig. 5 (continued)

Facet Joint Synovial Cyst

- Facet joint synovial cysts are a recognized cause of femoral and sciatic nerve root pain/compression or LBP and NP. They are cystic dilations of synovial sheaths with or without anatomical continuity within a joint space that occasionally involves the lumbar spine. Usually detected by using CT or MRI, at cervical level or thoracic spine are rare, while more frequent are at lumbar level presenting with myelopathic/radicular symptoms.
- Image-guided aspiration can be used successfully in the management of lumbar synovial cysts.
- The patient is placed in the prone position and skin fashion is recommended.

- With fluoroscopic guidance, a 20-gauge, 9-cm spinal needle is inserted vertically and parallel to the x-ray beam toward the inferior recess of the joint until the bone is reached. Return of fluid confirms the correct intra-articular position of the needle.
- An injection of 1 mL of contrast element can be used in order to opacify the superior recess, confirming correct intra-articular needle position, and fill the facet joint synovial cyst. No contrast material is withdrawn during arthrography. The steroid is injected (3.75 mg of cortivazol or 100 mg of prednisolone acetate without additional anesthetics).
- The CT-guided aspiration of the cyst can be performed using a double-needle technique: one needle is used to open up the epidural space while another aspirated the cyst, followed by epidural injection of local anesthetic and steroids.

Key Points

> Periradicular, epidural, and foraminal analgesic injection can be performed under CT or fluoroscopic guidance (DSA or C-arm) with patients in the prone position and with only local skin anesthesia.

> The rationale is to inject 1–2 cc of analgesic drug (Depo-Medrol 20–40 mq or Bentelan 4 mg or Solu-Medrol 20 mg steroid drug) in a selective manner at a specific level correlated by the clinical status of the patient to obtain an antalgic effect.

> All procedures can be performed at the cervical or lumbar level.

> Generally, for thoracic or lumbar level, a postero-oblique approach with a 17–20-gauge Chiba needle under CT or fluoroscopic guidance is recommended.

> For cervical level, a posterior or anterolateral approach with manual dislocation of the carotid axis is recommended with a 19–21-gauge Chiba needle.

> Patients do not require hospitalization and be mobilized after the procedure without needing any other medical treatment. Anesthetic agent is not injected into the cervical epidural space to avoid the risk of respiratory suppression resulting from high cervical anesthesia.

> Facet joint analgesic injection can be performed under fluoroscopy or CT guidance with patients in the prone position injecting steroid drugs (1 cc of Depo-Medrol 20–40 mq) plus 1 cc lidocaine 1 % directly into the facet joint with antalgic using an 18–20- or 22-gauge Chiba needle.

> The orientation of the needle depends on the orientation of each joint. CT guidance is easier than fluoroscopy to identify the correct orientation to approach to facet joint.

> Once the needle is placed into the joint capsule, arthrography may be performed with intra-articular injection of 0.2–0.5 of contrast drug.

> The CT-guided aspiration of the facet joint synovial cyst can be performed using a double-needle technique: one needle is used to open up the epidural space while another aspirated the cyst, followed by epidural injection of local anesthetic and steroids.

Suggested Reading

1. Abdi S, Datta S, Trescot AM, et al. Epidural steroids in the management of chronic spinal pain: a systematic review. Pain Physician. 2007;10:185–221.
2. Baum J, Hanley E. Intraspinal synovial cyst simulating spinal stenosis. Spine. 1986;11:487–9.
3. Bjorkengren A, Kurz L, Resnick D, Sartoris D, Garfin S. Symptomatic intraspinal synovial cysts: opacification and treatment by percutaneous injection. AJR Am J Roentgenol. 1987; 149:105–7.
4. Bratton RL. Assessment and management of acute low back pain. Am Fam Physician. 1990;60:2299–308.
5. Byrod G, Otani K, Brisby H, Olmarker K, et al. Methylprednisolone reduces the early vascular permeability increase in spinal nerve roots induced by epidural nucleus pulposus application. J Orthop Res. 2000;18:983–7.
6. Carette S, Marcoux S, Truchon R, et al. A controlled trial of corticosteroid injections into facet joints for chronic low back pain. N Engl J Med. 1991;325:1002–7.
7. Carrera G. Lumbar facet joint injection in low back pain and sciatica. Radiology. 1989;137: 665–7.
8. Davis R, Iliya A, Roque C, Pampati M. The advantage of magnetic resonance imaging in diagnosis of the lumbar synovial cyst. Spine. 1990;15:244–6.
9. Finkelstein S, Sayegh R, Watson P, Knuckey N. Juxta-facet cysts: report of two cases and review of clinicopathologic features. Spine. 1993;18:779–82.
10. Hayashi N, Weinstein JN, Meller ST, Lee HM, Spratt KF, Gebhart GF. The effect of epidural injection of betamethasone or bupivacaine in a rat model of lumbar radiculopathy. Spine. 1998;23:877–85.
11. Hemminghytt S, Daniels D, Williams A, Haughton V. Intrasynovial cysts: natural history and diagnosis by CT. Radiology. 1982;145:375–6.
12. Hua SY, Chen YZ. Membrane receptor-mediated electrophysiological effects of glucocorticoid on mammalian neurons. Endocrinology. 1989;124:687–91.
13. Jackson D, Atlas S, Mani J, Norman D. Intraspinal synovial cysts: MR imaging. Radiology. 1989;170:527–30.
14. Jacob J, Weisman M, Mink JH, et al. Reversible cause of back pain and sciatica in rheumatoid arthritis: an apophyseal joint cyst. Arthritis Rheum. 1986;29:431–5.
15. Johnson BA, Schellhas KP, Pollei SR. Epidurography and therapeutic epidural injections: technical considerations and experience with 5334 cases. AJNR Am J Neuroradiol. 1999;20: 697–705.
16. Kingery WS, Castellote JM, Maze M. Methylprednisolone prevents the development of autotomy and neuropathic edema in rats, but has no effect on nociceptive thresholds. Pain. 1999;80:555–66.
17. Lee HM, Weinstein JN, Meller ST, Hayashi N, Spratt KF, Gebhart GF. The role of steroids and their effects on phospholipase A2: an animal model of radiculopathy. Spine. 1998;23: 1191–6.
18. Lemish W, Apsimon T, Chakera T. Lumbar intraspinal synovial cysts: recognition and CT diagnosis. Spine. 1989;14:1378–83.
19. Lundin A, Magnuson A, Axelsson K, Nilsson O, Samuelsson L. Corticosteroids preoperatively diminishes damage to the C-fibers in microscopic lumbar disc surgery. Spine. 2005;30:2362–7.
20. Maldjian C, Mesgarzadeh M, Tehranzadeh J. Diagnostic and therapeutic features of facet and sacroiliac joint injection. Anatomy, pathophysiology, and technique. Radiol Clin North Am. 1998;36(3):497–508.

21. Minamide A, Tamaki T, Hashizume H, Hayashi N, et al. Effects of steroids and lipopolysaccharide on spontaneous resorption of herniated intervertebral discs: an experience study in the rabbit. Spine. 1998;23:870–6.

22. Nicol GD, Klingberg DK, Vasko MR. Prostaglandin E2 enhances calcium conductance and stimulates release of substance P in avian sensory neurons. J Neurosci. 1992;12:1917–27.

23. Parlier-Cuau C, Wybier M, Nizard R, Champsaur P, Le Hir P, et al. Symptomatic lumbar facet joint synovial cysts: clinical assessment of facet joint steroid injection after 1 and 6 months and long-term follow-up in 30 patients. Radiology. 1999;210:509–13.

24. Sowa G. Facet mediated pain. Dis Mon. 2005;51:18–31.

25. Vallee C, Chevrot A, Benhamouda M, Gires F, Wybier M. Aspects tomodensitometriques des kystes synoviaux articulaires lombaires à développement intrarachidien. J Radiol. 1987;68: 519–26.

26. Wybier M, Laredo JD. Facet joint arthrography and steroid injection. In: Bard M, Laredo JD, editors. Interventional radiology in bone and joint. Vienna: Springer; 1988. p. 157–74.

27. Yuh WT, Drew JM, Weinstein JN, et al. Intra spinal synovial cysts: magnetic resonance evaluation. Spine. 1991;16:740–5.

Periprocedural Anesthetic Care for Interventional Neuroradiological Procedures

Chris Taylor and Mary Newton

Abstract

Anesthetists have many important concerns while providing care to patients undergoing interventional neuroradiological (INR) procedures; these include maintenance of patient physiological stability, manipulating systemic or regional blood flow, ensuring patient immobility, managing anticoagulation, treating and managing sudden unexpected complications during the procedure, guiding the medical management of critical care patients during transport to and from the radiology suites, and rapid emergence from anesthesia or sedation following a procedure to facilitate neurological observations. To achieve these goals, anesthetists must be familiar with all the specific radiological procedures and their potential complications. Additionally they must be part of an integrated neuroradiological team and work in an appropriately equipped unit.

Keywords

Anesthetists • Physiological stability • Manipulating blood flow • Ensuring patient immobility • Managing anticoagulation • Managing sudden unexpected complications • Guiding the medical management of critical care patients during • Rapid emergence from anesthesia or sedation • Neurological observations

C. Taylor, BSc (Hons), MBBS, MRCP, FRCA, FFICM (✉)
Department of Neuroanesthesia and Neurocritical Care,
The National Hospital for Neurology and Neurosurgery, London, UK
e-mail: chris.taylor@uclh.nhs.uk

M. Newton, MD
Department of Anesthesia, The National Hospital
for Neurology and Neurosurgery, London, UK

K. Murphy, F. Robertson (eds.), *Interventional Neuroradiology,*
Techniques in Interventional Radiology,
DOI 10.1007/978-1-4471-4582-0_24, © Springer-Verlag London 2014

Introduction

Anesthetists have many important concerns while providing care to patients undergoing interventional neuroradiological (INR) procedures; these include the following: (1) maintenance of patient physiological stability, (2) manipulating systemic or regional blood flow, (3) ensuring patient immobility and managing anticoagulation, (4) treating and managing sudden unexpected complications during the procedure, (5) guiding the medical management of critical care patients during transport to and from the radiology suites, and (6) rapid emergence from anesthesia or sedation following a procedure to facilitate neurological observations. To achieve these goals, anesthetists must be familiar with all the specific radiological procedures and their potential complications. Additionally they must be part of an integrated neuroradiological team and work in an appropriately equipped unit.

Essential Features of the Interventional Neuroradiology Team and Suite

Essential Features of the Interventional Neuroradiology Team

- Consultant-led and consultant-delivered service.
- All staff fully trained and experienced in working in isolated sites.
- All staff fully trained and experienced in working in interventional neuroradiology.
- Immediate availability of a consultant neurovascular surgeon to advise or intervene for complications requiring surgical treatment.

Essential Features of the Interventional Neuroradiology Suite

- All anesthetic equipment to meet those of neurosurgical operating theatre standards.
- Immediate availability of specialized drugs (heparin, protamine, abciximab, etc.) and specialized equipment for near-patient testing (i.e., activated clotting time).
- Facilities for post-procedure recovery in suitable environment [Recovery Ward, Neurocritical Care Unit (HDU)] staffed by nurses experienced in the recovery of neurosurgical patients.

The anesthetic care of the patient undergoing INR procedures can be divided into pre-, intra-, and post-procedural care.

Pre-procedural Care

The first priority is to "triage" the timing of the procedure into:

- Elective (ward patients).
- Urgent.

- Emergency (critical care patients).

Followed by pre-assessment of all patients, to include:

- Review of the medical notes, correspondence, details of previous procedures, and any complications.
- Obtaining accurate medical history from the patient or relatives.
  - Clarification of the presenting complaint and reason for referral.
  - Review of relevant past medical history.
  - Clarification of medication history and allergies. Checking compliance with medication particularly important for patients taking "antiplatelet" agents.
  - Review of patient systems to establish organ reserves and potential problems, i.e., presence of ischemic heart disease, asthma, epilepsy, etc.
- Examination of the patient.
  - Cardiovascular assessment to determine cardiovascular reserve and assessment of hydration. To assess "baseline" blood pressure and pulse.
  - Respiratory assessment to identify and treat respiratory complications early (i.e., aspiration).
  - Neurological assessment [i.e., mini-mental state (MMSE), Glasgow Coma Score (GCS)], pupil responses and visual field defects, and limb power and sensation to accurately document "baseline" neurological function.
  - Airway assessment to identify and predict a potential difficult intubation. A known/predicted difficult airway may require availability of additional airway equipment or dictate an alternative "safer site" for anesthetic induction (i.e., an anesthetic room in the main theatre complex).
  - The patient's weight and height should be recorded to aid periprocedural drug dosing.
- Blood tests and other investigations.
  - Results for hemoglobin, white blood cell and platelet count, coagulation, electrolytes, and estimation of glomerular filtration rate should be obtained.
  - Blood should be sent for grouping and a specimen saved for crossmatching blood if necessary.
  - Review of investigations: electrocardiography (ECG) (abnormalities frequently present following subarachnoid hemorrhage), chest x-ray (CXR), and neuroimaging.
- Discussions.
  - Patient, family, and next of kin and informed consent for procedure obtained (Patients with GCS <15 will require consent form specifically for those with mental incapacity.)

Nonurgent cases may benefit from postponement of the procedure to allow for system optimization (i.e., blood pressure control, asthma control, renal function).

Appropriate transport monitoring and equipment must be available to ensure the safe transfer of critically ill patients by experienced neuroanesthetists from the Neurocritical Care Unit (NCCU) or HDU to the INR suite. Careful note should be taken of all medication doses, ventilator settings, etc. Monitoring of intracranial pressure (ICP) should be continued if an intraparenchymal pressure measuring device is in place. Ideally external ventricular drains (EVDs) should be clamped during transport to prevent over drainage of cerebral spinal fluid (CSF) which may precipitate aneurysm rupture.

Intra-procedural Care

Each patient's case detail should be discussed with the neuroradiologist before the commencement of anesthesia so that the aims and potential complications of treatment are understood.

Before arrival of the patient, the anesthetic machine and equipment must be checked. Emergency drugs should be readily available as should drugs which may be required during interventional neuroradiological procedures (aspirin, clopidogrel, nimodipine, glyceryl trinitrate, tissue plasminogen activator, abciximab, heparin, and protamine) together with appropriate dosage guidelines and details of administration.

The need for general anesthesia should be established; it is usually required:

- To aid physiological stability.
- For noncompliant patients.
- To provide immobility.
- For prolonged procedures.

For many patients, it is the continuation of the cardiorespiratory support initiated on NCCU.

Some procedures should ideally be performed under local anesthesia to aid continual assessment of neurological function (i.e., placement of internal carotid stent) and/or to maintain blood pressure where cerebral perfusion is critical (i.e., hyperacute stroke). An experienced anesthetist should always be in attendance.

Before induction of anesthesia, the "sign in" section of World Health Organization (WHO) Surgical Safety checklist (adapted for use in the interventional neuroradiology suite) (Fig. 1) must be checked with specific attention to:

- Correct identification of the patient (especially important in those with altered conscious state).
- MRSA status.
- Baseline creatinine/glomerular filtration rate (GFR) and adherence to precautions recommended by the Royal College of Radiologists.
- Pregnancy status.
- Medication and allergy history.
- Appropriate fasting prior to general anesthesia/sedation (6 h for food and 2 h for clear fluids).

Monitoring for all patients should include:

- 3-lead ECG, noninvasive blood pressure (BP), pulse oximetry, oxygen (O_2) and CO_2 analysis, inspired and expired concentration of volatile agent, and ventilator pressure recording (all monitoring equipment should be carefully positioned to avoid obscuring areas being visualized radiographically).

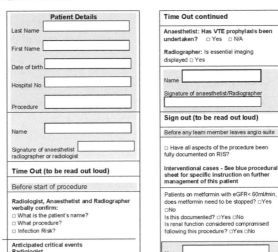

Fig. 1 World Health Organization (WHO) Surgical Safety checklist (Adapted for use in the Interventional Neuroradiology Suite, The National Hospital for Neurology and Neurosurgery)

- +/− Invasive arterial blood pressure (IABP) monitoring (most interventional procedures require this to provide immediate knowledge of changes in BP and to accurately monitor the response to pharmacological interventions in BP manipulation. Additionally IABP monitoring is useful for arterial blood gas (ABG) analysis, measurement of blood glucose, and monitoring anticoagulation following administration of heparin).
- ICP monitoring, if already initiated, should be continued especially if ICP is high as the inability to provide a reverse Trendelenburg position on the angiography table will result in a further increase in ICP.
- Central venous monitoring is not usually required but may be useful in the initiation of a triple-H therapy in patients with symptomatic vasospasm.
- Core body temperature measurement (i.e., nasopharyngeal).

Induction of Anesthesia

- The choice of anesthetic agent is guided primarily by cardiovascular and cerebral considerations.
- There is no "recommended" specific anesthetic drug technique.
- Total intravenous anesthetic (TIVA) techniques or combinations of inhalational and intravenous (IV) methods are popular choices.

- Theoretically N2O should be avoided because of the risk of expanding the volume of microemboli accidently introduced into the cerebral circulation through arterial flushing devices. There is no evidence to support this.
- Anesthesia should follow the general principles of neuroanesthesia and provide smooth induction with cardiovascular stability, avoidance of pressor response to laryngoscopy, etc.
- Intra-procedural BP should be tailored to the individual patient based on preoperative baseline values (especially in hypertensive patients who should be assumed to have right shift of the cerebral autoregulation curve) and adjusted for specific conditions:
  — For unprotected cerebral aneurysms, a systolic BP <160 mmHg (mean arterial pressure <110 mmHg) and the avoidance of hypotension are recommended.
  — For hyperacute stroke patients (presenting for endovascular treatment following intravenous thrombolysis), a systolic BP target of <185 mmHg and a diastolic BP <110 mmHg are required. High pressures are usually centrally driven to maintain a vital collateral circulation.
  — Maintenance of normoxia (PaO_2 of 13 kPa or SpO_2 between 94 and 98 % in acute situations where hyperoxia injury is a potential complication).
  — Maintenance of normocapnia ($PaCO_2$ between 4.5 and 5.0 kPa) to regulate intracranial pressures.
  — Maintenance of normoglycemia (5–9.5 mmol/l).
  — Maintenance of normothermia (avoid hyperthermia which is associated with worse outcomes).
- It is advisable to intubate all patients undergoing interventional procedures with a tracheal tube (TT):
  — This is the most reliable method of controlling the airway for ventilated patients.
  — This secures the airway especially if the patient requires emergency transfer to theatre for treatment of a complication arising during an INR procedure.
- Avoid using reinforced TTs for spinal angiography as the metallic spiral reinforcement may obscure spinal vessels. Additionally reinforced TTs will need to be changed if a post-procedural MRI scan is required.
- Secure intravenous (iv) access is essential:
  — With adequate extension tubing to allow drug and fluid administration at maximal distance from the image intensifier and an easily accessible injection port.
  — One IV line should be of "large-bore" calibre to allow rapid administration of fluids/drugs if necessary.

A fine-bore nasogastric feeding tube is often required to administer loading doses of antiplatelet drugs (aspirin and/or clopidogrel) for some INR procedures. Usually inserted at induction under direct vision and imaged by the radiologist to confirm position in the stomach before use.

- Bladder catheters are required for most procedures:
  — They assist in fluid management.
  — Useful to manage high urine output because of osmotic diuresis caused by contrast agent and high volumes of saline flush used to prevent clot formation in arterial catheters.

Positioning and Care of Patient

- Monitoring to be attached before transfer to angiography table.
- Head and neck in neutral position with no rotation; straight alignment of spinal column.
- Protection of eyes (taping).
- Careful positioning to prevent pressure areas developing during long procedures; pillow under knees to limit extension of lumbar spine.
- Mechanical thromboprophylaxis should be considered (graduated compression stockings and intermittent calf compression) for all patients.
- Maintenance of normothermia (warming of IV fluids and forced air warming blanket).
  - Perform "on table" baseline investigations, i.e., ABG, activated clotting time (ACT), and platelet function, as appropriate.
  - EVD (when present) should be firmly secured to prevent accidental removal by moving equipment, zeroed and opened at the predetermined height to allow drainage. Personnel must be warned not to alter the angiography table height without liaising with anesthetist.
  - Prior to sterile draping of the patient all connections of the ventilation circuit and vascular lines should be secured.
  - Sample blood for relevant baseline investigations, i.e., ABG, ACT, and platelet function.

Before the procedure begins the "time-out" section of WHO Surgical Safety checklist should be completed to include:

- Introduction of team members (neuroradiologist, neuroanesthetist, neuroradiographer, and neuroradiology nurses).
- Confirmation of immediate availability of named consultant neurosurgeon.
- Procedure to be undertaken and potential complications.
- Specific equipment requirements.
- Review of imaging.
- Patient issues (identity, pregnancy status, renal function, etc.).
- Post-procedural destination, i.e., NCCU/HDU/Recovery Ward.

Vital sign parameter targets:

Aim for "stable" general anesthetic conditions as detailed above so that changes in vital signs during the procedure can be attributed to the procedure (i.e., ruptured aneurysm) rather than a change in depth of anesthesia, etc.

The need for anticoagulation and/or antiplatelet agents and the timing of their administration should be discussed at the beginning of the case:

- If required, heparin (70 units/kg) is administered to achieve an ACT of two to three times baseline values (no consensus on "ideal" ACT).
- ACT checked hourly and maintained by continuous infusion or intermittent bolus of heparin.
- At the end of the procedure or in emergency situations, the heparin may need to be reversed with protamine sulfate.

The use of antiplatelet agents (aspirin, clopidogrel, and the glycoprotein IIb/IIIa receptor antagonists) varies considerably:

- Rapid reversal of antiplatelet activity can only be achieved by platelet transfusion.

Intra-procedural Complications and Their Management

Complications during interventional neuroradiological procures can be of rapid onset and life-threatening. Rapid and effective communication between the anesthesia, radiology, and other relevant teams is critical. Having a well thought-out plan for dealing with intra-cranial catastrophe can make the difference between an uneventful outcome and death. The three most serious complications are hemorrhage, thromboembolism, and vasospasm.

Hemorrhagic Complications

In the anesthetized patient, intra-procedural aneurysm rupture is usually heralded by cardiovascular disturbance:

- Arrhythmias (bradycardia or supraventricular tachycardia) and subtle relative hypertension are often picked up by the attentive anesthetist. More commonly rupture is associated with a huge sudden increase in BP (200 mmHg is not unusual).
- Administration of vasoactive drugs should be avoided during placement of the microcatheter and coils within the aneurysm as this may mask cardiovascular changes associated with rupture. For the same reason IABP monitoring should not be interrupted (for monitoring of ACT, etc.) while the aneurysm is being catheterized/coiled.
- Rarely, extravasation of contrast or coil from the aneurysm may be the only sign of hemorrhage.
- Hemorrhage must be dealt with rapidly. This usually involves the immediate reduction of BP. Propofol boluses are effective in rapidly reducing BP back to "baseline" values. Propofol also provides a degree of cerebral protection by lowering the cerebral meta-bolic rate of oxygen ($CMRO_2$).
- Reversal of heparinization using protamine sulfate may be necessary, at the request of the radiologist, in extreme circumstances. 1 mg protamine can be given for each 100 unit heparin total dosage during the case. The ACT can be used to "fine-tune" the final protamine dose.
- Platelet administration may be required to reverse the effect of antiplatelet drugs.
- While managing the acute situation, it is important for other team members to be made aware of the complication (i.e., neurovascular surgeon, radiographers in CT scan,

operating theatre personnel) in case further urgent scanning/surgical intervention is required.

- As soon as the aneurysm is secured, the pupils should be checked for size and response to light. BP should be maintained at "high normal" levels.
- If neurosurgical intervention is not required post-rupture, the authors' practice is to aim, where appropriate, for extubation of the patient to improve the quality of neurological observations and to transfer patient to an HDU or NCCU.

Thromboembolic Complications

The anesthetist can help the neuroradiologist manage thromboembolic complications in a variety of ways:

- Improve distal end-organ perfusion by elevating BP pharmacologically or with IV fluid infusions.
- Preparation of glycoprotein IIb/IIIa receptor antagonists for intra-arterial injection by the neuroradiologist +/− intravenous infusion by anesthetist or IV administration of aspirin.
- Discussing and planning thromboprophylactic management post-procedure.

Complications Secondary to Vasospasm

Vasospasm (catheter-induced or secondary to subarachnoid hemorrhage (SAH)) may also be problematic:

- Catheter-induced may require intra-arterial administration of GTN by the radiologist.
- Symptomatic vasospasm following SAH, unresponsive to medical management, may require intra-arterial administration of nimodipine infusion by the radiologist or balloon angioplasty.

Post-procedural Care

At the conclusion of the procedure, the "sign-out" section of the WHO Surgical Safety checklist should be completed following discussion with the INR team to include:

- A record of fluid balance (urine output, blood loss, volume of administered intravenous/ arterial fluids and contrast agents).

THE NATIONAL HOSPITAL FOR NEUROLOGY AND NEUROSURGERY
Post-care instructions for interventional neuroradiology

1. Puncture site   R   L
- pressure only   ☐   ☐
- sealing device   ☐   ☐

2. Mobilisation
- keep supine – 0 to 30 ^{0} _____ **hours**
  can then mobilise gently provided there are no contraindications

3. Thromboprophylaxis / drug intervention
ALL patients who have received heparin intra-
procedure need platelet count - Day 1/7/14
- aspirin   once only ☐   14 days☐   Other ☐ ____
- clopidogrel   once only☐   14 days☐   Other ☐ ____

(aspirin and clopidogrel together need H₂ antag cover - avoid PPI)
- Heparin infusion - maintain APTT @ 2 x normal (regime in UCLH Formulary). Continue until reviewed by neuroradiologist.

or,
- Dalteparin 100units /Kg (max 100,000 units) twice daily for ____ h
  (refer to 'Treatment dose of dalteparin laminate' for dosage guidance and platelet count monitoring *before* prescibing)

- Dalteparin – for VTE prophylaxis   Yes ☐   No ☐

4. Pathology
- cured/protected   ☐
- partially treated/protected   ☐
  (see BP guidelines below)
- other   ☐

5. Blood pressure parameters   Review frequently in relation to neurological
- _____ systolic   status, especially if change in BP or neurology
                                            (If vasopressors required and no CVP consider metaraminol infusion -
                                            see 'Guidelines for anaesthesia – Angiography Suite')

6. Neurological observations   1. **GCS plus pupillary signs and limb power**
                                            2. **Vision – can patient read?**
                                            3. **Other:**

7. Additional instructions
- If severe headache (Pain score 3/4 or 4/4 despite adequate analgesia) then immediate CT
- If new neurological deficit (new focal deficit, drop in GCS from baseline, new seizure, new pupillary signs or new cranial nerve signs) immediate CT.
- In either event, the clinical team must be contacted and informed of the change, and the clinical team must immediately review the CT.
- Between 08:30 and 17:30 Mon-Fri, contact angiography suite x 83444

All patients MUST be reviewed by a member of the admitting medical or surgical team on the day of the procedure. This must include a review of the post-care instructions (in particular point 7).

Name	Signature	Date

Please sign and date any changes made after this   MN /SB/FR/AT/BC/SF/IA/JG Sept. 2011

Fig. 2 Post-procedure care instructions

- Post-procedure care instructions [a pro forma is useful (Fig. 2) to include details on arterial puncture site, mobilization, thromboprophylaxis, BP parameters, status of aneurysm, additional neurological observations, etc.].
- Additionally, written documentation of the procedure should accompany the patient to their post-procedure destination.

An antiemetic and analgesia (if required) should be administered. Patients returning to Recovery Ward or HDU post-procedure are best extubated under "deep" anesthesia:

- Avoids coughing +/− gagging (detrimental in those with raised ICP).
- Reduces the risk of hypertension which may be significant in patients with partially treated aneurysms or arteriovenous malformations (AVM).

In our institution, patients who had a good GCS at the start of the procedure and who have received glycoprotein IIb/IIIa receptor antagonists with good effect are extubated very carefully under "deep" anesthesia in a non-isolated environment (i.e., main theatre complex). Great care is taken to prevent minor airway trauma (i.e., careful suctioning) which may precipitate bleeding. Waking of the patient post-procedure allows more sensitive neurological observation and earlier indication of deteriorating neurological status.

The ideal neuroanesthetic results in rapid, high-quality recovery. This enables early assessment of neurological function. Onset of "new" neurological signs should be investigated with early imaging. When imaging is negative, other conditions should be considered such as subclinical seizures.

Most procedures require the patient to lie relatively flat for 2–4 h following the procedure to reduce the chance of a femoral artery hematoma, especially since many patients are anticoagulated and/or on antiplatelet agents. Specialized femoral arterial sealing devices can reduce this risk.

Post-procedure guidelines for BP management should be closely adhered to and patients may require infusions of vasoactive drugs. Severe post-procedural pain is uncommon and needs to be carefully evaluated as it may herald the onset of complications (i.e., hemorrhage following venous escape during glue embolization of an AVM).

Dexamethasone is started following tumor embolization to minimize swelling. Patients who are at risk of decompensating because of swelling should ideally be nursed in an HDU environment.

Neurological assessment needs to be repeated at frequent intervals and may have to be extended to examine specific areas of concern (i.e., visual acuity, visual fields). Neurological deficits need to be recognized promptly to allow rapid diagnosis and initiation of treatment where appropriate.

Patients returning to NCCU post-procedure will require the same standard of care to ensure safe intrahospital transfer. Wherever possible a patient's sedation is reduced in a controlled manner to enable extubation or assessment of neurological status. Frequently, however, continued sedation is required to enable cardiorespiratory support.

Miscellaneous Considerations for Anesthetists During Interventional Neuroradiological Procedures

Radiation Safety

A fundamental knowledge of radiation safety is essential for all staff members working in an INR suite. These units should be designed so that personnel can work as far as possible from the source of radiation. All personnel should wear lead aprons, thyroid shields, and radiation exposure badges. Movable lead glass screens may provide additional protection for the anesthesia team. With correct precautions, the anesthesia team should be exposed to less than the annual recommended limit for health-care workers.

Contrast-Induced Nephropathy

Contrast-induced nephropathy is very common and can be limited by identifying patients with kidney disease in advance of an interventional procedure by calculation of estimated glomerular filtration rate (eGFR) and:

- Maintaining good hydration.
- Minimizing dose of contrast agent used.
- Use of low or iso-osmolar contrast agent.
- Avoiding hypotension.
- Patients with severe kidney disease may benefit from periprocedural 1.6 % $NaHCO_3$ infusion.
  - Maintaining good hydration following the procedure.

Post-procedure renal function should be monitored carefully for at least 48 h in at-risk patients (eGFR <60 ml/min). In moderate to severe kidney disease, medications that accumulate in renal failure (e.g., metformin) should be discontinued until renal function returns to pre-procedural levels.

Anaphylaxis

Life-threatening reactions to intravascular contrast agents are rare. The incidence of severe reactions with nonionic agents is 0.04 %. All staff working in this environment must be familiar with the symptoms and signs of anaphylaxis and its treatment. Resuscitation equipment and drugs must be immediately available.

Suggested Reading

1. Diringer M, Bleck T, Hemphill III J, et al. Critical Care management of patients following aneurysmal sub-arachnoid hemorrhage: recommendations from the Neurocritical Care Society's multidisciplinary consensus conference. Neurocrit Care. 2011;15:211–40.
2. The National Institute of Neurological Disorders and Stroke rt-PA Stroke Study Group. Tissue plasminogen activator for acute ischemic stroke. N Engl J Med. 1995;333:1581–8.
3. The Royal College of Radiologists. Standards for intravascular contrast agent administration to adult patients. 2nd ed. London: The Royal College of Radiologists; 2010. Ref No. BFCR(10)4© The Royal College of Radiologists. ISBN 978-1-905034-43-7.

Key Points

> Thorough pre-procedural assessment of patient and results of their investigations including relevant imaging are essential.

> Pre-procedural preparation should include communication with the radiologist to establish the plan of treatment and any anticipated complications, together with their management.

> The anesthetic technique must provide physiological stability and may require manipulation of systemic or regional blood flow.

> The anesthetic technique must also guarantee immobility at all stages of the procedure and include rapid emergence (where appropriate) to facilitate neurological observations.

> Post-procedure, the patient's clinical records should be updated immediately to include an account of the procedure and instructions for ongoing care.

Index

K. Murphy, F. Robertson (eds.), *Interventional Neuroradiology,*
Techniques in Interventional Radiology,
DOI 10.1007/978-1-4471-4582-0, © Springer-Verlag London 2014